PROLOG

Gynecology and Surgery

SEVENTH EDITION

Critique Book

The American College of
Obstetricians and Gynecologists
WOMEN'S HEALTH CARE PHYSICIANS

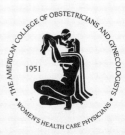

ISBN 978-1-934984-36-9

2345/876

The American College of Obstetricians and Gynecologists
409 12th Street, SW
PO Box 96920
Washington, DC 20090-6920

Contributors

PROLOG Editorial and Advisory Committee

CHAIR

Ronald T. Burkman, Jr, MD
   Professor of Obstetrics and Gynecology
   Tufts University School of Medicine
   Division of General Obstetrics and
      Gynecology
   Department of Obstetrics and
      Gynecology
   Baystate Medical Center
   Springfield, Massachusetts

MEMBERS

Louis Weinstein, MD
   Past Paul A. and Eloise B. Bowers
      Professor and Chair
   Department of Obstetrics and
      Gynecology
   Thomas Jefferson University
   Philadelphia, Pennsylvania

Linda Van Le, MD
   Leonard Palumbo Distinguished
      Professor
   Division of Gynecologic Oncology
   Department of Obstetrics and
      Gynecology
   University of North Carolina School of
      Medicine
   Chapel Hill, North Carolina

PROLOG Task Force for *Gynecology and Surgery*, Seventh Edition

COCHAIRS

John F. Greene, MD
   Chief Medical Officer
   MidState Medical Center
   Meriden, Connecticut
   Professor of Obstetrics and
      Gynecology
   The Frank H. Netter, MD, School of
      Medicine
   Quinnipiac University
   North Haven, Connecticut

James M. Shwayder, MD, JD
   Professor and Chair
   Department of Obstetrics and
      Gynecology
   University of Mississippi Medical
      Center
   Jackson, Mississippi

MEMBERS

Leslie R. DeMars, MD
   Associate Professor
   Division Director
   Gynecologic Oncology
   Geisel School of Medicine
   Dartmouth-Hitchcock Medical Center
   Lebanon, New Hampshire

Geri D. Hewitt, MD
   Associate Professor
   Department of Obstetrics and
      Gynecology
   Ohio State University Medical Center
   Columbus, Ohio

Fred M. Howard, MD
   Professor Emeritus
   Department of Obstetrics and
      Gynecology
   University of Rochester Medical Center
   Rochester, New York

Continued on next page

PROLOG Task Force for *Gynecology and Surgery*, Seventh Edition *(continued)*

CONFLICT OF INTEREST DISCLOSURE

This PROLOG unit was developed under the direction of the PROLOG Advisory Committee and the Task Force for *Gynecology and Surgery*, Seventh Edition. PROLOG is planned and produced in accordance with the Standards for Enduring Materials of the Accreditation Council for Continuing Medical Education. Any discussion of unapproved use of products is clearly cited in the appropriate critique.

Current guidelines state that continuing medical education (CME) providers must ensure that CME activities are free from the control of any commercial interest. The task force and advisory committee members declare that neither they nor any business associate nor any member of their immediate families has material interest, financial interest, or other relationships with any company manufacturing commercial products relative to the topics included in this publication or with any provider of commercial services discussed in the unit except for **Khaled Sakhel, MD**, who is a consultant for Hologic and a speaker for Conceptus; **James M. Shwayder, MD**, who receives royalties from Cook Ob-Gyn for an SIS catheter and who is a consultant for Philips Healthcare Ultrasound; and **Linda Van Le, MD**, who serves on the Advisory Board of Biologics, Inc. All potential conflicts have been resolved through the American College of Obstetricians and Gynecologist's mechanism for resolving potential and real conflicts of interest.

Preface

PROLOG (Personal Review of Learning in Obstetrics and Gynecology) is a voluntary, strictly confidential, self-evaluation program. PROLOG was developed specifically as a personal study resource for the practicing obstetrician–gynecologist. It is presented as a self-assessment mechanism that, with its accompanying performance information, should assist the physician in designing a personal, self-directed life-long learning program. It may be used as a valuable study tool, reference guide, and a means of attaining up-to-date information in the specialty. The content is carefully selected and presented in multiple-choice questions that are clinically oriented. The questions are designed to stimulate and challenge physicians in areas of medical care that they confront in their practices or when they work as consultant obstetrician–gynecologists.

PROLOG also provides the American College of Obstetricians and Gynecologists (the College) with one mechanism to identify the educational needs of the Fellows. Individual scores are reported only to the participant; however, cumulative performance data and evaluation comments obtained for each PROLOG unit help determine the direction for future educational programs offered by the College.

Process

The PROLOG series offers the most current information available in five areas of the specialty: obstetrics, gynecology and surgery, reproductive endocrinology and infertility, gynecologic oncology and critical care, and patient management in the office. A new PROLOG unit is produced annually, addressing one of those subject areas. Gynecology and Surgery, Seventh Edition, is the second unit in the seventh 5-year PROLOG series.

Each unit of PROLOG represents the efforts of a special task force of subject experts under the supervision of an advisory committee. PROLOG sets forth current information as viewed by recognized authorities in the field of women's health. This educational resource does not define a standard of care, nor is it intended to dictate an exclusive course of management. It presents recognized methods and techniques of clinical practice for consideration by obstetrician–gynecologists to incorporate in their practices. Variations of practice that take into account the needs of the individual patient, resources, and the limitations that are special to the institution or type of practice may be appropriate.

Each unit of PROLOG is presented as a two-part set, with performance information and cognate credit available to those who choose to submit their answer sheets for confidential scoring. The first part of the PROLOG set is the Assessment Book, which contains educational objectives for the unit and multiple-choice questions, and an answer sheet with return mailing envelope. Participants can work through the book at their own pace, choosing to use PROLOG as a closed- or open-book assessment. Return of the answer sheet for scoring is encouraged but voluntary.

The second part of PROLOG is the Critique Book, which reviews the educational objectives and items set forth in the Assessment Book and contains a discussion, or critique, of each item. The critique provides the rationale for correct and incorrect options. Current, accessible references are listed for each item.

Continuing Medical Education Credit

ACCME Accreditation
The American College of Obstetricians and Gynecologists is accredited by the Accreditation Council for Continuing Medical Education (ACCME) to provide continuing medical education for physicians.

AMA PRA Category 1 Credit(s)™
The American College of Obstetricians and Gynecologists designates this enduring material for a maximum of 25 *AMA PRA Category 1 Credits*™. Physicians should claim only the credit commensurate with the extent of their participation in the activity.

College Cognate Credit(s)

The American College of Obstetricians and Gynecologists designates this enduring material for a maximum of 25 Category 1 College Cognate Credits. The College has a reciprocity agreement with the American Medical Association that allows *AMA PRA Category 1 Credit(s)*™ to be equivalent to College Cognate Credits.

Fellows who submit their answer sheets for scoring will be credited with 25 CME credits. Participants who return their answer sheets for CME credit will receive a Performance Report that provides a comparison of their scores with the scores of a sample group of physicians who have taken the unit as an examination. An individual may request credit only once for each unit. *Please allow 4–6 weeks to process answer sheets.*

Credit for PROLOG *Gynecology and Surgery*, Seventh Edition, is initially available through December 2016. During that year, the unit will be reevaluated. If the content remains current, credit is extended for an additional 3 years, with credit for the unit automatically withdrawn after December 2019.

Conclusion

PROLOG was developed specifically as a personal study resource for the practicing obstetrician–gynecologist. It is presented as a self-assessment mechanism that, with its accompanying performance information, should assist the physician in designing a personal, self-directed learning program. The many quality resources developed by the College, as detailed each year in the College's *Publications and Educational Materials Catalog* are available to help fulfill the educational interests and needs that have been identified. PROLOG is not intended as a substitute for the certification or recertification programs of the American Board of Obstetrics and Gynecology.

PROLOG CME SCHEDULE

Reproductive Endocrinology and Infertility, Sixth Edition	Credit through 2015
Gynecologic Oncology and Critical Care, Sixth Edition	Credit through 2016
Patient Management in the Office, Sixth Edition	Reevaluated in 2014– Credit through 2017
Obstetrics, Seventh Edition	Reevaluated in 2015– Credit through 2018
Gynecology and Surgery, Seventh Edition	Reevaluated in 2016– Credit through 2019

PROLOG Objectives

PROLOG is a voluntary, strictly confidential, personal continuing education resource that is designed to be both stimulating and enjoyable. By participating in PROLOG, obstetrician–gynecologists will be able to do the following:

- Review and update clinical knowledge.
- Recognize areas of knowledge and practice in which they excel, be stimulated to explore other areas of the specialty, and identify areas requiring further study.
- Plan continuing education activities in light of identified strengths and deficiencies.
- Compare and relate present knowledge and skills with those of other participants.
- Obtain continuing medical education credit, if desired.
- Have complete personal control of the setting and of the pace of the experience.

The obstetrician–gynecologist who completes *Gynecology and Surgery*, Seventh Edition, will be able to:

- Establish a differential diagnosis and screen patients with appropriate diagnostic tests for specific gynecologic conditions.
- Determine the appropriate medical management for specific gynecologic conditions in adolescents and adult women.
- Identify appropriate surgical interventions for various gynecologic conditions and strategies to prevent and treat surgical complications.
- Apply concepts of anatomy, genetics, pathophysiology, and epidemiology to the understanding of diseases that affect women.
- Counsel women regarding treatment options and adjustment to crises that may alter their lifestyles.
- Apply professional medical ethics and the understanding of medical–legal issues relative to the practice of gynecology.

Gynecology and Surgery, Seventh Edition, includes the following topics (item numbers appear in parentheses):

SCREENING AND DIAGNOSIS
Abnormal cervical cytology results (71)
Abnormal uterine bleeding in an adolescent patient (81)
Atypical glandular cells Pap test result (34)
Cervical cancer screening and diagnosis (138–142)
Chronic pelvic pain (29)
Complications of uterine artery embolization (80)
Eating disorders and irregular menstruation (130)
Dysmenorrhea in an adolescent patient (116)
Frequent urination (108)
Intraoperative hypotension (96)
Levonorgestrel intrauterine device with missing strings (110)
Ovarian cancer screening (59)
Ovarian mass in an adolescent patient (2)
Pap test result in a patient older than 40 years that shows endometrial cells (1)
Pediatric vaginitis (154–158)
Perioperative cardiac evaluation (38)
Persistent vulvar pain (73)
Recurrent urinary incontinence (100)
Recurrent urinary tract infection (119)
Recurrent yeast infections (53)

Screening for vaginal intraepithelial neoplasia (75)
Severe dyspareunia (46)
Sexual dysfunction in menopausal women (10)
Tumor markers (150–153)
Thrombophilias and contraception (106)
Vaginal cancer screening after hysterectomy (68)
Vesicovaginal fistula (32)

MEDICAL MANAGEMENT
A patient with ductal carcinoma in situ (129)
A patient with sexual partner who has genital herpes (107)
Abnormal uterine bleeding in an adolescent patient (4)
Abnormal uterine bleeding in a reproductive-aged woman (40)
Adnexal mass in a postmenopausal woman (95)
Adverse effects of pharmacologic therapy for overactive bladder (61)
Appropriate treatment of sexually transmitted diseases (74)
Asymptomatic myomas (72)
Beta-blocker therapy in perioperative care (126)
Breast abscess (87)
Clinical depression (45)
Complex endometrial hyperplasia (104)
Contraception in a patient with gastric bypass (134)
Contraception in the morbidly obese patient (118)
Contraceptive options for a woman with diabetes mellitus and a seizure disorder (7)
Depot medroxyprogesterone acetate and bone loss (33)
Dysmenorrhea (13)
Ectopic pregnancy (44, 93)
Endometriosis (88)
Evaluation of urinary incontinence (20)
Extended-cycle combined oral contraceptives (122)
First-trimester pregnancy loss (114)
Fibrocystic breast disease (105)
Follow-up after loop electrosurgical procedure (15)
Heavy menstrual bleeding (113)
Heavy menstrual bleeding in a patient with a low platelet count (62)
Hormone therapy after hysterectomy for endometriosis (69)
Hormone therapy after hysterectomy (48)
Human immunodeficiency virus exposure and prophylaxis (18)
Hydrosalpinx (125)
Hysteroscopic complications (82)
Hysteroscopic sterilization (60)
Immunization (131)
Lichen sclerosus (92)
Mature cystic teratoma with recurrence (12)
Metformin hydrochloride and polycystic ovary syndrome (43)
Molar pregnancy (54)
Nonhormonal therapy for menopause (128)
Obesity (24)
Office hysteroscopy (65)
Outpatient management of pelvic inflammatory disease (84)
Ovarian cancer in *BRCA 1* and *BRCA 2* carriers (117)
Ovarian mass in an older reproductive-aged woman (25)
Ovarian remnant syndrome (17, 64)
Perioperative care of a patient with diabetes mellitus (89)

Postmenopausal bleeding (26)
Postmenopausal bleeding with hormone therapy (85)
Premalignant and in situ breast disease (102)
Recalcitrant condyloma (86)
Recommendations to prevent osteoporosis (97)
Recurrent bacterial vaginosis (36)
Recurrent breast mass (30)
Recurrent genital herpes (78)
Recurrent urinary tract infection (115)
Recurrent vaginal yeast infection (123)
Sexual dysfunction (58)
Single-rod implantable contraception (19)
Squamous dysplasia of the cervix (50)
Unplanned pregnancy (124)
Urinary retention after an antiincontinence procedure (3)
Use of levonorgestrel intrauterine device for heavy menstrual bleeding (83)
Vaginal intraepithelial neoplasia (94)
Wound management (5)

PHYSIOLOGY
Anterior abdominal wall anatomy and surgical complications (143–146)
Vascular supply of the pelvis (91)

SURGICAL MANAGEMENT
Adenocarcinoma in situ with positive margins (14)
Alternatives to hysterectomy for myomas (37)
Anterior abdominal wall anatomy and surgical complications (143–146)
An ovarian tumor of low malignant potential (6)
Bradycardia during minor gynecologic surgery (42)
Endometrial ablation (90)
Ethical management of unexpected surgical findings (51)
Incomplete abortion in the second trimester (132)
Indications for risk-reducing surgery (98)
Intraoperative hypotension (96)
Oliguria in the elderly patient (49)
Ovarian torsion (28)
Ovary preservation or removal at the time of hysterectomy (99)
Pelvic floor anatomy (41)
Pelvic organ prolapse (70)
Perioperative anticoagulants (63)
Perioperative pulmonary complications (35)
Postoperative delirium in an elderly patient (109)
Postoperative intestinal obstruction (47)
Postoperative management of nerve injury (8)
Postoperative oliguria (121)
Postoperative pelvic abscess (66)
Prophylactic antibiotics for abdominal surgery (101)
Surgery for uterovaginal prolapse (31)
Use of prophylactic antibiotics in surgery for patients allergic to penicillin (67)
Uterosacral ligament suspension for vaginal prolapse (16)
Vulvar vestibulitis (163–165)
Wound dehiscence (111)

EPIDEMIOLOGY AND BIOSTATISTICS

Atypical endometrial hyperplasia and endometrial cancer (76)
Carcinoma risk reduction (127)
Familial cancer syndromes (147–149)
Risk of acquiring human immunodeficiency virus after sexual assault (56)
Risk reduction factors for ovarian cancer (27)

COUNSELING

Atypical endometrial hyperplasia and endometrial cancer (76)
Complications of embolization (55)
Contraception in a patient with gastric bypass (134)
Contraception in the morbidly obese patient (118)
Eating disorders and irregular menstruation (130)
Emergency contraception (11, 112)
End-of-life counseling (133)
Etonogestrel subdermal implants (77)
Extended-cycle combined oral contraceptives (122)
Heavy menstrual bleeding (113)
Human papillomavirus vaccination (159–162)
Lynch II syndrome (39)
Obesity (103)
Ovary preservation or removal at the time of hysterectomy (99)
Patient with sexual partner who has genital herpes (107)
Perioperative cardiac evaluation (38)
Prevention of human papillomavirus transmission (52)
Recommendations to prevent osteoporosis (97)
Recurrent urinary tract infection (119)
Risk of acquiring human immunodeficiency virus after sexual assault (56)
Role of hormone therapy in menopause (120)
Smoking cessation (22)

ETHICAL AND LEGAL ISSUES

Discussion of medical errors (23)
Ethical management of unexpected surgical findings (51)
Patient privacy: electronic communication and office practice (21)
Peer review of operative complications (57)
Recognition of physician burnout (9)

OFFICE PROCEDURES

Coding for office-based procedures (79)
Patient privacy: electronic communication and office practice (21)
Patient safety in the office (135–137)
Recognition of physician burnout (9)

A complete subject matter index appears at the end of the Critique Book.

1

Pap test result in a patient older than 40 years that shows endometrial cells

A 52-year-old menopausal woman comes to your office for her annual examination. She has not experienced spotting or vaginal bleeding since menopause 18 months ago. Her sister has a history of cervical cancer. Her Pap test results are "satisfactory with no malignancy" with the notation of "endometrial cells present in a woman older than 40 years." The next step in her evaluation is

* (A) endometrial assessment
  (B) high-risk human papillomavirus testing
  (C) repeat cervical cytology in 6 months
  (D) colposcopy with endocervical curettage

The use of cytology as a screening tool has significantly reduced the incidence of cervical cancer since it was first described by Dr. George N. Papanicolaou. The 2001 Bethesda System recommends reporting benign endometrial cells found in cervical cytologic specimen of women aged 40 years and older, irrespective of menopausal status. This recommendation was upheld with the development of the 2012 Consensus Guidelines for the Management of Abnormal Cervical Cancer Screening Tests and Cancer Precursors. The 2001 Bethesda System continues to be recommended by organizations committed to the investigation and treatment of cervical cancer. The impetus behind these guidelines was to ensure that all postmenopausal women who were shedding endometrial cells would be identified. This finding in premenopausal women without signs or symptoms of abnormal uterine bleeding is not associated with any significant endometrial pathology and does not require further evaluation. Asymptomatic postmenopausal women with endometrial cells shown on cervical cytology have consistently been identified in pathologic reviews to have a significantly greater risk of uterine pathology. Therefore, the appropriate management for a postmenopausal woman with benign endometrial cells, such as the described patient, is endometrial assessment regardless of symptoms.

Uterine assessment with endometrial biopsy or dilation and curettage would be appropriate methods to begin the evaluation of benign endometrial cells in a postmenopausal woman. High-risk human papillomavirus testing and colposcopy with endocervical curettage would be appropriate for the assessment of atypical endocervical cells. However, these procedures would not be helpful in evaluating the presence of benign endometrial cells. Repeat cervical cytology is not appropriate because it is a screening test for cervical cancer. As such, simply repeating cervical cytology would not provide additional evaluation for concern of uterine pathology.

Beal HN, Stone J, Beckmann MK, McAsey ME. Endometrial cells identified in cervical cytology in women >40 years of age: criteria for appropriate endometrial evaluation. Am J Obstet Gynecol 2007; 196:568.e1–5; discussion 568.e5–6.

Sibers AG, Verbeek ALM, Massuger LF, Grefte JMM, Bulten J. Normal appearing endometrial cells in cervical smears of asymptomatic postmenopausal women have predictive value for significant endometrial pathology. Int J Gynecol Cancer 2006;16:1069–74.

Massad LS, Einstein MH, Huh WK, Katki HA, Kinney WK, Schiffman M, et al. 2012 updated consensus guidelines for the management of abnormal cervical cancer screening tests and cancer precursors. 2012 ASCCP Consensus Guidelines Conference. Obstet Gynecol 2013; 121:829–46.

* Indicates correct answer.
Note: See Appendix A for a table of normal values for laboratory tests.

1

2

Ovarian mass in an adolescent patient

A 16-year-old patient experienced acute back pain after a sports-related injury. The back pain resolved with physical therapy; however, imaging studies obtained during her evaluation suggested an adnexal mass. Ultrasonography is performed and reveals the image shown in Figure 2-1. The most likely diagnosis is

* (A) mature cystic teratoma
  (B) endometrioma
  (C) hydrosalpinx
  (D) ectopic pregnancy
  (E) hemorrhagic ovarian cyst

Figure 2-1 shows a mature cystic teratoma or dermoid tumor. Dermoids, the most frequent germ cell tumors and the most common neoplastic cysts observed in adolescents, are benign and sometimes bilateral (in 7% of cases). They contain cells from at least two germ cell layers and often contain hair, sebum, and teeth. Although dermoids have a wide range of appearance on ultrasonography, based on the type of tissue present, some common features include the following:

• A shadowing echodensity

• Diffuse or regional high amplitude echoes

• Fat-fluid levels

• Intracystic floating balls

The presence of two or more characteristic signs is associated with a high positive predictive value of correctly identifying a dermoid cyst. Additionally, the presence of ovarian calcification on abdominal flat plate, pelvic magnetic resonance imaging, or pelvic computed tomography studies should raise suspicion for a dermoid. Dermoid cysts typically have a cystic component. A solid adnexal mass in an adolescent should raise suspicion for immature teratomas or other germ cell tumors. Tumor markers are indicated in this scenario.

Dermoids can present with dull abdominal pain but are frequently asymptomatic and often found by examination or incidental imaging. Dermoids also may present acutely with ovarian torsion, from the weight of the contents of the cyst, their ability to enlarge rapidly, or their "floating" location in the pelvis caused by high fat content. Because ovarian dermoids are neoplastic and do not spontaneously regress, many cases require surgical intervention. The focus should be on fertility-sparing procedures for young women, most typically laparoscopic ovarian cystectomy. Dermoid cysts rarely rupture spon-

taneously, but, if they do, chemical peritonitis, foreign body reaction, or dense adhesions may result. Small, asymptomatic dermoids may be monitored with the use of ultrasonography.

Although endometriosis frequently is identified laparoscopically in adolescents with refractory dysmenorrhea, endometriomas are uncommon. The ultrasonographic appearance of an endometrioma includes a low, homogeneous echogenicity, often described as a "ground glass appearance." An endometrioma (Fig. 2-2) requires fertility-sparing surgical removal with complete removal of cyst wall to prevent recurrence.

A hydrosalpinx is a postinflammatory abnormality of the fallopian tube. Proximal and distal ends become scarred, which leads to accumulation of serous fluid and swelling. A hydrosalpinx (Fig. 2-3) can mimic a complex ovarian mass because the dilated tube folds on itself, which gives the impression of a septation within an ovarian cyst. Patients with hydrosalpinx typically are asymptomatic, and no intervention is indicated.

A hemorrhagic ovarian cyst (Fig. 2-4) typically is complex in nature and resolves over time. Although hemorrhagic ovarian cysts often can be the cause of lower abdominal discomfort, they can be monitored by ultrasonography unless intraperitoneal bleeding is identified.

Ectopic pregnancy (Fig. 2-5) is a diagnosis that should be considered in any young patient who has abdominal pain or abnormal bleeding. An ectopic pregnancy can be easily ruled out with a negative result of a pregnancy test. Ultrasonographic findings in ectopic pregnancy can include an extrauterine embryo with cardiac activity, adnexal fluid with a yolk sac or embryo, a tubal ring, or complex or solid adnexal masses. Ectopic pregnancy can be managed either surgically or medically, in appropriately chosen patients.

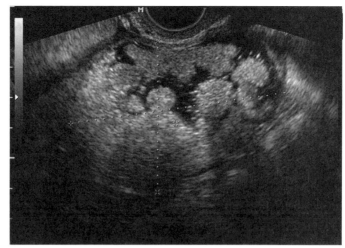

FIG. 2-1

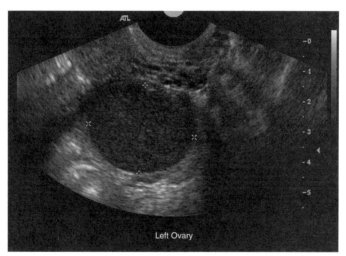

FIG. 2-2. Endometrioma.

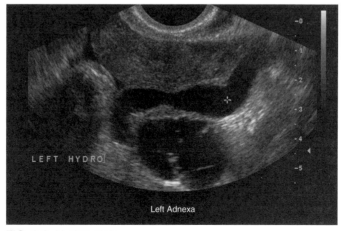

FIG. 2-3. Hydrosalpinx.

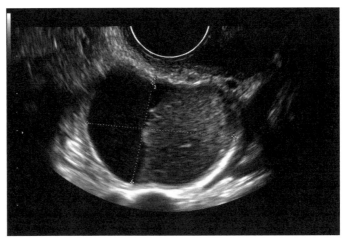

FIG. 2-4. Hemorrhagic ovarian cyst.

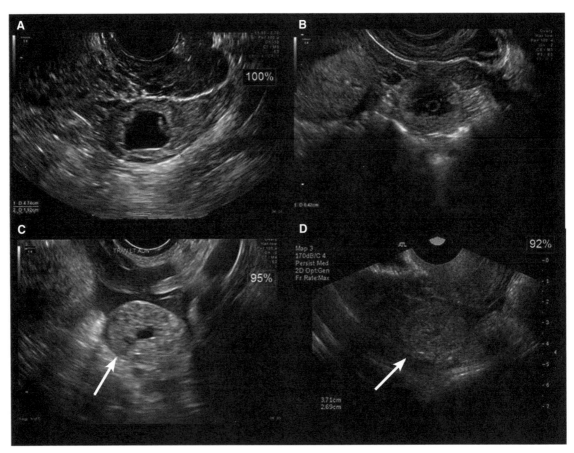

FIG. 2-5. Examples of ectopic pregnancy: **A.** Embryo without cardiac activity, **B.** adnexal mass with yolk sac (100%), **C.** tubal ring (95%), and **D.** right adnexa with complex mass (92%).

Liu JH, Zanotti KM. Management of the adnexal mass. Obstet Gynecol 2011;117:1413–28.

Management of adnexal masses. ACOG Practice Bulletin No. 83. American College of Obstetricians and Gynecologists. Obstet Gynecol 2007;110:201–14.

Pfeifer SM, Gosman GG. Evaluation of adnexal masses in adolescents. Pediatr Clin North Am 1999;46:573–92.

3

Urinary retention after an antiincontinence procedure

On postoperative day 4 after placement of a suburethral sling for urinary stress incontinence, your patient has a postvoid residual volume of 250 mL. Before discharge from the hospital, the postvoid residual volume was 300 mL, and the patient was discharged with an indwelling bladder catheter. The surgery and postoperative course were otherwise uncomplicated. The best next step in management is to

        (A) release the sling
        (B) start antibiotics
        (C) replace the indwelling bladder catheter
*   (D) start intermittent self-catheterization
        (E) perform urethral dilation

Voiding dysfunction with incomplete bladder emptying occurs in 20–45% of patients after placement of a retropubic suburethral sling. Slow preoperative urinary flow rate (less than 15 mL/s) may be a predictor of postoperative urinary retention. All patients should be counseled regarding this potential complication. No single, ideal management strategy exists for persistent urinary retention. Because most women resume adequate voiding within 4–6 weeks, conservative management with intermittent self-catheterization would offer the best option.

Sling release should not be the initial approach to management of urinary retention because of the risk of recurrence of stress incontinence. Sling release usually is performed only if urinary retention persists for 4–6 weeks.

Initiation of antibiotic therapy would be indicated only in the presence of a urinary tract infection. Antibiotic prophylaxis for short-or long-term catheter use is not beneficial and likely increases the risk of resistant organisms.

A high risk of urinary tract infection exists after placement of suburethral slings (approximately 30%). Therefore, a urine culture would be appropriate in the described case.

Replacing the indwelling bladder catheter is a reasonable management choice, but an indwelling bladder catheter carries a higher risk of urinary tract infection than does intermittent self-catheterization. Therefore, intermittent self-catheterization is the better option in this case.

Urethral dilation places downward traction on the sling, but it carries the theoretical risk of increasing the chance of mesh erosion into the urethra. Thus, urethral dilation is not the best option.

Glavind K, Glavind E. Treatment of prolonged voiding dysfunction after tension-free vaginal tape procedure. Acta Obstet Gynecol Scand 2007;86:357–60.

Niël-Weise BS, van den Broek, Peterhans J. Antibiotic policies for short-term catheter bladder drainage in adults. Cochrane Database of Systematic Reviews 2005, Issue 3. Art. No.: CD005428. DOI: 10.1002/14651858.CD005428.

4

Abnormal uterine bleeding in an adolescent patient

A 12-year-old girl is referred to your office by her pediatrician. She arrives with her mother. She experienced her first menstrual cycle 14 months ago and has had irregular, heavy menstrual periods since that time. She had no abnormal bleeding at the time of a tonsillectomy. She has no family history suggestive of blood disorders. Her vital signs are within normal limits: quantitative human chorionic gonadotropin level, less than 5 mIU/mL; hemoglobin level, 11.1 g/dL; hematocrit, 33.2%; mean corpuscular volume, 75 cubic micrometers; platelet count, 342×10^3 per microliter; prothrombin time, 12.2 seconds; partial thromboplastin time, 27.4 seconds; and thyroid-stimulating hormone level, 3.4 mIU/L. The best next step in management is

* (A) iron supplementation
  (B) office pelvic examination
  (C) additional coagulation studies
  (D) pelvic ultrasonography
  (E) oral contraceptives

Evaluation of abnormal uterine bleeding often is an adolescent patient's first encounter with a reproductive care physician. Preteens and teenagers should be educated regarding reproductive health. Current recommendations state that adolescents aged 13–15 years should undergo an initial introductory evaluation by a gynecologist with an emphasis on preventive care, including discussion of vaccinations, healthy eating and exercise, and, when applicable, safe sexual practices. Although the physician may conduct other aspects of the physical examination as needed, it is not vital to perform a pelvic examination at these visits.

Abnormal bleeding in an adolescent patient is approached in a different fashion than in the adult patient. In the described patient, the clinical history and laboratory findings suggest that she has anovulatory bleeding. Anovulatory bleeding is common in the adolescent population; it affects approximately 55–82% of girls for the first 24 months after menarche. This is thought primarily to be caused by the relative immaturity of the hypothalamic–pituitary–ovarian axis. Usually, it will resolve spontaneously in this time frame. Pelvic examination is not indicated.

Because the patient is only mildly anemic and the problem is a self-limited one, iron supplementation would be the best next step in management. Oral contraceptives would be initiated if she does not respond to iron therapy, if the bleeding becomes so frequent that it interferes with school and physical activities, or if contraception is desired. Box 4-1 outlines a generalized approach to the management of anemia caused by abnormal bleeding in an adolescent patient based on the results of an initial or subsequent laboratory evaluation.

Screening for coagulation deficits as performed in this case is appropriate because bleeding disorders can prove to be the causative pathology in adolescent patients with

---

BOX 4-1

BOX 4-1. General Approach to Managing Anemia Caused By Abnormal Uterine Bleeding in an Adolescent Patient

- Mild anemia
  Hematocrit greater than 33% or hemoglobin (Hg) level greater than 11 g/dL can be managed with iron supplementation. If contraception is needed, combined oral, transdermal, or intravaginal methods also can be prescribed to aid with anemia.

- Moderate anemia
  Hematocrit 27–33% or Hg level of 9–11 g/dL can be managed with oral contraceptives to control the abnormal uterine bleeding in addition to iron supplementation.

- Severe anemia
  Hematocrit less than 27% or Hg level less than 9 g/dL should be managed with oral contraceptives (one pill every 6 hours until bleeding decreases and then a tapered dose to complete a 21-day pill pack). This dosage of estrogen usually will require an additional antiemetic medication. For the following 3 months, the patient should receive oral contraceptives in the manner prescribed for contraception in addition to iron supplementation to treat anemia. The patient can then be reevaluated to determine whether the maintenance of therapy with oral contraceptives is necessary.

abnormal uterine bleeding. However, because these conditions are comparatively rare and because no symptoms exist that would raise concern for an inherited bleeding disorder and initial coagulation studies yield normal results, it is not cost effective to pursue extensive testing before treatment. Pelvic ultrasonography or other imaging is not indicated for the described patient and should be reserved for patients with atypical presentations or patients who did not respond to empiric therapy.

American College of Obstetricians and Gynecologists. Management of anovulatory bleeding. ACOG Practice Bulletin 14. Washington, DC: ACOG; 2000.

The initial reproductive health visit. Committee Opinion No. 460. American College of Obstetricians and Gynecologists. Obstet Gynecol 2010;116:240–3.

Menstruation in girls and adolescents: using the menstrual cycle as a vital sign. ACOG Committee Opinion No. 349. American College of Obstetricians and Gynecologists. Obstet Gynecol 2006;108:1323–8.

Strickland JL, Wall JW. Abnormal uterine bleeding in adolescents. Obstet Gynecol Clin North Am 2003;30:321–35.

5

Wound management

A 29-year-old obese nulliparous woman underwent an open myomectomy through a vertical midline incision. Two weeks after the surgery, she comes to your office to have the incision inspected. She has not experienced fever, but reports incisional pain, redness, and warmth. The bowel and bladder functions are normal. Her vital signs are unremarkable and the incision is intact with moderate periumbilical drainage, erythema, and tenderness. The best next step in her management is

      (A) intravenous antibiotics
      (B) oral antibiotics
      (C) computerized tomography of the abdomen and pelvis
*   (D) explore the incision

Wound infections represent one of the most common complications for the practicing obstetrician–gynecologist with reported rates of approximately 12% in the postoperative period. Aggressive early identification and management can limit systemic impact and improve overall outcome. Wound infections from organisms typically originate at three sites:

1. Gram-positive organisms on the skin
2. Gram-negative organisms in the genitourinary tract
3. Anaerobic organisms in the pelvic and colorectal regions

The polymicrobial component of wound infections during gynecologic surgery underscores the importance of early treatment with broad-spectrum antibiotics.

Myomectomy and postcesarean incisions have been characterized as clean-contaminated incisions. Patients may have a pelvic or abdominal process associated with a local wound complication that may require an aggressive surgical approach. Computerized tomography of the abdomen and pelvis may be helpful, but delay of local wound care in this setting would not be indicated and may lead to progression of the local wound infection.

Oral antibiotics for patients with local wound infections should cover a broad spectrum of potential microbes.

Reasonable options for antibiotics include oral cephalosporins, such as amoxicillin clavulanate and sulfamethoxazole–trimethoprim. It is important to consider methicillin-resistant *Staphylococcus aureus* in a patient with signs of a moderate infection. Initiation of oral antibiotics without exploration of the patient's incision is not indicated. Inappropriate use of antibiotics may lead to drug-resistant infections without affecting the local wound care.

The first step in the management of patients with local wound infection is identification of the depth and breadth of infection. A complete examination of a surgical wound should assess for tenderness, swelling, redness, and warmth. Identification of an area amenable to drainage and local wound care is essential to limit progression and worsening of a wound infection. In instances of minimal drainage or suspected wound infection, a cotton swab can be used for inspection without opening the entire wound. Patients may require wet to dry dressing changes, vacuum-assisted wound closure, or operative intervention. It is important to monitor patients for potential necrotizing fasciitis and fascial dehiscence, although both conditions are rare. If such conditions develop, it is a surgical emergency. Patients with local infections that are not complicated by serious wound breakdown may be treated in the office with close follow-up until improvement is noted.

Antibiotic prophylaxis for gynecologic procedures. ACOG Practice Bulletin No. 104. American College of Obstetricians and Gynecologists. Obstet Gynecol 2009;113:1180–9.

Larsen JW, Hager WD, Livengood CH, Hoyme U. Guidelines for the diagnosis, treatment and prevention of postoperative infections. Infect Dis Obstet Gynecol 2003;11:65–70.

Rivlin ME, Carroll CS, Morrison JC. Conservative surgery for uterine incisional necrosis complicating cesarean delivery. Obstet Gynecol 2004;103:1105–8.

6

An ovarian tumor of low malignant potential

A 25-year-old woman is taken to the operating room for removal of an 8-cm complex adnexal mass (Fig. 6-1). Inspection at the time of laparoscopy shows normal appearing diaphragms, peritoneal surfaces, and omentum. The contralateral ovary has a 2-cm cyst and no excrescences. Pelvic washings and laparoscopic cystectomy are completed, and the cyst is removed without rupture. The frozen-section diagnosis reveals a serous tumor of low malignant potential. The most appropriate surgical procedure for this patient is

       (A) no other procedure
       (B) cystectomy of contralateral ovary
       (C) peritoneal biopsies
  *   (D) omentectomy and peritoneal biopsies
       (E) omentectomy plus pelvic and paraaortic lymphadenectomy

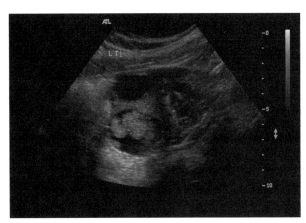

FIG. 6-1

A young woman with a persistent complex adnexal mass requires surgical evaluation. In addition to the common benign adnexal masses, such as mature teratomas, persistent hemorrhagic corpus luteum cysts, or endometriomas, the differential diagnosis includes malignant germ cell tumors, sex cord–stromal tumors, epithelial cancer, and epithelial tumors of low malignant potential. The purpose of surgical evaluation is to make an accurate diagnosis and to perform comprehensive staging or debulking in the event of malignancy. Fertility-sparing surgery (unilateral oophorectomy or salpingo-oophorectomy with preservation of normal contralateral ovary and uterus) and comprehensive surgical staging are indicated when a frozen-section diagnosis reveals an ovarian malignancy or a tumor of low malignant potential. The preoperative imaging study result (Fig. 6-1) is concerning for malignancy because the solid mural nodule within the cyst is greater than 1 cm. Other findings concerning for malignancy would be a thick septation (greater than 3 mm) or abnormal vascular flow to the ovary or nodule.

Ovarian tumors of low malignant potential represent approximately 10–15% of all cases of ovarian cancer. They are commonly serous but also can be mucinous. Most are confined to the ovary at the time of diagnosis, but extraovarian disease in the form of invasive or noninvasive implants is seen in 30% of patients.

When an ovarian tumor of low malignant potential is diagnosed, age-appropriate surgical staging is indicated. For a young woman with invasive epithelial ovarian cancer, comprehensive surgical staging includes abdominal washings, removal of the affected ovary, peritoneal biopsies, omentectomy, and ipsilateral pelvic and paraaortic lymphadenectomy. Lymphadenectomy is not required for women with a tumor of low malignant potential that is grossly confined to the ovary because the incidence of metastasis is low, and presence of metastasis would not affect adjuvant therapy decisions. Stage I tumors of low malignant potential have a nearly 100% cure rate. Women found to have noninvasive peritoneal implants have a 20–40% recurrence rate, but this risk is not decreased by adjuvant chemotherapy. Although microscopic disease found in a lymph node would increase the patient's risk of recurrence, no data suggest that she should receive adjuvant therapy.

In accordance with the 2012 National Comprehensive Cancer Network Guidelines, the general gynecologist confronted with a low malignant potential tumor at the time of laparoscopic cystectomy should perform the additional fertility-sparing surgery required. A general survey of the abdomen should be performed to exclude gross extraovarian disease. Oophorectomy alone is inappropriate because the patient does not undergo staging and the recurrence rate is high. The contralateral ovary has a 2-cm cyst. Serous tumors of low malignant potential can be bilateral in 50% of cases, but this should be detectable on preoperative imaging. Biopsy or cystectomy of the contralateral ovary is inappropriate in the absence of clinical suspicion and will potentially affect fertility. Because the patient has no gross extraovarian disease, she should have fertility-sparing comprehensive staging, which includes unilateral oophorectomy, peritoneal biopsies, and omentectomy.

Gershenson DM. Treatment of ovarian cancer in young women. Clin Obstet Gynecol 2012;55:65–74.

Morgan RJ Jr, Alvarez RD, Armstrong DK, Boston B, Burger RA, Chen LM, et al. Epithelial ovarian cancer. National Comprehensive Cancer Network. J Natl Compr Canc Netw 2011;9:82–113.

Rao GG, Skinner E, Gehrig PA, Duska LR, Coleman RL, Schorge JO. Surgical staging of ovarian low malignant potential tumors. Obstet Gynecol 2004;104:261–6.

Gershenson DM. Treatment of ovarian cancer in young women. Clin Obstet Gynecol 2012;55:65–74.

7

Contraceptive options for a woman with diabetes mellitus and a seizure disorder

A 33-year-old woman, gravida 1, para 1, recently stopped breastfeeding. She comes to your office to inquire about interval contraception. She had a normal spontaneous vaginal delivery and gave birth to a healthy, term infant 12 months ago. The pregnancy was complicated by gestational diabetes mellitus (GDM) and a seizure disorder. She is currently taking carbamazepine. Her past surgical history includes a laparoscopic salpingostomy for ectopic pregnancy 5 years ago and malabsorptive bariatric surgery. In the past, she has used only condoms and wishes to avoid irregular anovulatory bleeding, but does not want to use an injectable contraceptive method. You counsel that her best choice for contraception is

* (A) levonorgestrel intrauterine device (IUD)
  (B) cyclic combination oral contraceptive pills
  (C) contraceptive rod
  (D) extended-cycle oral contraceptive pills
  (E) hysteroscopic bilateral tubal occlusion

The World Health Organization and the Centers for Disease Control and Prevention have issued comprehensive, evidence-based guidelines for use of contraceptives. Several medical conditions are listed with categories or scores associated with the use of different contraceptive methods (Appendix B). This patient has several medical factors that affect her choice of contraceptive method. Discontinuation of breastfeeding has no bearing on her contraceptive choice.

The levonorgestrel IUD is the best method for this patient based on the medical eligibility scoring system. The method has a medical eligibility score of 1, which indicates no restriction of use for patients with a past history of GDM, use of carbamazepine, past history of ectopic pregnancy, and history of either restrictive or malabsorptive bariatric surgery.

Neither cyclic combination oral contraceptive pills nor extended-cycle oral contraceptive pills would be the best choice for this patient. History of GDM and prior ectopic pregnancy both have a medical eligibility score of 1. Carbamazepine use and a malabsorptive bariatric surgery procedure have a score of 3, which indicates that the risk of using these contraceptives outweighs benefit in a patient with these concomitant medical conditions. Therefore, an alternative, safer method should be chosen.

The contraceptive rod, despite a medical eligibility score of 1 in this setting, is not a good choice for this patient because she has expressed a desire to avoid anovulatory bleeding, a common adverse effect with this method. Bilateral tubal occlusion is a permanent, not interval, method and, therefore, does not meet this patient's contraceptive needs.

Understanding and using the U.S. Medical Eligibility Criteria for Contraceptive Use, 2010. Committee Opinion No. 505. American College of Obstetricians and Gynecologists. Obstet Gynecol 2011;118:754–60.

Update to CDC's U.S. Medical Eligibility Criteria for Contraceptive Use, 2010: revised recommendations for the use of contraceptive methods during the postpartum period. Centers for Disease Control and Prevention. MMWR Morb Mortal Wkly Rep 2011;60:878–83.

World Health Organization. Medical eligibility criteria for contraceptive use. 4th ed. Geneva: WHO; 2009. Available at: http://whqlibdoc.who.int/publications/2010/9789241563888_eng.pdf. Retrieved June 7, 2013.

8

Postoperative management of nerve injury

A 65-year-old woman undergoes robotic-assisted laparoscopic abdominal–sacral colpopexy and transobturator tension-free vaginal tape procedure for symptomatic pelvic organ prolapse and urinary incontinence. The surgical time was 4.5 hours and estimated blood loss was 100 mL. On postoperative day 1, her vital signs are stable and urine output is 40 mL/hr. The Foley catheter is removed. On ambulating to the toilet, she experiences right foot drop, gait instability, and numbness over her lateral leg and dorsum of the foot. The most appropriate next step in managing her gait instability is

* (A) physical therapy
 (B) electromyography of the right leg
 (C) magnetic resonance imaging of the pelvis
 (D) duplex ultrasonography of the right leg

Nerve injury during pelvic surgery occurs with stretching or compression of the nerve, entrapment caused by suture placement, transection, or electrocautery thermal injury. Typically, a patient will present with motor weakness and a sensory deficit in the distribution of the affected nerve. A patient might present with pain in the case of a transection or ligation injury. With pelvic surgery, the most common neuropathies are seen with the femoral, ilioinguinal, iliohypogastric, genitofemoral, lateral femoral cutaneous, obturator, and pudendal nerves. With advanced laparoscopic procedures and robotic-assisted procedures, the brachial plexus and peroneal nerves also are at risk of injury caused by pressure, stretching, or compression. Patients who undergo most laparoscopic gynecologic surgical procedures are placed in a low lithotomy position, and stirrups are used that support the legs and are adjustable during surgery to improve access to the vagina (Fig. 8-1). It is important to minimize tension on the femoral, sciatic, and peroneal nerves.

The described patient has signs of a peroneal nerve injury. This compression nerve injury was most likely caused by improper positioning of the patient's leg in the stirrup in the operating room. Pressure on the lateral aspect of the fibula will compress the common peroneal nerve. In proper lithotomy position, the weight of the patient's legs should be on the feet; the knees and ankles should be aligned to the contralateral shoulder with minimal abduction and external hip rotation, and the knees and

hips should not be flexed more than 90 degrees. Hips, lateral fibulas, posterior thighs, and heels should be padded.

The patient should have physical therapy for training in gait stabilization and ankle bracing if appropriate. The duration of the neuropathy depends on the degree to which the nerve was affected by a hypoxic insult, but with time the injury should spontaneously resolve without sequelae. The risk of peroneal nerve injury increases with prolonged lithotomy position.

In procedures that last longer than 4 hours, the surgeon can consider repositioning the patient to remove stretching and compression on nerves. In addition to direct compression from positioning, nerve injury associated with gynecologic surgery also can occur with retractor placement or as a direct surgical injury during dissection.

The most common nerve injury related to retractor use is a femoral neurapraxia that occurs with direct compression of the femoral nerve by a long retractor blade. Femoral nerve injury also may occur as the result of hyperflexion of the hips in exaggerated lithotomy position. Femoral neuropathy is characterized by inability to straighten the leg or extend the knee and by knee instability. Hyperflexion also can result in a stretch injury of the sciatic nerve. Obturator nerve injury occurs most commonly as the result of direct surgical injury during pelvic lymphadenectomy or paravaginal repair. Obturator neuropathy is characterized by inability to adduct the leg. Brachial plexus neuropathy occurs as a result of stretching

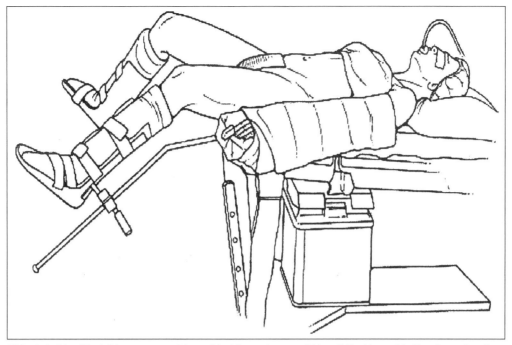

FIG. 8-1. Modified lithotomy position with Allen stirrups. (Trivedi P, Abreo M. Predisposing factors for fibroids and outcome of laparoscopic myomectomy in infertility. J Gynecol Endosc Surg 2009;1:47–56.)

of the brachial plexus if a patient slides cephalad when she is in steep Trendelenburg position with her arms fixed to her sides. Shoulder blocks can place direct pressure on the nerves if placed too medially; therefore, the blocks should have pressure directed on the acromial processes.

Because this patient has a peroneal neuropathy that is diagnosed based on her clinical findings (ie, foot drop), pelvic magnetic resonance imaging and duplex ultrasonography are unnecessary. Electromyographic studies can be helpful to distinguish a transection injury from a severe stretch or traction injury, but the peroneal nerve was not at risk of transection in this patient.

Bohrer JC, Walters MD, Park A, Polston D, Barber MD. Pelvic nerve injury following gynecologic surgery: a prospective cohort study. Am J Obstet Gynecol 2009;201:531.e1–7.

Chan JK, Manetta A. Prevention of femoral nerve injuries in gynecologic surgery. Am J Obstet Gynecol 2002;186:1–7.

Phong SV, Koh LK. Anaesthesia for robotic-assisted radical prostatectomy: considerations for laparoscopy in the Trendelenburg position. Anaesth Intensive Care 2007;35:281–5.

Trivedi P, Abreo M. Predisposing factors for fibroids and outcome of laparoscopic myomectomy in infertility. J Gynecol Endosc Surg 2009;1:47–56.

9

Recognition of physician burnout

Your office staff expresses concern when a colleague becomes increasingly more irritated after patient encounters. This behavior escalated after the practice administrator added ten additional new patient slots per week and has opened the office an hour earlier to accommodate these additional appointments. The staff worries that the physician's "bad attitude" might have a negative effect on patient care, satisfaction, and safety. When you discuss the staff's concerns with the physician, the physician expresses indifference toward work and patient care. You suspect physician burnout. The factor most strongly linked to avoiding physician burnout is

* (A) control over one's schedule and hours worked
  (B) earlier retirement age
  (C) specialty choice
  (D) level of financial compensation

The burnout syndrome is characterized by losing enthusiasm for work (emotional exhaustion), treating people as if they are objects (depersonalization), and having a sense that work is no longer meaningful (low personal accomplishment). Burnout represents a deterioration of values, dignity, spirit, and will. Numerous studies suggest that physician burnout is common, affecting one out of three physicians at any given time.

Recognizing and addressing physician burnout is important because burnout leads to a change in the physician–patient relationship and the quality of care that physicians provide. The symptoms of burnout can increase the likelihood of medical errors, which can further contribute to burnout. Other factors associated with burnout include poor health, including headaches; sleep disturbances; irritability; marital difficulties; fatigue; hypertension; anxiety; depression; and myocardial infarction. Burnout may contribute to alcoholism and drug addiction. Physician burnout also can affect the ability to recruit and retain staff and the likelihood of professional liability actions. It has been observed that burnout is more common in professions that involve extensive care of other people than in other professions.

Inability to control one's schedule and the number of hours worked is the strongest risk factor linked to physician burnout. Other worksite-related risk factors include perceived work demands, lack of social support from colleagues, and dissatisfaction with available resources. Many physicians share personality factors that may increase the likelihood of burnout, including compulsiveness, doubt, guilt feelings, and an exaggerated sense of responsibility. Healthy personal relationships can serve as a protection against burnout.

Burnout affects all medical and surgical specialties; thus, choice of specialty is not a factor strongly linked to

physician burnout. Longevity of career and physician age are protective factors with respect to physician burnout. Younger age at time of retirement has no bearing on burnout, although younger retirement age may be either a marker or a result of physician burnout. Level of compensation has not been shown to have any effect on the rate of physician burnout.

Strategies to address and prevent physician burnout need to examine personal and work-related issues. Physicians with greater flexibility and control over their schedule are less likely to experience burnout than others. This involves developing innovative practice models that provide satisfaction to patients and physicians and enable safe patient care. Some studies suggest physician mindfulness and self-awareness help identify what the physicians value and help them connect with what is most meaningful in their workplace, decreasing rates of burnout. Physicians are less likely to develop burnout if they have efficiency, autonomy, and meaning in their work. On a personal level, physicians who spend time with family and friends, have a religious or spiritual activity, practice self-care, find meaning in their work, set limits at work, and practice a healthy philosophical outlook, such as being positive or focusing on success, are less likely to experience burnout.

Chopra SS, Sotile WM, Sotile MO. STUDENTJAMA. Physician burnout. JAMA 2004;291:633.

Keeton K, Fenner DE, Johnson TR, Hayward RA. Predictors of physician career satisfaction, work-life balance, and burnout. Obstet Gynecol 2007;109:949–55.

Shanafelt TD. Enhancing meaning in work: a prescription for preventing physician burnout and promoting patient-centered care. JAMA 2009;302:1338–40.

Spickard A Jr, Gabbe SG, Christensen JF. Mid-career burnout in generalist and specialist physicians. JAMA 2002;288:1447–50.

10

Sexual dysfunction in menopausal women

A 67-year-old woman comes to your office with dyspareunia and vaginal dryness. She has been sexually abstinent for the past 10 years because of her late husband's chronic health concerns. Previously, she enjoyed sexual activities, including vaginal penetration. She is recently widowed and has a new partner. However, she finds she is unable to tolerate vaginal penetration because of severe pain. Her history is notable for urinary incontinence, postherpetic neuropathy, and constipation controlled by medication. Vulvar and vaginal examinations reveal smooth, pale epithelium (Fig. 10-1; see color plate). Microscopic examination shows scant small, round, immature parabasal cells. Vaginal pH is 5. You do not observe clue cells, candidiasis, or increased inflamed cells. The most likely diagnosis is

    *   (A) vaginal atrophy
        (B) lichen sclerosus
        (C) lichen planus
        (D) desquamative inflammatory vaginitis
        (E) pemphigus vulgaris

Sexual dysfunction caused by dyspareunia is common among postmenopausal women. Although 15% of all gynecologic visits are for vulvar pain syndromes, including dyspareunia, evidence suggests that it is underreported and underdiagnosed in postmenopausal women. Dyspareunia may be a symptom of a number of disorders, including organic etiologies (eg, atrophic vaginitis, lichen sclerosus, lichen planus, desquamative inflammatory vaginitis, and pemphigus vulgaris), and disorders with no identifiable cause, such as vulvodynia (Box 10-1).

The most likely cause of vaginal dryness and dyspareunia in the described patient is vaginal atrophy. Many women do not recognize symptoms of vaginal atrophy, especially if they are not sexually active. The diagnosis of vaginal atrophy is made with examination findings, such as smooth, pale epithelium (diminished rugae), a urethral caruncle, immature parabasal cells on microscopy, and an elevated vaginal pH (greater than 4.7) with no evidence of infectious vaginitis. Although lichen sclerosus, lichen planus, desquamative inflammatory vaginitis, and pemphigus vulgaris may each result in dyspareunia, they are less common than vaginal atrophy and are not supported by the examination findings.

Women with lichen sclerosus typically present with pruritus. Examination findings reveal anatomic changes not present with atrophy, including involution of the labia minora (diminished or absent labia), phimosis of the clitoral hood, and scarring or narrowing of the introitus. The skin typically has thin, pale, hypopigmented plaques and may have areas of ecchymoses or purpura.

Lichen planus demonstrates a wide range of morphologic features. The most common form is erosive lichen planus, which classically presents on mucous membranes

as painful, erythematous erosions with white, lacy, reticulate striae (Wickham striae). Erosive lichen planus also

BOX 10-1

Conditions Associated with Dyspareunia

Superficial
- Atrophy
- Condyloma
- Vulvitis or vulvovaginitis
- Dermatologic disease (infectious or noninfectious)
- Dermatoses
- Epithelial defects
- Labial hypertrophy
- Urethritis, cystitis
- Bartholinitis
- Vulvodynia
- Vaginismus

Deep
- Endometriosis
- Interstitial cystitis
- Irritable bowel syndrome
- Levator ani muscle myalgia
- Uterine retroversion
- Pelvic inflammatory disease
- Pelvic adhesion disease
- Pelvic congestion syndrome
- Ovarian remnant syndrome
- History of sexual abuse

Stockdale CK, Boardman LA. Evaluation and treatment of postmenopausal dyspareunia. Case study and commentary. J Clin Outcomes Manage 2011;18:414–23.

may result in anatomic changes to the vulva and vagina, including involution and asymmetry of the labia minora, scarring or narrowing of the introitus, and coaptation of the vagina. As with atrophic changes, microscopic findings confirm immature epithelium (basal and parabasal cells). However, inflammation is marked.

Desquamative inflammatory vaginitis also may present with dyspareunia. However, the hallmark finding is non-infectious vaginitis along with profuse discharge, with marked inflammation, abundant immature squamous cells, and absent lactobacilli on wet mount (similar to erosive lichen planus). The vestibule and vagina typically are erythematous with areas of desquamation (superficial erosions). The anatomy is otherwise normal in appearance.

Pemphigus vulgaris is a rare immunobullous disease that generally occurs during the fourth to fifth decade of life. As with erosive lichen planus, it affects mucous membranes and often presents with pain secondary to erosive changes. Coaptation of opposing surfaces results in vaginal agglutination and scarring. Vaginal wet mount shows increased inflammation, basal and parabasal cells, and absent lactobacilli.

Vaginal atrophy and desquamative inflammatory vaginitis are clinical diagnoses. A biopsy may assist in the diagnosis of lichen sclerosus, erosive lichen planus, and pemphigus vulgaris.

Diagnosis and management of vulvar skin disorders. ACOG Practice Bulletin No. 93. American College of Obstetricians and Gynecologists. Obstet Gynecol 2008;111:1243–53.

Edwards L. Dermatologic causes of vaginitis: a clinical review. Dermatol Clin 2010;28:727–35.

Female sexual dysfunction. Practice Bulletin No. 119. American College of Obstetricians and Gynecologists. Obstet Gynecol 2011; 117:996–1007.

Stockdale CK, Boardman LA. Evaluation and treatment of postmenopausal dyspareunia. Case study and commentary. J Clin Outcomes Manage 2011;18:414–23.

11

Emergency contraception

A 19-year-old woman telephones your office to report that she had unprotected intercourse 4 days ago. Her last menstrual period was 10 days ago and she is concerned that she may become pregnant. You counsel her that the most effective recommended emergency contraception for her is

* (A) copper intrauterine device (IUD)
  (B) oral levonorgestrel
  (C) levonorgestrel IUD
  (D) oral mifepristone
  (E) oral ulipristal acetate

Emergency contraception is indicated in women who have had unprotected intercourse or failure of a barrier method within the past 5 days. Various forms of effective emergency contraception are currently available. With the exception of the levonorgestrel IUD, the contraceptive options listed have all been shown to be reliable means of emergency contraception. However, each method varies in its overall effectiveness, side effects and adverse effects, and appropriate time period of use. Insertion of the copper IUD within 120 hours (5 days) of unprotected intercourse has been shown to have the lowest subsequent pregnancy rates (0–0.2%). The method has the added benefit of long-term reversible birth control.

Oral levonorgestrel can be given as either a single-dose regimen or double-dose regimen. It has become the preferred method over earlier combination estrogen–progestin regimens because it is more effective in preventing pregnancy (risk reduction rate, 0.51) and less likely to result in nausea and vomiting. Pregnancy rates after the use of oral levonorgestrel up to 72 hours after unprotected intercourse are reported to be 1.7–2.4%. Although the efficacy appears to decrease after 72 hours, several studies have shown a moderate reduction in subsequent pregnancies; therefore, use is advised up to 120 hours after intercourse.

The levonorgestrel IUD has not been fully evaluated as a method for emergency contraception. Therefore, the levonorgestrel IUD is not currently a recommended option for emergency contraception, although investigational studies are underway.

Mifepristone, a progesterone receptor modulator, has been shown to be effective for emergency contraception. In one study of more than 2,000 women, single-dose oral mifepristone was found to be as effective as oral levonorgestrel when used within 5 days of unprotected intercourse (pregnancy rates of 1.3% and 2.0%, respectively). Both methods were found to have minimal adverse effects, most commonly menstrual delay.

Ulipristal acetate, a second-generation progesterone receptor modulator, has been shown to prevent ovulation even after the luteinizing hormone surge. Several studies have shown single-dose ulipristal acetate (0.9%) to be at least as effective as oral levonorgestrel (1.7%) for the prevention of pregnancy. In addition, it appears that unlike oral levonorgestrel, the effect does not seem to decrease between 72 hours and 120 hours after intercourse. In 2010, the U.S. Food and Drug Administration approved the use of ulipristal acetate for emergency contraception up to 120 hours after unprotected intercourse. Adverse effects most commonly include headache, nausea, and menstrual delay, similar to the adverse effects of levonorgestrel.

Creinin MD, Schlaff W, Archer DF, Wan L, Frezieres R, Thomas M, et al. Progesterone receptor modulator for emergency contraception: a randomized controlled trial. Obstet Gynecol 2006;108:1089–97.

Emergency contraception. ACOG Practice Bulletin No. 112. American College of Obstetricians and Gynecologists. Obstet Gynecol 2010; 115:1100–9.

Fine P, Mathe H, Ginde S, Cullins V, Morfesis J, Gainer E. Ulipristal acetate taken 48–120 hours after intercourse for emergency contraception. Obstet Gynecol 2010;115:257–63.

Hamoda H, Ashok PW, Stalder C, Flett GM, Kennedy E, Templeton A. A randomized trial of mifepristone (10 mg) and levonorgestrel for emergency contraception. Obstet Gynecol 2004;104:1307–13.

Long-acting reversible contraception: implants and intrauterine devices. ACOG Practice Bulletin No. 121. American College of Obstetricians and Gynecologists. Obstet Gynecol 2011;118:184–96.

Wu S, Godfrey EM, Wojdyla D, Dong J, Cong J, Wang C, et al. Copper T380A intrauterine device for emergency contraception: a prospective, multicentre, cohort clinical trial. BJOG 2010;117:1205–10.

12

Mature cystic teratoma with recurrence

An 18-year-old woman comes to the office for follow-up of a right adnexal mass noted on computed tomography of the abdomen and pelvis after a motor vehicle accident. She reports neither abdominal nor pelvic pain. She has regular menstrual cycles and is using oral contraceptives. A urine pregnancy test result is negative. Ultrasonography reveals a right adnexal mass of 3 cm in largest diameter (Fig. 12-1) with ovarian volume of 25 cm^3. She has a history of laparoscopic right ovarian cystectomy for a mature cystic teratoma 3 years ago. The best next step in the management of this mass is

        (A) CA 125 testing
        (B) laparoscopic resection
*   (C) observation
        (D) magnetic resonance imaging (MRI)

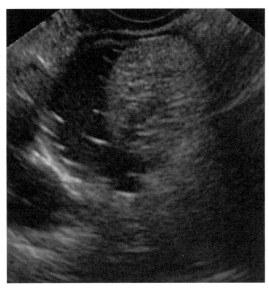

FIG. 12-1

This patient most likely has a recurrence of the mature cystic teratoma that was removed a few years earlier. Ovarian dermoid tumors are classified as mature cystic teratomas if they are cystic with mature elements and as immature teratomas if they are solid with immature malignant elements. In women younger than 30 years, mature cystic teratomas are the most common neoplasms and account for approximately 70% of benign ovarian tumors and 50% of pediatric tumors. They are bilateral in approximately 10–20% of cases.

At the time of diagnosis, 60% of mature cystic teratomas are asymptomatic. The most common symptom is abdominal pain. Other symptoms are rare and include increased abdominal girth, a palpable abdominal mass, constipation, nausea, vomiting, and anorexia.

Complications of mature cystic teratomas include:

- Torsion in 16% of cases
- Rupture in 1–2% of cases
- Infection in 1% of cases
- Malignant transformation in 2% of cases

The major indications for surgical resection of an mature cystic teratoma are clinical symptoms. Other indications are large size (usually greater than 5–10 cm), an enlarging mass over time, or a mass that is considered to be suspicious of malignancy.

The risk of malignancy among pediatric and adolescent patients who undergo a resection of a mature cystic teratoma is 1–2%. It can be a challenge to distinguish benign tumors from malignant tumors based solely on radiologic findings. Hence conservative management is an option especially in adolescent women, in whom ovarian preservation is important. In two studies, no malignant transformations were noted with conservative management. In these studies, surgical resection was performed if the patients developed symptoms or if the cysts grew by more than 2 cm/y. The risk of recurrence at 2 years is estimated to be 3–4% after cystectomy. The risk may be higher if the prior surgical excision was performed by laparoscopy compared with laparotomy. The value of CA 125 testing in differentiating benign from malignant masses in premenopausal patients has not been established. In a prospective study of patients who underwent surgery for a pelvic mass, the positive predictive value of an elevated CA 125 level was 98% in postmenopausal women and 49% in premenopausal women. Therefore, in the described case, a CA 125 test is not indicated.

Additional imaging of a pelvic mass after an adequate transvaginal ultrasound evaluation is of limited use.

Although MRI has an overall lower sensitivity in detecting ovarian masses compared with transvaginal ultrasonography, it has been shown to be superior in correctly classifying masses as malignant. In addition, MRI is helpful in differentiating the origin of nonadnexal pelvic masses, such as uterine myomas. However, in the case under discussion, ultrasound evaluation was adequate, and MRI would not offer additional information that would alter the patient's management.

The described patient is a young woman with the need to conserve her ovaries. The mature cystic teratoma is an incidental finding and is currently not symptomatic. In addition, it is small with no other ultrasonographic indicators of malignancy. After she has been counseled, the patient may be offered conservative management with ultrasonographic follow-up to conserve the ovary.

Benoit MF, Hannigan EV, Strickland JL. Recurrent mature cystic ovarian teratoma in adolescence: atypical case of the growing teratoma syndrome. Obstet Gynecol 2005;105:1264–6.

Management of adnexal masses. ACOG Practice Bulletin No. 83. American College of Obstetricians and Gynecologists. Obstet Gynecol 2007;110:201–14.

O'Neill KE, Cooper AR. The approach to ovarian dermoids in adolescents and young women. J Pediatr Adolesc Gynecol 2011;24:176–80.

13

Dysmenorrhea

A 24-year-old nulliparous woman is referred to you with severe dysmenorrhea for the past 3 years. She is incapacitated for 1–3 days at each menses. Trials of combined oral contraceptives, ibuprofen, naproxen, and celecoxib have not relieved the pain. She has been married for 2 years and has been trying to conceive for almost 1 year without success. The most appropriate management is

    (A) laparoscopic uterine nerve ablation
    (B) depot leuprolide
    (C) noncyclic combined oral contraceptives
*   (D) diagnostic laparoscopy
    (E) opioid analgesic

Survey data suggest that more than 50% of women of reproductive age experience pain at the time of menses. Younger women, especially adolescents, most often have primary dysmenorrhea or lower abdominal pain at the time of menses in the absence of any demonstrable disease that would account for the pain. With increasing age, secondary dysmenorrhea or abdominopelvic pain at the time of menses is more common and may be attributed to disorders, such as endometriosis, adenomyosis, or uterine myomas. The symptoms can significantly affect a woman's quality of life, including attendance at school, work, exercise, or social activities. It is vital that the patient's symptoms are evaluated and treated. If the symptoms are consistent with primary dysmenorrhea, and physical examination and laboratory or imaging study results are normal, it is appropriate to treat the patient empirically for primary dysmenorrhea.

If contraception is not desired, initial treatment with nonsteroidal antiinflammatory drugs is appropriate; a trial of at least 3 months is usual. It is also reasonable to try more than one drug of this type before concluding lack of efficacy. Combined oral contraceptives also have shown significant efficacy in the treatment of dysmenorrhea. An alternative to cyclical administration is to provide continuous combined oral contraceptives. However, this may result in an increase of breakthrough bleeding. Combined oral contraceptives would not be an appropriate choice for the described woman because she is trying to conceive. Evidence from randomized clinical trials supports the empiric use of gonadotropin-releasing hormone agonists when endometriosis is suspected. However, gonadotropin-releasing hormone agonists would impede conception.

With failed therapy for dysmenorrhea it is important that the patient be evaluated for any underlying cause of menstrual pain. Ultrasonography can be especially helpful in identifying uterine myomas, adenomyosis, and adnexal abnormalities, such as endometriomas. Generally, it is appropriate to proceed to a laparoscopic evaluation for a definitive diagnosis of endometriosis. In the case of the described woman with a history of severe dysmenorrhea and infertility, a diagnostic laparoscopy would be the most appropriate intervention. It is crucial that the laparoscopy be performed by a gynecologic surgeon who is experienced in the recognition of the variety of appearances of endometriosis and that this surgeon have the ability to surgically resect or destroy the endometriosis at the time of diagnostic laparoscopy. Laparoscopy also may be an important tool in the evaluation and treatment of infertility.

Based on a small randomized trial and anecdotal experience, laparoscopic uterine nerve ablation has been performed for the treatment of primary dysmenorrhea and secondary dysmenorrhea associated with endometriosis. Multiple, large clinical trials have subsequently shown that laparoscopic uterine nerve ablation is not efficacious for the treatment of primary or secondary dysmenorrhea. Thus, it is not a recommended procedure and is not an appropriate choice for this patient.

Although there may be certain cases in which short-term use of opioid analgesics is appropriate for the treatment of severe dysmenorrhea, generally, this is not an accepted regimen for treatment. In addition to the known risks of addiction and diversion, the sedating effects of opioid analgesics are not likely to accomplish the goal of returning the patient to normal function at the time of menses.

Bettendorf B, Shay S, Tu F. Dysmenorrhea: contemporary perspectives. Obstet Gynecol Surv 2008;63:597–603.

Daniels J, Gray R, Hills RK, Latthe P, Buckley L, Gupta J, et al. Laparoscopic uterosacral nerve ablation for alleviating chronic pelvic pain: a randomized controlled trial. LUNA Trial Collaboration. JAMA 2009;302:955–61.

Howard FM. Surgical treatment of endometriosis. Obstet Gynecol Clin North Am 2011;38:677–86.

Parker MA, Sneddon AE, Arbon P. The menstrual disorder of teenagers (MDOT) study: determining typical menstrual patterns and menstrual disturbance in a large population-based study of Australian teenagers. BJOG 2010;117:185–92.

14

Adenocarcinoma in situ with positive margins

A 29-year-old woman, gravida 2, para 2, presents to discuss management after a cervical loop electrosurgical excision procedure. The pathology report reveals adenocarcinoma in situ (AIS) with a positive endocervical margin. She desires to maintain fertility. The best next step in management for this patient is

*   (A) colposcopy with biopsy
    (B) cytology and high-risk human papillomavirus (HPV) in 4–6 months
    (C) endocervical curettage
    (D) cold knife cone biopsy
    (E) simple hysterectomy

Although adenocarcinoma is less common than cervical intraepithelial neoplasia (CIN), its incidence has increased nearly fivefold in recent decades. In the 1950s and 1960s, adenocarcinoma accounted for only 5% of all types of cervical cancer. In the 1990s, adenocarcinoma increased to account for 25% of all types of cervical cancer. Although the prevalence of AIS has increased, the prevalence of squamous cell cervical cancer decreased simultaneously. As with all types of cervical cancer and cervical dysplasia, AIS is associated with high-risk HPV (primarily HPV serotype 18).

Many of the assumptions that justify conservative management in women with CIN 2,3 (now termed high-grade squamous intraepithelial lesion [HSIL]) do not apply to AIS. The colposcopic changes associated with AIS can be minimal. Thus, it can be difficult to determine the extent of a lesion or to recognize recurrent disease.

Risk factors for residual disease include the number of quadrants involved with AIS, length of the cone specimen, and disease-free margin of less than 10 mm. Margin status is one of the most clinically useful predictors of residual disease; thus, interpretability of the margins is important for future treatment planning and management. Unlike HSIL, management of AIS has been difficult to define. Because AIS frequently extends for a considerable distance into the endocervical canal, complete excision often is difficult. The disease frequently is multifocal and can contain skip lesions, ie, noncontagious lesions. Thus, hysterectomy is the preferred treatment for women with AIS confirmed by an excisional procedure in those patients who have completed childbearing.

Conservative management is acceptable if future fertility is desired in appropriately counseled women. If conservative management is planned and the margins of the specimen are involved or endocervical sampling obtained at the time of excision contains CIN 2,3 (HSIL) or AIS, reexcision to increase the likelihood of complete excision is preferred. A number of studies demonstrate that complete excisional procedure with cold knife cone is curative in most patients, with recurrent or persistent AIS or invasive adenocarcinoma, which occurs in up to 9% of patients. Conversely, a small study demonstrated residual AIS in 45% of subsequent hysterectomy specimens despite negative margins after loop electrosurgical excision procedure.

Although long-term follow-up is recommended for women who do not undergo a hysterectomy, evaluation is limited by an inability to reliably predict the risk of residual disease or recurrence with the conventional clinicopathologic features that are applied to squamous dysplasia of the cervix. Reevaluation at 6 months with a combination of cervical cytology, high-risk HPV DNA testing, and colposcopy with endocervical sampling would be acceptable for the described patient, although it would not be the preferred next step (Fig. 14-1).

Close clinical follow-up is advocated for all patients with AIS because of the potential for recurrence or development of invasive disease. Once childbearing is complete, a simple hysterectomy should be recommended.

DeSimone CP, Day ME, Dietrich CS 3rd, Tovar MM, Modesitt SC. Risk for residual adenocarcinoma in situ or cervical adenocarcinoma in women undergoing loop electrosurgical excision procedure/conization for adenocarcinoma in situ. J Reprod Med 2011;56:376–80.

Massad LS, Einstein MH, Huh WK, Katki HA, Kinney WK, Schiffman M, et al. 2012 updated consensus guidelines for the management of abnormal cervical cancer screening tests and cancer precursors. 2012 ASCCP Consensus Guidelines Conference. Obstet Gynecol 2013;121:829–46.

Salani R, Puri I, Bristow RE. Adenocarcinoma in situ of the uterine cervix: a metaanalysis of 1278 patients evaluating the predictive value of conization margin status. Am J Obstet Gynecol 2009;200:182.e1–5.

van Hanegem N, Barroilhet LM, Nucci MR, Bernstein M, Feldman S. Fertility-sparing treatment in younger women with adenocarcinoma in situ of the cervix. Gynecol Oncol 2012;124:72–7.

Management of Women Diagnosed with Adenocarcinoma in-situ (AIS) during a Diagnostic Excisional Procedure

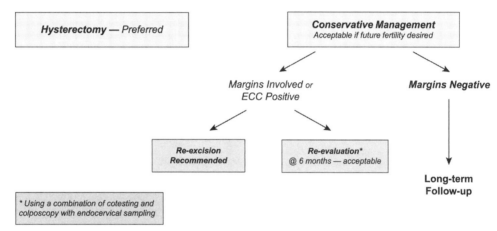

FIG. 14-1. Management of women diagnosed with adenocarcinoma in situ during a diagnostic excisional procedure. (Reprinted from the *Journal of Lower Genital Tract Disease* Volume 17, Number 5, with the permission of ASCCP © American Society for Colposcopy and Cervical Pathology 2013. No copies of the algorithms may be made without the prior consent of ASCCP. Massad LS, Einstein MH, Huh WK, Katki HA, Kinney WK, Schiffman M, et al. 2012 updated consensus guidelines for the management of abnormal cervical cancer screening tests and cancer precursors. 2012 ASCCP Consensus Guidelines Conference. J Low Genit Tract Dis 2013;17[5 Suppl 1]:S1–S27.)

15

Follow-up after loop electrosurgical procedure

A 38-year-old woman, gravida 3, para 3, comes to your office for follow-up of a loop electro-surgical excision procedure (LEEP). She has no significant past medical history but smokes five cigarettes per day. She has had seven lifetime sexual partners. Currently, her only sexual partner is her husband of 5 years. She has undergone a bilateral tubal ligation. The result of her last human immunodeficiency virus (HIV) test was negative 2 years ago during prenatal care. She also had normal Pap test results until the most recent one, which was positive for a high-grade squamous intraepithelial lesion (HSIL). Colposcopic biopsy confirms cervical intraepithelial neoplasia (CIN) 3. Endocervical curettage result is negative. The LEEP test result is CIN 3 with positive ectocervical margins. The best next step in this patient's management is

* (A) hysterectomy
* * (B) Pap test in 4–6 months
* (C) cryotherapy
* (D) treatment with topical imiquimod

Risk factors for cervical dysplasia include age at first sexual intercourse, number of lifetime sexual partners, tobacco use, and immunosuppression. Women should begin routine cervical cancer screening at age 21 years. Women who receive the diagnosis of CIN 3 after satisfactory colposcopy are recommended to receive follow-up treatment with a diagnostic excisional procedure, such as LEEP, cold-knife cone biopsy, or ablation of the cervical transformation zone by means of cryotherapy or laser. Exceptions may be made in certain circumstances, eg, pregnancy and young age.

Follow-up options after an excisional procedure with negative margins include human papillomavirus DNA testing at 6–12 months, cytology alone, or combination of cytology and colposcopy at 6-month intervals. After two consecutive negative results, the patient may return to routine screening. However, if CIN 2,3 is present at biopsy specimen margins or in an immediate postprocedure endocervical curettage specimen, the preferred management is cytology in 4–6 months. If CIN 2,3 result recurs, a repeat excisional procedure or hysterectomy also is acceptable. Patients who have excisional biopsy results with positive margins (dysplasia extending to edge of cervical specimen), particularly if they are endocervical margins, may be at an increased risk of disease recurrence.

To date, no nonsurgical therapy is available for CIN. Several topical therapies, such as imiquimod, and therapeutic human papillomavirus vaccination are being researched but, to date, none is as effective as excision or ablation.

Bell MC, Alvarez RD. Chemoprevention and vaccines: a review of the nonsurgical options for the treatment of cervical dysplasia. Int J Gynecol Cancer 2005;15:4–12.

Cervical cancer in adolescents: screening, evaluation, and management. Committee Opinion No. 463. American College of Obstetricians and Gynecologists. Obstet Gynecol 2010;116:469–72.

Massad LS, Einstein MH, Huh WK, Katki HA, Kinney WK, Schiffman M, et al. 2012 updated consensus guidelines for the management of abnormal cervical cancer screening tests and cancer precursors. 2012 ASCCP Consensus Guidelines Conference. J Obstet Gynecol 2013;121:829–46.

16

Uterosacral ligament suspension for vaginal prolapse

You perform a cystoscopy on a 65-year-old woman after you complete a total vaginal hysterectomy and uterosacral ligament suspension for vaginal prolapse. The patient received intravenous (IV) indigo carmine, and now you observe an immediate efflux of dye from the right ureter. After 30 minutes, no efflux is observed from the left ureter. The next step in management should be to

      (A) continue observation for another 15 minutes
      (B) administer IV furosemide
      (C) place a ureteral stent on the left side
*   (D) remove the most lateral and posterior suture on the left

Uterosacral ligament suspension for treatment of vaginal apex prolapse has become a popular procedure. It may be performed vaginally or laparoscopically. The surgical procedure consists of placing two, three, or four sutures into the high and posterior portions of the uterosacral ligaments on each side, respectively, and then placing the sutures into the anterior and posterior vaginal musculature to accomplish suspension of the vaginal apex. This procedure results in normal anatomic positioning of the vaginal apex. It is preferred over sacrospinous ligament fixation by many gynecologic surgeons because of ease of the procedure and the decreased risk of complications, such as hematoma or nerve injury. The most common complications of uterosacral ligament suspension are ureteral obstruction, pelvic nerve injury, hemorrhage that requires transfusion, and pelvic organ injury, especially injury to the rectosigmoid colon.

Ureteral obstruction is the most common complication, having been found during intraoperative cystoscopy in up to 11% of reported cases. For this reason, intraoperative cystoscopy after IV administration of indigo carmine is recommended at the completion of a uterosacral ligament suspension. Obstruction is most often caused by kinking of the ureter by the uterosacral ligament sutures. If obstruction occurs, the most appropriate intervention is to remove the ipsilateral, most lateral uterosacral ligament suture and then repeat the cystoscopy. Sutures on the ipsilateral side should be sequentially removed until normal efflux of dye from the ureter occurs.

For the described patient, to continue observation for at least 15 minutes longer is not advisable. Although some variability exists in the rapidity of clearance of dye between the two kidneys, it almost never differs by 45 minutes. This observation clearly suggests that ureteral obstruction exists on the left side. To administer IV furosemide and continue observation also is not recommended. The immediate efflux from the right ureter indicates sufficient hydration and renal function; therefore, the administration of furosemide will not change the observation.

Placing a ureteral stent on the left side is not appropriate management for this patient intraoperatively. In almost all cases, removal of one or more sutures on the side of the obstructed ureter results in rapid return of ureteral function. The increased risks of potential complications by placement of a ureteral stent are not justified unless the ureter does not function after removal of all sutures.

Barber MD, Visco AG, Weidner AC, Amundsen CL, Bump RC. Bilateral uterosacral ligament vaginal vault suspension with site-specific endopelvic fascia defect repair for treatment of pelvic organ prolapse. Am J Obstet Gynecol 2000;183:1402–10; discussion 1410–1.

Karram M, Goldwasser S, Kleeman S, Steele A, Vassallo B, Walsh P. High uterosacral vaginal vault suspension with fascial reconstruction for vaginal repair of enterocele and vaginal vault prolapse. Am J Obstet Gynecol 2001;185:1339–42; discussion 1342–3.

17

Ovarian remnant syndrome

A 40-year-old woman, gravida 2, para 2, returns to your office 3 years after you performed a total abdominal hysterectomy and bilateral salpingo-oophorectomy for stage IV endometriosis with severe adhesive disease. She has been experiencing right-sided abdominopelvic pain that is severe and similar to the pain she had before the hysterectomy. Her only medication is an estradiol patch. On examination, she has tenderness in the right lower quadrant and at the right vaginal apex. Ultrasonography suggests a 2 cm × 1.5 cm cyst at the right vaginal apex. The patient requests surgery. The most appropriate next step is

     (A) laparoscopic removal of the pelvic cyst
     (B) depot leuprolide treatment for 6 months
     (C) colonoscopy
*   (D) stop estradiol therapy and obtain follicle-stimulating hormone (FSH) level
     (E) referral to a chronic pain clinic

Ovarian remnant syndrome is the presence of ovarian tissue after an oophorectomy. Most often, it occurs after a difficult hysterectomy and bilateral salpingo-oophorectomy during which one or both fallopian tubes and ovaries are densely adhered to the pelvic sidewall. It has been shown that even small remnants of ovarian tissue may remain viable and subsequently enlarge in size, usually resulting in pelvic pain, a pelvic mass, or both.

Ovarian remnant syndrome is one of several diagnoses that should be considered with recurrent pelvic pain after a hysterectomy and bilateral salpingo-oophorectomy. Other possible diagnoses include interstitial cystitis, irritable bowel syndrome, abdominal myofascial pain syndrome, pelvic floor tension myalgia, and vaginal apex neuroma. Thus, it is important that a full evaluation be performed before surgery.

Recurrent endometriosis is a possible diagnosis, but it is rare after a hysterectomy and bilateral salpingo-oophorectomy with removal of all endometriosis. If no ovarian tissue remains, treatment with a gonadotropin-releasing hormone (GnRH) agonist is not likely to be effective for endometriosis. The GnRH agonists work by suppressing the hypothalamic–pituitary–ovarian axis. That is, GnRH agonists do not work directly on endometriosis lesions, but rather work by suppression of gonadotropins. Therefore, depot leuprolide treatment is not the correct choice if the intention is to treat endometriosis in the absence of ovarian remnant syndrome. Treatment with a GnRH agonist is likely to be effective for the treatment of ovarian remnant syndrome and would be an option for treatment once this diagnosis has been established.

Unless gastrointestinal symptoms suggestive of organic pathology are present, such as inflammatory bowel disease or diverticulitis, referral for colonoscopy is unlikely to help with the differential diagnosis.

The diagnosis of ovarian remnant syndrome can be established in a number of ways. The first approach is to discontinue hormone therapy and obtain an FSH level in approximately 4 weeks. If this patient has premenopausal levels of FSH, the diagnosis is ovarian remnant syndrome. If the hormonal levels are borderline for premenopausal status, then a GnRH agonist stimulation test can be performed. Imaging studies, especially ultrasonography, often will reveal the presence of a pelvic mass consistent with persistence of ovarian tissue and will localize the anatomic location of the ovarian remnant. Because of the complexity of surgery, a trial of medical management may be warranted. Discussion of the risks and benefits of medical and surgical treatments with the patient is imperative.

Referral to a chronic pain clinic without further evaluation for gynecologic and nongynecologic etiologies would rarely be appropriate. If a thorough evaluation is performed and no diagnosis other than chronic pelvic pain is found, then such a referral would be reasonable.

Magtibay PM, Magrina JF. Ovarian remnant syndrome. Clin Obstet Gynecol 2006;49:526–34.

Redwine DB. Endometriosis persisting after castration: clinical characteristics and results of surgical management. Obstet Gynecol 1994;83:405–13.

Steege JF. Ovarian remnant syndrome. Obstet Gynecol 1987;70:64–7.

18

Human immunodeficiency virus exposure and prophylaxis

A woman who is known to have human immunodeficiency virus (HIV) is undergoing an emergency cesarean delivery. Her viral titer is greater than 1,500 copies per milliliter. Postexposure prophylaxis should be offered for

* (A) a penetrating finger injury with a visibly bloody scalpel
(B) a blood splash onto the surgeon's unprotected forehead
(C) amniotic fluid saturating through the surgeon's sleeve
(D) a nonpenetrating needlestick through glove during myometrial closure
(E) unprotected skin exposure to sputum during extubation

Obstetrician–gynecologists frequently are involved in procedures with a clear risk of transmission of bloodborne pathogens. These procedures include deep suturing to arrest hemorrhage, cesarean delivery, hysterectomy, forceps delivery, episiotomy, cone biopsy, ovarian cystectomy, and other transvaginal or open surgical procedures that last more than 3 hours. The risk of HIV seroconversion after exposure to body fluids from an HIV-infected patient is low, approximately 0.33%.

As of 2005, 57 health care providers in the United States had seroconverted after occupational exposure to an HIV-infected individual. Most health care providers who have had seroconversion after occupational exposure have been nurses; no documented seroconversion among surgeons has been reported. The risk of seroconversion is dependent on the type of exposure and the viral load of the patient. Hollow-bore needlestick injuries are a recognized mechanism for health care provider seroconversion. A case–control study by the Centers for Disease Control and Prevention (CDC) found that deeply penetrating injuries have the highest risk of seroconversion (odds ratio [OR] = 15), followed by a visibly contaminated hollow needle (OR = 6.2), terminal illness in the source patient (OR = 5.6), and needle placement in a vein or artery (OR = 4.3).

The CDC has defined the types of exposure that merit consideration for postexposure prophylaxis to include a percutaneous injury and contact with mucous membrane or nonintact skin. Body fluids of concern are semen, vaginal secretions, and blood. Potentially infectious fluids include cerebrospinal, synovial, pleural, peritoneal, pericardial, and amniotic fluids. Nasal secretions, saliva, sputum, sweat, and tears are not infectious unless contaminated with blood.

All institutions should have a readily available policy for managing bloodborne pathogen exposure. The initial response to occupational exposure to potentially infectious body fluids is immediate cleansing of the exposed site with soap and water and a virucidal antiseptic. Exposed mucous membranes should be flushed with water.

The CDC has published recommendations regarding who should receive postexposure prophylaxis based on the type of exposure (percutaneous, mucous membrane, or nonintact skin), the likelihood that the source is HIV infected, and the stage of HIV infection (Table 18-1 and Table 18-2). The risk is highest when the source has a high viral load, the volume of blood is large, and the exposure is deep. Intact skin is an effective barrier against HIV infection, and contamination of intact skin does not require postexposure prophylaxis.

A health care provider who experiences a penetrating injury is at highest risk of HIV seroconversion and should be offered three-drug prophylaxis. A health care provider who experiences a breach of protective equipment during myometrial closure is at risk only if blood comes into contact with nonintact skin or in case of a percutaneous injury. In those scenarios, the health care provider should be offered two-drug prophylaxis. With a percutaneous exposure, the average risk of seroconversion is 3 to 1,000 but varies with viral load and volume of blood. Blood or body fluid contact with intact skin has not been associated with HIV infection; therefore, none of the other clinical scenarios warrant postexposure prophylaxis.

Postexposure prophylaxis reduces the risk of seroconversion by at least 80%, and the newest multi-agent prophylaxis might afford greater reduction. Postexposure prophylaxis should be started within 1–2 hours of exposure. The drugs should have a rapid onset of action. A single agent, zidovudine, has been shown to be effective in preventing HIV transmission in health care providers, but failures have been documented. Current CDC recommendations call for two nucleosides for low-risk exposure and two nucleosides plus a boosted protease

TABLE 18-1. Recommended Human Immunodeficiency Virus Postexposure Prophylaxis for Percutaneous Injuries

Exposure Type	Human Immunodeficiency Virus-Positive (HIV-RNA Count Less Than 1,500 Copies per Milliliter)	Human Immunodeficiency Virus-Positive (HIV-RNA Count Greater Than 1,500 Copies per Milliliter)	Source of Unknown HIV Status	Unknown Source*
Low risk[†]	Basic two-drug postexposure prophylaxis recommended	Expanded three-drug postexposure prophylaxis recommended	Generally, no postexposure prophylaxis warranted; however, consider basic two-drug postexposure prophylaxis[§] for source with HIV risk factors[‖]	Generally, no postexposure prophylaxis warranted; however, consider basic two-drug postexposure prophylaxis[§] in settings where exposure to HIV-infected persons is likely
High risk[‡]	Expanded three-drug postexposure prophylaxis recommended	Expanded three-drug postexposure prophylaxis recommended	Generally, no postexposure prophylaxis warranted; however, consider basic two-drug postexposure prophylaxis[§] for source with HIV risk factors[‖]	Generally, no postexposure prophylaxis warranted; however, consider basic two-drug postexposure prophylaxis[§] in settings where exposure to HIV-infected persons is likely

Abbreviation: HIV indicates human immunodeficiency virus.

*Unknown source (eg, a needle from a sharps disposal container).

[†]Injury of low severity (eg, solid needle or superficial injury).

[‡]Injury of increased severity (eg, large-bore hollow needle, deep puncture, or needle used in patient's artery or vein).

[§]The designation "consider postexposure prophylaxis" indicates that postexposure prophylaxis is optional and should be based on an individualized decision between the exposed person and the treating clinician.

[‖]If postexposure prophylaxis is offered and taken, and the source is later determined to be HIV-negative, postexposure prophylaxis should be discontinued.

Modified from Panlilio AL, Cardo DM, Grohskopf LA, Heneine W, Ross CS. Updated U.S. Public Health Service guidelines for the management of occupational exposures to HIV and recommendations for postexposure prophylaxis. U.S. Public Health Service. MMWR Recomm Rep 2005;54:1–17.

TABLE 18-2. Recommended Human Immunodeficiency Virus Postexposure Prophylaxis for Mucous Membrane and Nonintact Skin Exposure*

Exposure Type	Human Immunodeficiency Virus-Positive (HIV-RNA Count Less Than 1,500 Copies per Milliliter)	Human Immunodeficiency Virus-Positive (HIV-RNA Count Greater Than 1,500 Copies per Milliliter)	Source of Unknown HIV Status	Unknown Source[†]	Human Immunodeficiency Virus-Negative
Small volume[‡]	Consider basic two-drug postexposure prophylaxis[§]	Basic two-drug post-exposure prophylaxis recommended	Generally, no postexposure prophylaxis warranted	Generally, no postexposure prophylaxis warranted	No postexposure prophylaxis warranted
Large volume[∥]	Basic two-drug post-exposure prophylaxis recommended	Expanded three-drug postexposure prophylaxis recommended	Generally, no postexposure prophylaxis warranted; however, consider basic two-drug postexposure prophylaxis[∥] for source with HIV risk factors[¶]	Generally, no postexposure prophylaxis warranted; however, consider basic two-drug postexposure prophylaxis[∥] in settings where exposure to HIV-infected persons is likely	No postexposure prophylaxis warranted

Abbreviation: HIV indicates human immunodeficiency virus.

*For skin exposure, follow-up is indicated only if evidence exists of compromised skin integrity (eg, dermatitis, abrasion, or open wound).

[†]Unknown source (eg, splash from inappropriately disposed blood)

[‡]Small volume (ie, a few drops)

[§]The designation "consider postexposure prophylaxis" indicates that postexposure prophylaxis is optional and should be based on an individualized decision between the exposed person and the treating clinician.

[∥]Large volume (eg, major blood, amniotic fluid, or peritoneal fluid splash)

[¶]If postexposure prophylaxis is offered and taken and the source is later determined to be HIV-negative, postexposure prophylaxis should be discontinued.

Modified from Panlilio AL, Cardo DM, Grohskopf LA, Heneine W, Ross CS. Updated U.S. Public Health Service guidelines for the management of occupational exposures to HIV and recommendations for postexposure prophylaxis. U.S. Public Health Service. MMWR Recomm Rep 2005;54:1–17.

inhibitor for high-risk exposure. Common adverse effects of these regimens are gastrointestinal toxicity, asthenia, peripheral neuropathy, and headache.

Cardo DM, Culver DH, Ciesielski CA, Srivastava PU, Marcus R, Abiteboul D, et al. A case-control study of HIV seroconversion in health care workers after percutaneous exposure. Centers for Disease Control and Prevention Needlestick Surveillance Group. N Engl J Med 1997;337:1485–90.

Hepatitis B, hepatitis C, and human immunodeficiency virus infections in obstetrician-gynecologists. Committee Opinion No. 489. American College of Obstetricians and Gynecologists. Obstet Gynecol 2011; 117:1242–6.

Panlilio AL, Cardo DM, Grohskopf LA, Heneine W, Ross CS. Updated U.S. Public Health Service guidelines for the management of occupational exposures to HIV and recommendations for postexposure prophylaxis. U.S. Public Health Service. MMWR Recomm Rep 2005; 54:1–17.

19

Single-rod implantable contraception

A 23-year-old woman comes to the office and requests removal of her radioopaque single-rod implantable contraceptive 2 months after insertion because she wishes to conceive with a new partner. Palpation at the site of insertion is unsuccessful at localizing the rod. The patient reports neither infection nor trauma at the insertion site. Her pregnancy test result is negative. The best next step in the care of this patient is

      (A) serum etonogestrel level measurement
      (B) follow-up in 6 months if not pregnant
      (C) incision and exploration
*   (D) X-ray of the arm

The etonogestrel subdermal implant is an effective, long-acting reversible contraceptive that provides protection for up to 3 years. It consists of a core that contains the progestin etonogestrel and ethylene vinyl acetate copolymer. The implant measures 4 cm in length and 2 mm in diameter. The implant is placed in the needle of a prepackaged disposable applicator. It is placed subdermally in the medial aspect of the nondominant upper arm between the biceps and triceps muscles approximately 8–10 cm above the level of the medial epicondyle of the humerus.

Approximately 40% of implants show some degree of migration, which in most cases is in a caudal direction toward the insertion site, but rarely by more than 2 cm. The first etonogestrel implant approved by the U.S. Food and Drug Administration was not radioopaque. The options for visualization of this implant include ultrasonography with a high-frequency (10–15 MHz), high-resolution linear array transducer. The ultrasonographic image commonly reveals this type of implant as a highly echogenic linear image. Most transabdominal ultrasonographic probes used in an obstetrician–gynecologist's office are low frequency (3–5 MHz), and thus are not suitable for localization. The best place to begin looking for the device is at the insertion scar. The optimal plane is the

transverse plane with the implant, which is recognizable as an echogenic focus that casts a posterior acoustic shadow. Once the implant is found, the probe can be moved along the transverse plane in cross-section to ensure that the echogenic focus approximates the length of an implant. The length of the implant can also be determined along its long axis by rotating the probe into the longitudinal plane. If ultrasonography is unable to identify the implant, then magnetic resonance imagining should be considered.

The newer etonogestrel implant is radioopaque because it contains barium sulfate. Imaging studies such as X-ray should localize most nonpalpable rods. In cases where the actual presence of an implant in the patient's arm is in question, measurement of serum etonogestrel level would be appropriate. However, this will not localize its position.

In patients who use the etonogestrel implant for contraception, the risk of pregnancy is 0.05%. Therefore, it would be inappropriate to observe patients who are planning to conceive and in whom the etonogestrel implant was not palpated and removed, as in this case. It is not recommended to proceed with exploration without first localizing the implant. Blind exploration can be unsuccessful and can result in bleeding, pain, and scarring at the incision site.

Ismail H, Mansour D, Singh M. Migration of Implanon. J Fam Plann Reprod Health Care 2006;32:157–9.

Shulman LP, Gabriel H. Management and localization strategies for the nonpalpable Implanon rod. Contraception 2006;73:325–30.

Singh M, Mansour D, Richardson D. Location and removal of non-palpable Implanon implants with the aid of ultrasound guidance. J Fam Plann Reprod Health Care 2006;32:153–6.

20

Evaluation of urinary incontinence

A 69-year-old woman comes to your office and reports increasing urinary incontinence over the past year. The episodes have occurred with coughing or when she has been unable to make it to the bathroom in time. She has been menopausal for 12 years and has no chronic medical problems. The answers on The 3 Incontinence Questions (3 IQ) assessment tool suggests she may have mixed incontinence. In addition to the screening questionnaire, a complete history, physical examination, urinalysis, and urine culture, the next step in this patient's management should be

*   (A) a voiding diary
     (B) anticholinergic therapy
     (C) urodynamic testing
     (D) Kegel exercises
     (E) a pessary

Initial evaluation of urinary incontinence is designed to elucidate severity and classification of symptoms. All types of urinary incontinence (stress, urge, overflow, and mixed) have different patterns of symptomatology, although often they are not initially recognized by either the health care provider or the patient. Stress urinary incontinence is characterized by leakage only when the intraabdominal pressure exceeds that of the urethral sphincter. Thus, urinary leakage is associated with coughing, sneezing, and other events that increase intraabdominal pressure. In contrast, urge urinary incontinence or overactive bladder syndrome is caused by uncontrolled bladder contractions that are not predictable and often not associated with Valsalva maneuvers. Mixed incontinence may have elements of either of these conditions and overflow incontinence typically is seen in the presence of other neurogenic conditions, such as spinal cord injury or multiple sclerosis.

A useful tool is a voiding diary kept in real time by the patient. Such a diary can prove helpful in assessing symptoms. Often, patient histories or screening questionnaires will not fully reveal the cause of urinary incontinence even when combined with a complete examination. Most authors recommend documenting symptoms in a diary for 2–7 days; the patient is asked to note the frequency of diurnal and nocturnal voids and details related to incontinence episodes. Box 20-1 shows an example of a voiding diary.

Initiation of any therapy without additional information to determine the cause of incontinence is not appropriate. Therefore, starting medication, Kegel exercises, or inserting a pessary would not be correct choices. Although urodynamic testing may be helpful in many cases, it may not be necessary once a voiding diary has been obtained.

Although a complete history and physical examination may narrow the differential, other tools may help. The 3 Incontinence Questions questionnaire (Box 20-2) has been evaluated in a study of 300 middle-aged women. Although the sensitivity for diagnosing urge and stress incontinence was reasonable in this age group, the performance of this tool in older women, such as the described patient, has not been established.

Brown JS, Bradley CS, Subak LL, Richter HE, Kraus SR, Brubaker L, et al. The sensitivity and specificity of a simple test to distinguish between urge and stress urinary incontinence. Diagnostic Aspects of Incontinence Study (DAISy) Research Group. Ann Intern Med 2006;144:715–23.

DuBeau CE. Clinical presentation and diagnosis of urinary incontinence. In: Basow DS, editor. UpToDate. Waltham (MA): UpToDate; 2013.

Wyman JF, Choi SC, Harkins SW, Wilson MS, Fantl JA. The urinary diary in evaluation of incontinent women: a test-retest analysis. Obstet Gynecol 1988;71:812–7.

BOX 20-1

Example of a Voiding Diary

Your name _____   Started on Date _____

Date	Time	Measured amount of urine	Did you have leakage, yes or no?	Approximate amount of leakage	Time you went to bed and got up, drank coffee or soda, or any other comments

- This diary will help us determine why you have trouble holding your urine or why you go to the bathroom very often.
- **Keep this record for at least 2 days.**
- Please write down these four things every time you pass or leak urine:
  1. The time (for example, "10:30 AM")
  2. The amount of urine that you pass.
  3. Whether you leaked any urine (were "wet") or not (were "dry").
  4. Whether anything special may have caused you to leak urine (for example, "just had coffee", "coughed", "was running to the bathroom", or "just took my water pill").
- Start the record in the morning the first time you go to the bathroom after you get up. **Please write on the form the time you got up and the time you went to bed.**
- To measure the amount of urine you pass, we will give you a special receptacle (called a "hat"). Place the hat in the toilet to catch the urine every time you urinate. Look at the numbers on the inside of the hat to see how high the urine fills the hat. Write down the number that corresponds to the level of urine. Remember to empty the hat after each time you use it.

BOX 20-2

The 3 Incontinence Questions (3 IQ) Questionnaire to Assess Urinary Incontinence

1. During the past 3 months, have you leaked urine (even a small amount)?

❑ Yes   ❑ No

                                 ↓

            Questionnaire completed

2. During the past 3 months, did you leak urine:
(Check all that apply)

❑ a. When you were performing some physical activity, such as coughing, sneezing, lifting, or exercise?

❑ b. When you had the urge or the feeling that you needed to empty your bladder, but you could not get to the toilet fast enough?

❑ c. Without physical activity and without sense of urgency?

3. During the past 3 months, did you leak urine:
(Check only one)

❑ a. When you were performing some physical activity, such as coughing, sneezing, lifting, or exercise?

❑ b. When you had the urge or the feeling that you needed to empty your bladder, but you could not get to the toilet fast enough?

❑ c. Without physical activity and without sense of urgency?

❑ d. About equally as often with physical activity as with a sense of urgency?

Definitions of type of urinary incontinence are based on responses to question 3:

Response to Question 3	Type of Incontinence
Most often with physical activity	Stress only or stress predominant
Most often with the urge to empty the bladder	Urge only or urge predominant
Without physical activity or sense of urgency	Other cause only or other cause predominant
About equally with physical activity and sense	Mixed

Brown JS, Bradley CS, Subak LL, Richter HE, Kraus SR, Brubaker L, et al. The sensitivity and specificity of a simple test to distinguish between urge and stress urinary incontinence. Diagnostic Aspects of Incontinence Study (DAISy) Research Group. Ann Intern Med 2006;144:715–23.

21

Patient privacy: electronic communication and office practice

You were recently notified about a possible legal action that might be filed against you regarding a patient who had a serious complication after surgery. You have kept numerous e-mail messages with this patient during her difficult postoperative recovery. Her attorney has sent a letter, which includes her signed consent, for release of her medical records. Regarding the e-mail communication between you and the patient, the proper course of action is to

(A) delete them from your computer
(B) supply them only if specifically requested
(C) supply them only to your attorney
* (D) send them with the medical records

The medical profession has been slow to incorporate e-mail as a means to improve patient communication. Concerns include the security of transmitting sensitive medical information, a lack of reimbursement, and the potential volume of messages. The American Medical Association has stated that the provider needs to take on an explicit measure of responsibility for the patient's care in health care provider–patient e-mail communication. Health care providers who choose to use e-mail for patient and medical practice communication are required to follow these communication, medical–legal, and administrative guidelines. The guidelines apply to electronic communication within an established partnership. Attention must be given to informed consent, confidentiality, and record keeping of e-mail exchanges. E-mail messages should be retained as part of the patient's medical record.

Security and privacy concerns regarding patient e-mail communication can be improved by using a secure server, an integrated web system, or a secure web-based portal for physician–patient communication. Confidentiality is at risk when multiple individuals share the same e-mail address or when access passwords are not used or are not kept secured. Practices that use e-mail communication with patients should disseminate formal guidelines regarding e-mail use to ensure that health care providers and patients effectively use e-mail for health care communication while being fully aware of possible risks. Any system developed by a practice must address the needs of the patient and ensure privacy and security. Efforts need to be made to educate patients and health care providers regarding the appropriate and effective use of e-mail communication.

In the described scenario, the most appropriate response is to forward the e-mail messages as part of the medical record. Because they are considered part of the medical record, they do not require a special request. Because no part of the medical records should be destroyed or concealed these e-mail messages should not be deleted from the computer. They should be supplied to the patient and the physician's legal representatives in total as part of the complete medical record. Before releasing any medical records, patient-written consent should be obtained. Any request from a plaintiff's attorney for medical records should prompt contact with your medical liability carrier.

American Medical Association. Ethical guidelines for the use of electronic mail between patients and physicians. Report of the Council on Ethical and Judicial Affairs. Chicago (IL): AMA; 2002. Available at: http://www.ama-assn.org/resources/doc/code-medical-ethics/5026a.pdf. Retrieved June 6, 2013.

Freed DH. Patient-physician e-mail: passion or fashion? Health Care Manag (Frederick) 2003;22:265–74.

Shwayder JM. Cybermedicine: medicine and e-mail: what evil web we weave! Preventive L Rep 2000-2001;19:20–4.

U.S. Department of Health and Human Services. Does the HIPAA Privacy Rule permit health care providers to use e-mail to discuss health issues and treatment with their patients? Health Information Privacy. Washington, DC: HHS; 2008. Available at: http://www.hhs.gov/ocr/privacy/hipaa/faq/health_information_technology/570.html. Retrieved June 6, 2013.

Ye J, Rust G, Fry-Johnson Y, Strothers H. E-mail in patient-provider communication: a systematic review. Patient Educ Couns 2010;80:266–73.

22

Smoking cessation

A 34-year-old woman comes to your office for her annual health maintenance examination. She has been smoking one pack of cigarettes per day for the past 7 years. During the interview, she mentions that she has been thinking about the effect of smoking on her health and is considering quitting. She has tried to quit in the past. The patient's current stage of readiness to change her smoking behavior is

    (A) precontemplation
*   (B) contemplation
    (C) action
    (D) maintenance
    (E) relapse

Smoking is one of the most important types of modifiable risk-taking behavior. In addition to its negative effects on fertility and fetal development, smoking has been linked to 90% of lung cancer cases and a dose-related increased risk of colon cancer. Also, it has been linked to an increased risk of gynecologic cancer (ovarian and cervical) cancer of the head and neck, lung, gastrointestinal system, bladder, kidney, and pancreas. It is the single greatest modifiable risk factor for cardiovascular disease; women who smoke have a sixfold increase in myocardial infarction. The risk of stroke is doubled in smokers. Smokers also are at risk of early menopause with an increased risk of osteoporotic fracture.

It has been estimated that health-related economic losses from tobacco use cost the United States $193 billion dollars during the period 2000–2004, with 50% dedicated to direct medical costs. In 2009, 18% of women older than 18 years smoked, and more than 80% of current smokers began smoking before age 18 years. Among current smokers, 70% say they want to quit smoking and 40% say they try to quit each year.

It is the responsibility of the clinician to evaluate and counsel patients regarding potentially modifiable risk-taking behavior. Numerous opportunities are available to initiate discussion of a patient's smoking, eg, especially when preparing for surgery, during pregnancy, and at the annual health maintenance visit. The "5 A's" intervention model is an evidence-based model that is used for substance use counseling. The 5 A's stand for 1) **A**sk, 2) **A**dvise, 3) **A**ssess, 4) **A**ssist, and 5) **A**rrange. Part of the assessment is to identify the patient's current stage of readiness for change in behavior. The transtheoretical model with the stages of readiness for change is shown in Box 22-1. The fact that the described patient is considering smoking cessation puts her at the contemplation stage of readiness for change in behavior.

Once the stage of readiness for change is established, the purpose of the discussion would be to move the patient toward action and then maintenance. This has to be viewed as a process of engaging the patient in multiple discussions rather than a single event. At times, these discussions can be met by a strong resistance to change. Motivational interviewing technique has shown much promise in assisting patients to alter risk-taking behavior in a number of clinical settings, including weight reduction, exercise, safe sex, use of contraception, and

---

BOX 22-1

Stages of Readiness for Change in Terms of Instituting Smoking Cessation

- Precontemplation—The patient does not believe a problem exists. ("Smoking is not harmful to my health.")
- Contemplation—The patient recognized a problem exists and is considering treatment or a behavior change. ("Smoking might be harmful to me and there are things I can do to stop smoking."
- Action—The patient begins treatment or behavior change. ("I will take the prescription for the nicotine patch.")
- Maintenance—The patient incorporates new behavior into daily life. ("I will wear the nicotine patch as directed.")
- Relapse—The patient returns to the undesired behavior. ("I'm tired of using the patch. I miss my cigarettes.")

Modified from Motivational interviewing: a tool for behavioral change. ACOG Committee Opinion No. 423. American College of Obstetricians and Gynecologists. Obstet Gynecol 2009;113:243–6.

smoking. The definition of motivational interviewing is "a directive client-centered style for eliciting behavior change by helping clients explore and resolve ambivalence." The purpose is to help patients identify and alter risk-taking behavior to move them along the phases of readiness for change. One example of motivational interviewing is FRAMES, ie, Feedback, Responsibility, Advice, Menu, Empathy, and Self-Efficacy (Box 22-2).

The American College of Obstetricians and Gynecologists encourages the use of motivational interviewing for change in behavior. When the discussion is performed by a physician or a qualified staff member, it can be coded and reimbursed. The Affordable Care Act requires that smoking cessation counseling be covered as a U.S. Preventive Services Task Force Grade A preventive service. Current Procedural Terminology codes 99406 (smoking and tobacco use cessation counseling visit; intermediate, greater than 3 minutes up to 10 minutes) and 99407 (smoking and tobacco use cessation counseling visit; intensive, greater than 10 minutes) can be used.

Motivational interviewing: a tool for behavioral change. ACOG Committee Opinion No. 423. American College of Obstetricians and Gynecologists. Obstet Gynecol 2009;113:243–6.

Prochaska JO, DiClemente CC, Norcross JC. In search of how people change. Applications to addictive behaviors. Am Psychol 1992;47:1102–14.

Tobacco use and women's health. Committee Opinion No. 503. American College of Obstetricians and Gynecologists. Obstet Gynecol 2011;118:746–50.

BOX 22-2

Motivational Interviewing FRAMES

Feedback	Compare the patient's risk-taking behavior with non-risk-taking behavior because she may not be aware of the risks.
Responsibility	Emphasize to the patient that it is her responsibility to make the change in behavior
Advice	Give direct advice to change behavior
Menu	Identify risk situations and offer ways to cope
Empathy	Use a style of communication that is understanding and involved
Self-Efficacy	Elicit and reinforce self-motivating statements, such as "I am confident that I can stop smoking." Help the patient develop strategies and implement them.

Modified from Motivational interviewing: a tool for behavioral change. ACOG Committee Opinion No. 423. American College of Obstetricians and Gynecologists. Obstet Gynecol 2009;113:243–6.

23

Discussion of medical errors

Your hospital administrator asks you to give a presentation to the medical staff on the topic of medical liability. During the question-and-answer period, audience members ask if full disclosure will decrease the number of professional liability suits, reduce average settlement amounts, improve patient ratings of quality of care, or produce negative publicity about the care provided by the hospital. You reply that, of those questions, full disclosure has been shown to

*   (A) decrease the number of professional liability suits
          (B) have no effect on the average settlement amount
          (C) decrease the patient's rating of quality of care
          (D) increase the number of negative media reports

The Institute of Medicine reports that each year in the United States, 98,000 deaths occur secondary to medical errors. Approximately 400,000 drug-related injuries occur annually in U.S. hospitals that result in approximately 7,000 deaths. Decreasing the number of medical errors and improving quality of care has become a major focus of the U.S. federal government and various medical organizations.

In 2011 the American College of Obstetricians and Gynecologists' Committee on Patient Safety and Quality Improvement published a Committee Opinion that discusses the appropriate steps to disclose and positively manage medical errors. After recognizing that an error has occurred, every attempt should be made to gather the contributing factors that surround the error. Facts should be gathered promptly so that the provider can discuss or disclose the error to the patient, her family, or both as soon as possible. This allows the parties involved to not only maintain open and honest lines of communication, but also to answer questions whenever possible. The error should be disclosed in a confidential and timely manner by the treating physician or necessary health care providers. When possible, the health care provider should assure the patient that if they do not know the answer to a question then the necessary steps will be taken to provide a response in the near future. All information should be delivered in a manner that is easily understood by the patient and family members. The focus of the discussion should be on the patient's condition and future treatment plans. The health care providers should express their regret and concern for the patient and their family's position. Ongoing and open communication should be maintained.

Disclosure of medical errors has been shown to have several beneficial outcomes. Studies indicate that when an adverse medical event occurs, patients and their families want timely and factual information. In addition, such studies show that patients not only expect a statement of regret, but also want to hear what will be done to prevent such an occurrence in the future. Several studies have reported that patients are more likely to sue if they feel that the information is being withheld.

In addition, research shows that disclosure is associated with improved patient recovery, improved patient ratings of the quality of care, and a decrease in the number of professional liability actions and settlement amounts. Disclosure likely improves the patient–health care provider relationship and development of trust and helps to decrease patient and health care provider emotional distress.

Coping with the stress of medical professional liability litigation. ACOG Committee Opinion No. 551. American College of Obstetricians and Gynecologists. Obstet Gynecol 2013;121:220–2.

Disclosure and discussion of adverse events. ACOG Committee Opinion No. 520. American College of Obstetricians and Gynecologists. Obstet Gynecol 2012;119:686–9.

Improving medication safety. Committee Opinion No. 531. American College of Obstetricians and Gynecologists. Obstet Gynecol 2012;120: 406–10.

24
Obesity

A 44-year-old woman, gravida 2, para 2, comes to your office for a well-woman examination. Her body mass index (BMI) is 35 (calculated as weight in kilograms divided by height in meters squared). You note that the patient has gained 10 kg (22 lb) over the past 2 years. She has no illnesses, but her family history is significant for diabetes mellitus, coronary artery disease, and hypertension. The first intervention to facilitate weight loss in this patient should be

*   (A) counsel aboout the importance of weight loss
    (B) refer for bariatric surgery
    (C) prescribe weight loss medication
    (D) screen for metabolic risk

One of the most significant public health concerns facing the U.S. population is obesity. *Obesity* is defined as a BMI of 30 or greater and overweight is defined as BMI of 25–29.9. Obesity is classified by the World Health Organization as Class I, BMI of 30–34.9; Class II, BMI of 35–39.9; and Class III, BMI of 40 or greater. The prevalence of obesity nationwide has increased by approximately 15% in the past 15 years. Currently, more than two thirds of women in the United States are overweight, of which one third are obese.

Obesity is a complex, multifactorial condition that affects multiple adverse health conditions; eg, hypertension; type 2 diabetes mellitus; sleep apnea; other respiratory problems; coronary heart disease; and numerous psychologic problems, including depression, anxiety, low self-esteem, and eating disorders. The metabolic syndrome is a group of factors that increase the risk of developing diabetes mellitus, heart disease, and stroke (Box 24-1).

Obstetrician–gynecologists can address obesity through screening, counseling, and offering appropriate treatment and referral for weight loss for overweight and obese women. Behavioral motivation and change is paramount for the initiation and success of weight loss. Studies suggest that individuals who receive advice from health care providers regarding weight loss and physical activity are more likely to try to lose weight, consume fewer calories, and increase their physical activity.

Further steps in promoting weight loss may include screening to further demonstrate the actual impact obesity plays in individual health risks, referral for additional counseling, and consideration of weight loss medication approved by the U.S. Food and Drug Administration to improve the induction or continuation of weight loss. Currently, several medications are approved by the Food and Drug Administration for short-term weight loss and chronic weight management; information regarding these medications can be found at http://www.fda.gov/drugs/drugsafety/informationbydrugclass/default.htm.

Generally, bariatric surgery is reserved for individuals with Class III obesity (BMI of 40 or greater or Class II obesity (BMI 35–39.9) with obesity-associated comorbidities, such as diabetes mellitus, hypertension, and dyslipidemia. It is the most effective therapy available for morbid obesity. Two primary approaches to bariatric surgery exist: 1) restrictive operations and 2) combination of restrictive and malabsorptive operations.

The basic treatment of overweight and obese patients requires a comprehensive approach with an emphasis on long-term weight management, rather than short-term extreme weight reduction. Obstetrician–gynecologists often develop strong relationships with their patients.

BOX 24-1

Risk Factors for Metabolic Syndrome

A patient can have any one of these risk factors by itself, but they tend to occur together. The patient must have at least three of the following risk factors to receive the diagnosis of metabolic syndrome:

*   A large waistline—Males: 102 cm (40 in) or more; females: 89 cm (35 in) or more

*   A high triglyceride level—Either 150 mg/dL or higher or using a cholesterol-lowering medication

*   Low high density lipoprotein cholesterol level

*   High blood pressure—Either blood pressure of 135 mm Hg or greater systolic and 85 mm Hg or greater diastolic or using an antihypertensive medication

*   High fasting glucose level—100 mg/dL or higher

Modified from National Heart, Lung and Blood Institute. What is metabolic syndrome? Available at http://www.nhlbi.nih.gov/health/health-topics/topics/ms. Retrieved March 29, 2013.

Gynecology and Surgery

Thus, they have significant influence regarding patient behavior and improved wellness, such as weight loss and smoking cessation. By assessing readiness to change and reinforcing the importance of weight loss, the health care provider may move the patient forward in the process of behavioral change. The health care provider may then target strategies most likely to provide benefit to the patient. For the described patient, the first intervention to facilitate weight loss should be to reinforce the importance of weight loss.

Bariatric surgery and pregnancy. ACOG Practice Bulletin No. 105. American College of Obstetricians and Gynecologists. Obstet Gynecol 2009;113:1405–13.

Cogswell ME, Power ML, Sharma AJ, Schulkin J. Prevention and management of obesity in nonpregnant women and adolescents: beliefs and practices of U.S. obstetricians and gynecologists. J Womens Health (Larchmt) 2010;19:1625–34.

Lyznicki JM, Young DC, Riggs JA, Davis RM. Obesity: assessment and management in primary care. Council on Scientific Affairs, American Medical Association. Am Fam Physician 2001;63:2185–96.

25

Ovarian mass in an older reproductive-aged woman

A 48-year-old woman comes to your office after a visit to the emergency department for severe left flank pain during which ultrasonography showed a 3.96-cm left ovarian mass (Fig. 25-1). She has not experienced any change in appetite, early satiety, or increased abdominal girth. The ultrasonographic marker that is most concerning for an ovarian neoplasm in this patient is

    (A) cyst size
    (B) fluid echogenicity
    (C) cyst wall thickness
*   (D) solid excrescence

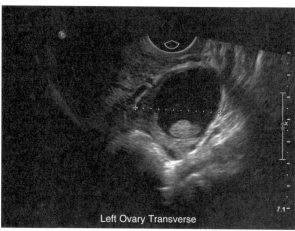

FIG. 25-1

Adnexal masses are a common finding in women. Physicians face a diagnostic dilemma in trying to differentiate benign masses from malignant masses. Women have an approximately 5–10% lifetime risk of undergoing surgery for a suspected ovarian mass. A woman's lifetime risk of developing ovarian cancer is 1 in 70. The 5-year survival of stage 1 disease is approximately 90%, whereas it is only 30–55% for advanced stage disease. However, only 20% of ovarian cancers are detected at an early stage.

Ultrasonographic evaluation of asymptomatic ovarian masses has become the standard of care although the utility of ultrasonography as a screening tool for ovarian cancer has not been established. In an attempt to differentiate benign masses from malignant masses, many ovarian tumor ultrasonographic scoring systems that combine morphologic markers have been developed. Their clinical utility remains to be proved. However, scoring systems agree that a smooth, thin wall, anechoic, simple cyst should receive a low score; whereas a large, complex mass, with solid areas, thickened wall, and peritoneal fluid should receive a high score.

The ovarian tumor ultrasonographic markers most predictive of a malignant neoplasm are papillations or solid excrescences, defined as a focal echoic structure protruding inside the cystic portion of the mass that is greater than 3 mm; tumor septum that is greater than 3 mm; or tumors that are mostly solid. Using such morphologic criteria, the sensitivity of detecting ovarian malignancy can be as high as 91%.

Cyst wall thickness greater than 3 mm also is an ultrasonographic marker of malignancy; however, it is less predictive than a solid excrescence. The cyst wall may be involved in the excrescence and at times may be difficult to distinguish.

Asymptomatic, unilocular, simple cysts less than 10 cm in diameter rarely are associated with malignancy irrespective of the menopausal status. In addition, cyst size as an ultrasonographic marker by itself is of limited use in distinguishing benign masses from malignant masses. Often, other ultrasonographic markers can be present that are more predictive than size alone.

Fluid echogenicity is not prognostic of malignancy. However, echogenic foci inside the cystic component of the tumor, which indicate solid areas, are important prognostic factors. In addition, the ultrasonographic finding of ascites increases the suspicion of malignancy.

Vascular flow parameters using color Doppler ultrasonography, including resistive index, pulsatility index, and maximum systolic velocity, also are used for differentiation of benign masses from malignant masses. A resistive index greater than 0.5–0.6 has been used as a cut-off to differentiate benign masses from malignant masses; a mass with a resistive index higher than 0.5–0.6 is regarded as benign. In this patient, the ultrasonographic finding of a solid excrescence that contains vascular flow is suspicious for a malignancy.

Bromley B, Goodman H, Benacerraf BR. Comparison between sonographic morphology and Doppler waveform for the diagnosis of ovarian malignancy. Obstet Gynecol 1994;83:434–7.

Levine D, Brown DL, Andreotti RF, Benacerraf B, Benson CB, Brewster WR, et al. Management of asymptomatic ovarian and other adnexal cysts imaged at US: Society of Radiologists in Ultrasound Consensus Conference Statement. Radiology 2010;256:943–54.

Management of adnexal masses. ACOG Practice Bulletin No. 83. American College of Obstetricians and Gynecologists. Obstet Gynecol 2007;110:201–14.

Sassone AM, Timor-Tritsch IE, Artner A, Westhoff C, Warren WB. Transvaginal sonographic characterization of ovarian disease: evaluation of a new scoring system to predict ovarian malignancy. Obstet Gynecol 1991;78:70–6.

van Nagell JR Jr, Miller RW, DeSimone CP, Ueland FR, Podzielinski I, Goodrich ST, et al. Long-term survival of women with epithelial ovarian cancer detected by ultrasonographic screening. Obstet Gynecol 2011;118:1212–21.

26

Postmenopausal bleeding

A 62-year-old woman, gravida 2, para 2, is referred to you for recurrent postmenopausal bleeding. She reports a history of light bleeding 6 months ago. At that time, her primary care physician ordered pelvic ultrasonography that demonstrated a 4-mm endometrial thickness. The patient tells you that she had no further bleeding until 3 weeks ago. She reports that she has no other medical problems and that she is not taking any prescription medications. Her last Pap test was approximately 1 year ago and the result was normal. She has no history of cervical dysplasia. Her body mass index is 36 (calculated as weight in kilograms divided by height in meters squared) and the pelvic examination is notable only for vaginal atrophy. You counsel her that the best next step is to perform

  (A) pelvic examination in 6 months
  (B) hysteroscopy with dilation and curettage
  (C) saline sonohysterography
 * (D) an endometrial biopsy

Endometrial cancer is observed in approximately 1–15% of patients with postmenopausal bleeding. Although many benign and malignant causes exist, experts agree that pelvic ultrasonography is the appropriate first step in evaluation. Women found to have an endometrial thickness of 4 mm or less are considered to be at low risk of endometrial cancer (negative predictive value 98–100%) and may forego endometrial sampling as part of their initial evaluation. However, patients who present with recurrent postmenopausal bleeding need a more thorough evaluation; therefore, an endometrial biopsy would be indicated.

Despite prior pelvic ultrasonography with a thin endometrium 6 months earlier, women who have recurrent bleeding should not defer further evaluation for another 6 months. Therefore, to repeat a pelvic examination in 6 months would be inappropriate because it may falsely reassure the patient and potentially miss a malignant or premalignant lesion.

Saline sonohysterography is a valuable tool in the evaluation of bleeding in postmenopausal women because it can help to identify endometrial polyps and submucosal myomas. However, saline sonohysterography alone cannot reliably eliminate the concern for malignancy and should be used in conjunction with endometrial sampling.

A meta-analysis has shown that endometrial biopsy yielded endometrial cancer detection rates of 83–99.6% in postmenopausal women. The biopsy can be performed in an expeditious fashion in the office without anesthesia or delay, and the risk of uterine perforation is minimal. Hysteroscopy with dilation and curettage may be subsequently warranted in patients with either sampling failures or inadequate sampling. However, such procedures would not be the first step in evaluating this patient.

The described patient has no history of cervical dysplasia and she recently had a normal Pap test result. Therefore, cervical cancer is an unlikely cause of her bleeding and repeat cytology is not warranted.

Dijkhuizen FP, Mol BW, Brolmann HA, Heintz AP. The accuracy of endometrial sampling in the diagnosis of patients with endometrial carcinoma and hyperplasia: a meta-analysis. Cancer 2000;89:1765–72.

Gull B, Karlsson B, Milsom I, Granberg S. Can ultrasound replace dilation and curettage? A longitudinal evaluation of postmenopausal bleeding and transvaginal sonographic measurement of the endometrium as predictors of endometrial cancer. Am J Obstet Gynecol 2003;188:401–8.

The role of transvaginal ultrasonography in the evaluation of postmenopausal bleeding. ACOG Committee Opinion No. 426. American College of Obstetricians and Gynecologists. Obstet Gynecol 2009;113:462–4.

Ronghe R, Gaudoin M. Women with recurrent postmenopausal bleeding should be re-investigated but are not more likely to have endometrial cancer. Menopause Int 2010;16:9–11.

27

Risk reduction factors for ovarian cancer

A 30-year-old multiparous woman with a *BRCA 2* mutation comes to your office for her annual gynecologic examination. She wishes to decrease her risk of developing ovarian cancer over the next 10 years. She does not desire pregnancy now or in the future. You advise her that the most appropriate contraceptive management is

      (A) bilateral salpingo-oophorectomy
      (B) levonorgestrel intrauterine device
*   (C) combined oral contraceptives
      (D) bilateral tubal ligation

Women who carry *BRCA 1* and *BRCA 2* mutations have a 56–87% lifetime risk of breast cancer, and a 10–40% lifetime risk of ovarian cancer, which is more than a 10-fold increase in risk compared with the general population. Two theories have been proposed to explain the pathogenesis of ovarian cancer. The first theory, based on epidemiologic data, suggests that ovarian cancer risk is proportional to the number of ovulatory cycles a woman has during her reproductive life. Mutations arising within the epithelium that is undergoing damage and repair from ovulation lead to nests of cells with malignant potential. Epidemiologic evidence supports that suppression of ovulation by hormonal contraception, such as oral contraceptives, will decrease the risk of developing ovarian cancer by 50%. However, it is unclear whether this same degree of protection exists for a woman with a *BRCA* mutation. The second theory suggests that ovarian cancer and primary peritoneal cancer arise from a progenitor in the fallopian tube. Women with *BRCA* mutations have been found to have serous tubal intraepithelial carcinomas within the distal end of the fallopian tube. To date, only salpingectomy is an effective prevention strategy under this theory.

Factors associated with a decreased risk of ovarian cancer are multiple pregnancies and bilateral tubal ligation. Pregnancy and hormonal contraception decrease ovarian cancer risk by reducing the number of ovulatory cycles. Bilateral tubal ligation is thought to decrease the risk of ovarian cancer by isolating the ovary from potential environmental carcinogens and perhaps by altering the blood supply to the ovary in a subtle fashion.

For a patient with a *BRCA* mutation, surgical removal of the ovaries and tubes remains the most effective method for prevention of ovarian cancer. Combined oral contraceptives will decrease her risk of ovarian cancer and will not change her risk of breast cancer.

Risk-reducing bilateral salpingo-oophorectomy (BSO) reduces the risk of ovarian and fallopian tube cancer by approximately 96%. Bilateral salpingo-oophorectomy approaches the 100% prevention rate against ovarian cancer when the entire ovary, fallopian tube, and mesosalpinx are removed together with ligation and transection of the ovarian artery and vein near the pelvic sidewall. Approximately 2% of women with *BRCA* mutations will have an occult ovarian or tubal carcinoma at the time of risk-reducing BSO, and 1% will develop peritoneal carcinomatosis after risk-reducing BSO. Nevertheless, *BRCA* mutation carriers are advised to undergo risk-reducing BSO when their childbearing is complete and after age 35 years. In addition to decreasing a woman's risk of ovarian cancer, risk-reducing BSO also will decrease her risk of breast cancer by nearly 50%. For women with *BRCA* mutations, the timing of risk-reducing BSO has practical and personal considerations. Women who undergo surgical menopause prematurely are at risk of menopausal symptoms, such as hot flushes, vaginal dryness, decreased libido, dyspareunia, osteoporosis, and cardiovascular disease. Women with severe menopausal symptoms can consider the use of hormone therapy (HT) at the lowest effective dose.

Before undergoing risk-reducing BSO, women with *BRCA* mutations should consider annual or semiannual screening with transvaginal ultrasonography and CA 125 test. Suppression of ovulation should be the contraceptive method of choice. Oral contraceptive use has a stronger protective effect than tubal ligation. Unless a woman has a prior history of breast cancer or has a relative in whom ovarian cancer was diagnosed before age 50 years, she has a low risk of ovarian cancer over the next 10 years. Estimates of the risk of ovarian cancer from age 40 years to age 50 years are 6.9% for *BRCA 1* mutation carriers and 1.9% for *BRCA 2* mutation carriers, respectively.

The described patient should consider risk-reducing BSO when nearing the age 40 years. Women with *BRCA* mutations who undergo risk-reducing BSO also can consider HT until age 50 years. Observational studies indicate that the risk of breast cancer in *BRCA* mutation carriers who take HT is not increased over that of *BRCA* mutation carriers who do not receive HT.

Oral contraceptives provide the most appropriate contraceptive management for this patient because they are associated with a decreased risk of ovarian cancer. The levonorgestrel intrauterine device has not been shown to decrease the risk of ovarian cancer because it does not prevent ovulation.

Erickson BK, Conner MG, Landen CN Jr. The role of the fallopian tube in the origin of ovarian cancer. Am J Obstet Gynecol 2013;209:409–14.

Guillem JG, Wood WC, Moley JF, Berchuck A, Karlan BY, Mutch DG, et al. ASCO/SSO review of current role of risk-reducing surgery in common hereditary cancer syndromes. ASCO and SSO. J Clin Oncol 2006;24:4642–60.

Iodice S, Barile M, Rotmensz N, Feroce I, Bonanni B, Radice P, et al. Oral contraceptive use and breast or ovarian cancer risk in BRCA1/2 carriers: a meta-analysis. Eur J Cancer 2010;46:2275–84.

Rebbeck TR, Kauff ND, Domchek SM. Meta-analysis of risk reduction estimates associated with risk-reducing salpingo-oophorectomy in BRCA1 or BRCA2 mutation carriers. J Natl Cancer Inst 2009;101:80–7.

Rebbeck TR, Friebel T, Wagner T, Lynch HT, Garber JE, Daly MB, et al. Effect of short-term hormone replacement therapy on breast cancer risk reduction after bilateral prophylactic oophorectomy in BRCA1 and BRCA2 mutation carriers: the PROSE Study Group. PROSE Study Group. J Clin Oncol 2005;23:7804–10.

28

Ovarian torsion

An 18-year-old woman comes to the emergency department with an 8-hour history of severe right lower quadrant pain. She has a history of a prior left salpingo-oophorectomy performed for ovarian torsion 3 years ago. Ultrasonography shows a 3-cm simple ovarian cyst and concern for adnexal torsion. Intraoperatively, the remaining ovary appears ischemic with a blue-black color. The most appropriate surgical intervention is

- (A) proceed with removal of the right fallopian tube and ovary
- (B) perform ovarian cystectomy
- * (C) detorse the ovary and perform an oophoropexy
- (D) perform hysterectomy and right salpingo-oophorectomy

Historically, removal of a torsed fallopian tube and ovary was carried out with great care to avoid intraoperative detorsion because of a theoretical concern regarding dislodging a clot in the ovarian vein. Numerous published series over the past 15–20 years have demonstrated that minimally invasive surgical techniques with detorsion and preservation of the fallopian tube and ovary can be safely performed even with the appearance of a seemingly necrotic ovary. In almost all cases, normal hormonal function returns and fertility is preserved. Experimental studies suggest that although the ovary may remain dusky and hemorrhagic after detorsion, usually arterial occlusion is not total and reperfusion occurs. The recommended treatment in young women is detorsion and preservation of the adnexa as opposed to salpingo-oophorectomy. Thus, removal of the right fallopian tube and ovary with or without a hysterectomy is not an appropriate intervention, especially in an 18-year-old woman with only one ovary.

Rapid diagnosis and expeditious treatment are important. Animal studies have suggested that intervention within the first 24 hours after torsion reliably resulted in normal reperfusion, whereas delay greater than 24 hours often resulted in significant congestion and necrosis. It is important to recognize that after detorsion and preservation of the adnexa, reversible ischemic damage may lead to peritonitis and infection if the ovary remains necrotic. Careful postoperative observation and rapid intervention are essential if any concern exists for postoperative peritonitis or infection.

The other concern with ovarian preservation is the possible inadvertent retention of malignant ovarian tumors. If a significant concern exists that cancer may be present, then salpingo-oophorectomy is indicated. If the ovary appears to be so necrotic that pathologic evaluation may be inaccurate, then serum tumor marker levels, including human chorionic gonadotropin, alpha-fetoprotein, lactate dehydrogenase, and CA 125, should be obtained.

Prevention of recurrence of ovarian torsion always should be considered. Many cases of ovarian torsion are associated with ovarian cysts, although a simple cyst of the described size rarely requires removal. It has been thought that ovarian suppression with oral contraceptives would decrease the development of functional ovarian cysts and, therefore, the likelihood of recurrent torsion. However, this has not been demonstrated with current low-dose oral contraceptives. Most experts recommend that oophoropexy be performed, especially in young women with one remaining ovary. This is especially important because normal adnexae are sometimes liable to torsion.

Abes M, Sarihan H. Oophoropexy in children with ovarian torsion. Eur J Pediatr Surg 2004;14:168–71.

Oelsner G, Shashar D. Adnexal torsion. Clin Obstet Gynecol 2006; 49:459–63.

Taskin O, Birincioglu M, Aydin A, Buhur A, Burak F, Yilmaz I, et al. The effects of twisted ischaemic adnexa managed by detorsion on ovarian viability and histology: an ischaemia-reperfusion rodent model. Hum Reprod 1998;13:2823–7.

29

Chronic pelvic pain

A 38-year-old nulligravid woman comes to your office with lower abdominal cramping pain for the past 2 years. The pain is noted to be worse during her menses, which are regular in frequency, duration, and amount. Her last menstrual period was 3 weeks ago. She reports bloating and rectal pressure that is partially relieved by defecation, occasional diarrhea, and passage of mucus for 2 years. She has experienced occasional pain with urination for 2 months. Urinalysis results are negative for white blood cells and leukocyte esterase. Pelvic examination reveals a 5-cm left pelvic mass. The next diagnostic test for this patient should be

      (A) laparoscopy
      (B) computed tomography (CT)
      (C) colonoscopy
*   (D) ultrasonography
      (E) magnetic resonance imaging (MRI)

Chronic pelvic pain is defined as noncyclic pain for 6 months or longer that is localized to the pelvis, the anterior abdominal wall at or below the umbilicus, the lumbosacral back, or buttocks. The pain is of sufficient severity to cause functional disability or lead to seeking medical care.

Chronic pelvic pain affects approximately 15–20% of women aged 18–50 years. It has many etiologic factors and is a symptom not a diagnosis. Conditions that have been shown to be causally related to chronic pelvic pain are listed in Box 29-1 and include irritable bowel syndrome (IBS), interstitial cystitis–bladder pain syndrome, and endometriosis. Several causes of pelvic pain may coexist. Diagnostic studies should be based on the patient's history and the results of physical examination.

The patient's gastrointestinal symptoms are consistent with IBS, a condition that occurs in 50–80% of women who experience chronic pelvic pain. The diagnosis of IBS is clinical and is based on the Rome III criteria (Box 29-2). In patients with IBS, the colonoscopy result is most commonly normal with a 10% yield for organic disease.

Interstitial cystitis is a chronic noninfectious inflammatory condition of the bladder and is characterized by urgency and frequency, in the absence of objective evidence of another disease that could cause the symptoms.

Pelvic pain is reported in up to 70% of these women and can be the presenting symptom or chief problem. It has been reported that 38–85% of women with chronic pelvic pain may have interstitial cystitis. The diagnosis is based on a validated questionnaire that can be used to determine whether cystoscopy is indicated. When the patient's history is significant for urinary symptoms, and urinalysis yields negative results, the interstitial cystitis questionnaire should be administered.

Endometriosis, diagnosed by laparoscopy, is present in 33% of patients with chronic pelvic pain. However, it is important to first exclude and treat, where necessary, other causes of pain. In this patient whose symptoms are likely related to other disease entities, laparoscopy is not immediately indicated.

The described patient is in the luteal phase of her menstrual cycle and the left-sided fullness is likely to be caused by a corpus luteum. Ultrasonography is a relatively inexpensive and practical imaging modality that is readily available in the office. It is considered the first-line imaging modality in the evaluation of an adnexal mass. In combination with a pelvic examination, transvaginal ultrasonography can accurately diagnose advanced stage pelvic endometriosis. Computed tomography and MRI are relatively expensive. Neither is considered a first-line

BOX 29-1

Conditions That Can Cause Chronic Pelvic Pain

Malignant
- Bladder
- Gynecologic
- Colon

Gynecologic
- Endometriomas
- Ovarian remnant syndrome
- Pelvic congestion syndrome
- Pelvic inflammatory disease
- Tuberculous salpingitis

Urinary
- Urinary tract disease
- Interstitial cystitis
- Radiation cystitis
- Urethral syndrome

Gastrointestinal
- Chronic constipation
- Inflammatory bowel disease
- Irritable bowel syndrome

Musculoskeletal
- Abdominal wall myofascial pain
- Low back pain
- Fibromyalgia
- Iliopsoas bursitis (syndrome)
- Neuralgia of iliohypogastric, ilioinguinal, or genitofemoral nerves
- Pelvic floor myalgia (levator ani or piriformis syndrome)
- Peripartum pelvic pain syndrome
- Vaginismus

Other
- Abdominal cutaneous nerve entrapment in a surgical scar
- Depression
- Somatization disorder

BOX 29-2

Rome III Criteria for the Diagnosis of Irritable Bowel Syndrome

Recurrent abdominal pain or discomfort and a marked change in bowel habit for at least 6 months, with symptoms experienced on at least 3 days of at least 3 months and two or more of the following:

- Pain is relieved by a bowel movement
- Onset of pain is related to a change in frequency of stool
- Onset of pain is related to a change in the appearance of stool

With kind permission from Springer Science+Media: *Journal of Gastroenterology*, Prevalence of organic colonic lesions in patients meeting Rome III criteria for diagnosis of IBS: a prospective multi-center study utilizing colonoscopy, volume 47, 2012, pages 1084–90, Ishihara S, Yashima K, Kushiyama Y, Izumi A, Kawashima K, Fujishiro H, et al.

imaging modality for chronic pelvic pain or the evaluation of an adnexal mass. However, CT or MRI scan may be useful if the ultrasonographic findings are abnormal.

Hudelist G, Oberwinkler KH, Singer CF, Tuttlies F, Rauter G, Ritter O, et al. Combination of transvaginal sonography and clinical examination for preoperative diagnosis of pelvic endometriosis. Hum Reprod 2009;24:1018–24.

Ishihara S, Yashima K, Kushiyama Y, Izumi A, Kawashima K, Fujishiro H, et al. Prevalence of organic colonic lesions in patients meeting Rome III criteria for diagnosis of IBS: a prospective multi-center study utilizing colonoscopy. J Gastroenterol 2012;47:1084–90.

Longstreth GF, Thompson WG, Chey WD, Houghton LA, Mearin F, Spiller RC. Functional bowel disorders [published erratum appears in Gastroenterology 2006;131:688]. Gastroenterology 2006;130:1480–91.

Vercellini P, Somigliana E, Viganò P, Abbiati A, Barbara G, Fedele L. Chronic pelvic pain in women: etiology, pathogenesis and diagnostic approach. Gynecol Endocrinol 2009;25:149–58.

30

Recurrent breast mass

A 34-year-old woman comes to your office after feeling a lump in her left breast for the past 4 weeks. A breast examination reveals a mobile, cystic 2-cm mass. The patient agrees to a fine-needle aspiration that yields straw-colored fluid. Four months later, the patient returns and reports that the mass has reoccurred. Your examination confirms a 3-cm soft, mobile cystic lesion in the area of the prior aspiration site. The best next step in evaluation of this mass is

(A) reassurance with repeat examination in 6 months
* (B) ultrasonography
(C) repeat aspiration
(D) mammography
(E) dietary modification

Differentiating between benign breast lesions and breast cancer is a crucial part of women's health care. Although patient history and physical examination can provide important information, considerable overlap can exist between benign lesions and malignant lesions. Patients who present with a palpable lesion should be queried regarding pain, mass size, duration, skin changes, and nipple discharge. In addition, risk factors for breast cancer, such as family history, should be elicited. Age is an important risk factor for breast cancer because incidence increases significantly in the fifth and sixth decades of life.

Benign breast disease can be divided into three main categories:

1. Nonproliferative disorders
2. Proliferative disorders without atypia
3. Atypical hyperplasias

Categorizing lesions in this fashion correlates with the individual's future risk of developing breast cancer. Nonproliferative diseases, such as simple cysts, infer no substantial increased future risk. Proliferative disorders without atypia (eg, fibroadenomas and intraductal papillomas) are associated with a relative risk of 1.3–1.9. By comparison, the relative risk of future breast cancer with the finding of atypical hyperplasia is 4.1–5.3.

Typically, simple cysts are benign, and the first step in evaluation often includes aspiration. If the fluid aspirate is nonbloody it can be discarded and the patient can be monitored clinically. If the fluid is bloody, the National Cancer Comprehensive Network (NCCN) recommends sending the fluid for cytology and placing a tissue marker if possible. If the aspirate cytology result is negative,

the patient should return in 6 months for evaluation. The NCCN also recommends that women who have a recurrent cystic mass after a nonbloody aspirate should undergo ultrasonography for further evaluation. If that result is consistent with a simple cyst, the patient can be monitored clinically. However, if ultrasonography demonstrates a solid lesion or a complex cyst or if it fails to locate a lesion, further investigation is warranted.

Although the risk of a malignancy is still low with a recurrent cystic breast mass, imaging is indicated. Therefore, reassurance with repeat examination in 6 months would not be appropriate. Mammography is recommended for women older than 30 years who have palpable breast masses; however, the NCCN notes that ultrasonography is the preferred modality if the lesion is suspected to be a simple cyst, as in the described patient.

Dietary modification often is recommended for the treatment of mastalgia, but not in the case of breast cysts. To date, research has failed to show that dietary modification, such as decreasing consumption of caffeine or salt or supplementation with vitamin E, helps to reduce breast pain.

Chang YW, Kwon KH, Goo DE, Choi DL, Lee HK, Yang SB. Sonographic differentiation of benign and malignant cystic lesions of the breast. J Ultrasound Med 2007;26:47–53.

Dixon JM, McDonald C, Elton RA, Miller WR. Risk of breast cancer in women with palpable breast cysts: a prospective study. Edinburgh Breast Group. Lancet 1999;353:1742–5.

National Comprehensive Cancer Network. NCCN guidelines. Fort Washington (PA): NCCN; 2013. Available at: http://www.nccn.org/professionals/physician_gls/f_guidelines.asp. Retrieved June 7, 2013.

Pearlman MD, Griffin JL. Benign breast disease. Obstet Gynecol 2010; 116:747–58.

31

Surgery for uterovaginal prolapse

A 77-year-old woman, gravida 3, para 3, comes to your office with a vaginal bulge and urinary obstruction that requires a Foley catheter for bladder drainage. She has a history of severe coronary artery disease and chronic obstructive pulmonary disease. She underwent a total vaginal hysterectomy with anterior repair for prolapse at age 40 years. Recently, she had an unsuccessful pessary trial because of expulsion of the pessary with defecation. She was continent of urine without urinary obstruction or leakage when the pessary was in place. She has been widowed for 10 years and is not sexually active. A preoperative evaluation confirms that she is a poor surgical candidate with significant risk for surgical anesthesia. On examination, she has a large central defect. The best surgical option is

       (A) paravaginal repair
       (B) traditional midline colporrhaphy
       (C) uterosacral ligament suspension
       (D) sacrospinous ligament fixation
  * (E) Le Fort partial colpocleisis

Pelvic floor disorders, including pelvic organ prolapse, urinary dysfunction, and fecal incontinence, are common problems with increasing incidence during women's lifetimes. The prevalence of pelvic organ prolapse stage II or greater increases to 64.8% in women aged 68 years. The etiology of pelvic organ prolapse is complex and involves potential injury to the many ligaments, muscles, tissues, and innervation of the pelvis. Contributing factors include age, parity, abdominal circumference, and body mass index.

Some clinicians use the Pelvic Organ Prolapse Quantification technique, in which the support defects of the vagina and perineum are systematically measured including the anterior, posterior, and apical dimensions, along with the genital hiatus and perineal body measurements (Appendix C). It is common for women to be affected by more than one pelvic floor condition and, for this reason, women should be screened for other associated conditions before surgery.

The lifetime risk of having surgery for pelvic organ prolapse or urinary incontinence up to age 80 years is approximately 11%. Women who have undergone a pelvic prolapse repair procedure are at risk for recurrence with reoperation rates up to 29%.

The ideal procedure repairs symptomatic pelvic floor defects, is performed efficiently, allows for rapid recovery, and adheres to the sexual activity desires of the patient. Additionally, the approach must take into consideration the patient's overall health and physical activity status.

Surgical techniques to address anterior defects include anterior colporrhaphy and paravaginal repair. As with the described patient, repair of the anterior wall is associated with the highest long-term failure rates (37–100%). The most efficacious technique to repair posterior defects is traditional midline colporrhaphy. Although this may be performed along with the anterior colporrhaphy in this patient, apical support would necessitate uterosacral ligament suspension, sacrospinous fixation, or ileococcygeus fixation. However, long-term follow-up data demonstrate prolapse recurrence in up to 16% of patients, and apical procedures typically require increased operative time. Abdominal sacral colpopexy has less apical failure, but is associated with more complications.

Given the described patient's poor cardiovascular and pulmonary function, colpocleisis is the best option. It has a shorter operative time and fewer perioperative complications compared with reconstructive repair. A Le Fort partial colpocleisis (Fig. 31-1) is sufficient for the needs of the described patient. She does not require a complete colpocleisis. In a Le Fort partial colpocleisis, the cut edges of the anterior and posterior vaginal wall are sewn together with interrupted delayed absorbable sutures. The knot should be turned into the epithelium-lined tunnels that were created bilaterally. The uterus and vaginal apex are gradually turned inward. After the vagina has been inverted, the superior and inferior margins of the rectangle can be sutured.

Before consideration of closure of the vaginal tissue, a discussion of sexual function is imperative. Patient satisfaction is high and prolapse recurrence is rare after obliterative procedures.

Gerten KA, Richter HE. Pelvic floor surgery in the older woman. Clin Obstet Gynecol 2007;50:826–43.

Pelvic organ prolapse. ACOG Practice Bulletin No. 85. American College of Obstetricians and Gynecologists. Obstet Gynecol 2007;110:717–29.

Toh VV, Bogne V, Bako A. Management of recurrent vault prolapse. Int Urogynecol J 2012;23:29–34.

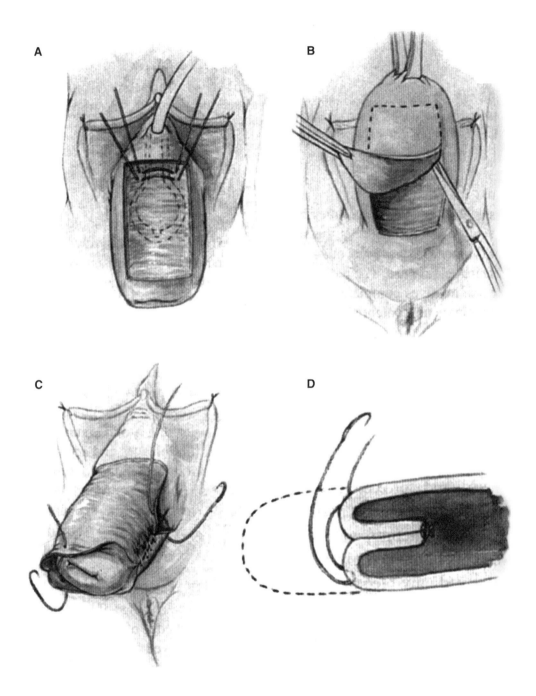

FIG. 31-1. Le Fort partial colpocleisis. **A.** The anterior vaginal wall has been removed and a plication stitch is placed at the bladder neck. **B.** The posterior vaginal wall is removed. **C** and **D.** The cut edge of the anterior vaginal wall is sewn in the cut edge of the posterior vaginal wall in such a way that the uterus and vagina are inverted. (This figure was published in Atlas of pelvic anatomy and gynecologic surgery, Baggish MS, Karram MM. Copyright Elsevier 2001).

32

Vesicovaginal fistula

A 42-year-old woman underwent a total vaginal hysterectomy 10 days ago. Yesterday she began to experience vaginal fluid leakage that requires the use of pads. She has no vaginal bleeding, fever, chills, dysuria, or urinary frequency. The most appropriate next step is

      (A) urine culture
      (B) urodynamic testing
  *   (C) office instillation of dye into bladder
      (D) check a postvoid residual

The patient's medical history suggests a genitourinary fistula. In the United States, genitourinary fistulas occur in more than 80% of women after gynecologic surgery, although in many other countries obstetric complications account for most cases. Urinary tract injuries at the time of hysterectomy have been reported in approximately 0.2–1.4% of cases. Direct injury by laceration or puncture usually presents with symptoms of immediate leakage of urine. Thermal, occlusive, or pressure injuries generally present as delayed complications, often with the development of genitourinary fistulas. Fistulas usually present within days after surgery. Occasionally, presentation is more delayed.

Postoperative infections also may contribute to the development of fistulas. Surgery for cancer or surgery after radiation increases the risk of genitourinary fistulas by up to 10%. Genitourinary fistulas cause leakage of urine from the vagina. Vesicovaginal fistulas are characterized by continuous leakage of urine, as in this clinical scenario, whereas ureterovaginal fistulas are characterized by intermittent leakage that is usually related to activity or position.

A vesicovaginal fistula may or may not be readily visible at the time of physical examination but can be confirmed by instilling sterile infant formula or methylene blue dye into the bladder through a transurethral catheter. Careful inspection while the patient coughs or bears down will almost always allow identification of one or more sites of extravasation of the instilled fluid.

A tampon test also can be performed in which, after instillation of methylene blue dye, a tampon is placed in the vagina and the patient is asked to get up and ambulate. The tampon is then removed and assessed for blue staining.

Although acute cystitis can lead to incontinence, it is usually intermittent and associated with symptoms of dysuria or frequency. To obtain a urine culture in this case is not inappropriate because infection is not the most likely cause of the leakage.

New onset urinary incontinence after vaginal hysterectomy without any reconstructive procedures is uncommon, so urodynamic evaluation to diagnose overactive bladder or stress incontinence is not indicated. Urinary retention occurs after surgical procedures, but onset is almost always immediately postoperatively, not 10 days later. Overflow incontinence is unlikely in this case; therefore, checking a postvoid residual is not useful.

Gilmour DT, Das S, Flowerdew G. Rates of urinary tract injury from gynecologic surgery and the role of intraoperative cystoscopy. Obstet Gynecol 2006;107:1366–72.

Lee RA, Symmonds RE, Williams TJ. Current status of genitourinary fistula. Obstet Gynecol 1988;72:313–9.

33

Depot medroxyprogesterone acetate and bone loss

A 17-year-old sexually active female comes to your office with her mother for contraceptive counseling. She has been using depot medroxyprogesterone acetate (DMPA) for birth control over the past 18 months. She wishes to continue the DMPA. She has no history of bone fractures and is in good health. Currently, she does not take any prescription medications, but in the past she had a difficult time remembering to take oral medications. Her mother has read about the thinning of bones associated with DMPA and inquires about bone mineral density (BMD) testing. After discussion of her risk factors for bone loss, the best next step in her management is

       (A) dual energy X-ray absorptiometry (DXA)
       (B) treat with bisphosphonates
   * (C) continue with DMPA
       (D) switch to oral contraceptives
       (E) check bone-turnover metabolites

Depot medroxyprogesterone acetate is a highly effective long-acting contraceptive injection that is approved in either intramuscular and subcutaneous formulations. It is used annually by more than 2 million women in the United States, including 400,000 adolescents. Evidence suggests that use of DMPA has contributed to the decrease of teenage pregnancy rates.

Most adult bone mass is achieved by age 19 years, and estrogen is required for its maintenance. Pituitary gonadotropin secretion is inhibited by DMPA, which results in anovulation, decreased ovarian estrogen production, and, in some cases, amenorrhea. A decrease in adult estrogen levels has been associated with loss of BMD in a number of conditions, such as anorexia nervosa, lactation, menopause, hypogonadism, and prolonged use of medications (DMPA, gonadotropin-releasing hormone agonists, and aromatase inhibitors).

In older women, osteopenia and osteoporosis are associated with an increased risk of bone fractures. This association has not been confirmed in adolescents and young women. In addition, studies have shown that after discontinuing DMPA, BMD will return to baseline or exceed it in most women by 2–5 years. In adolescents who receive DMPA, evidence is insufficient to support routine screening of BMD. The American College of Obstetricians and Gynecologists recommends that concerns regarding the effect of DMPA on BMD should neither prevent practitioners from prescribing DMPA nor limit its use to 2 consecutive years. Continued assessment of overall health and contraceptive needs should be performed annually while using DMPA.

All major health guidelines agree that screening for osteoporosis should commence at age 65 years. Screening for BMD can be initiated in postmenopausal women aged 50–64 years in the presence of other risk factors for osteoporosis (Box 33-1). Although other methods exist, the most common method of BMD screening for osteoporosis is dual-energy X-ray absorptiometry (DXA). This test should not be repeated in less than 2 years because of the inherent precision of the test.

The World Health Organization's online Fracture Risk Assessment Tool can be used in women younger than 65 years to determine which women should undergo DXA (Appendix D). Women with a 10-year risk of major osteoporotic fracture of 9.3% determined by the Fracture Risk Assessment Tool could be referred for DXA because that is the risk of fracture found in a 65-year-old Caucasian woman with no risk factors.

Urine and serum bone-turnover metabolites are byproducts of resorption (deoxypyridinoline, N-telopeptides, and

---

BOX 33-1

When to Screen for Bone Mineral Density Before Age 65 Years?

Bone mineral density should be assessed in postmenopausal women younger than 65 years if any of the following risk factors are noted:

• Medical history of a fragility fracture
• Body weight less than 57.6 kg (127 lb)
• Medical causes of bone loss (medications or diseases)
• Parental medical history of hip fracture
• Current smoker
• Alcoholism
• Rheumatoid arthritis

Osteoporosis. Practice Bulletin No. 129. American College of Obstetricians and Gynecologists. Obstet Gynecol 2012;120:718–34.

C-telopeptides from the breakdown of type I collagen) and formation (osteocalcin, bone-specific alkaline phosphatase, and procollagen type I N-terminal propeptide associated with bone matrix synthesis). They are used in clinical trials on osteoporosis to monitor patients' responses to treatment. Their utility in the clinical setting is controversial and cannot be used to screen for or diagnose osteoporosis.

Given the patient's history, she is not a candidate for BMD screening. The patient is in need of contraception and has been using DMPA thus far. She reports that she has a problem remembering to take oral medications, which makes a user-dependent contraceptive option, such as oral contraceptives, less desirable. Although other options in her case would be long-acting reversible contraceptives, such as the implant or the intrauterine device, she desires to continue to take DMPA.

Depot medroxyprogesterone acetate and bone effects. ACOG Committee Opinion No. 415. American College of Obstetricians and Gynecologists. Obstet Gynecol 2008;112:727–30.

Harel Z, Johnson CC, Gold MA, Cromer B, Peterson E, Burkman R, et al. Recovery of bone mineral density in adolescents following the use of depot medroxyprogesterone acetate contraceptive injections. Contraception 2010;81:281–91.

Osteoporosis. Practice Bulletin No. 129. American College of Obstetricians and Gynecologists. Obstet Gynecol 2012;120:718–34.

Scholes D, LaCroix AZ, Ichikawa LE, Barlow WE, Ott SM. Change in bone mineral density among adolescent women using and discontinuing depot medroxyprogesterone acetate contraception. Arch Pediatr Adolesc Med 2005;159:139–44.

Screening for osteoporosis: U.S. preventive services task force recommendation statement. U.S. Preventive Services Task Force. Ann Intern Med 2011;154:356–64.

World Health Organization Collaborating Centre for Metabolic Bone Diseases. WHO Fracture Risk Assessment Tool (FRAX). Sheffield, United Kingdom: University of Sheffield; 2013. Available at: http://www.shef.ac.uk/FRAX/. Retrieved June 21, 2013.

34

Atypical glandular cells Pap test result

A 33-year-old nulligravid woman comes to your office with Pap test results reported as atypical glandular cells, not otherwise specified (AGC–NOS). She has a history of irregular menses every 7–10 weeks. She has no medical problems and is not currently in a sexual relationship. Her last Pap test 3 years ago yielded a normal result; human papillomavirus (HPV) testing also yielded a normal result. Her family history is significant for colon cancer (it was diagnosed in her father at age 51 years). On physical examination, her height is 1.6 m (64 in), weight 106.6 kg (235 lb), blood pressure 125 mm Hg systolic, 75 mm Hg diastolic, and pulse 84 beats per minute. Pelvic examination yields a normal result. The best next step in management is

      (A) repeat Pap test with reflex HPV testing in 6 months
      (B) repeat HPV testing in 12 months
      (C) loop electrosurgical excision procedure (LEEP)
*   (D) colposcopy, endocervical curettage, and endometrial biopsy

Pap test results that show a finding of AGC are uncommon. Such findings merit follow-up diagnostic procedures. The screening result can be associated with underlying neoplastic processes, such as adenocarcinoma of the cervix or other types of reproductive tract cancer. However, the workup must rule out squamous lesions because these are the most common neoplasias of the cervix associated with AGC.

In women with an AGC–NOS result, colposcopic evaluation with endocervical curettage is recommended. Endometrial sampling should be performed in women older than 35 years and women younger than 35 years who are at risk of endometrial hyperplasia or cancer. Women with chronic anovulation, such as the described patient, should have an endometrial biopsy as should women with

unexplained vaginal bleeding. Follow-up with Pap test and HPV testing is inadequate. Pregnant women with AGC results should not undergo endocervical or endometrial sampling.

Testing for HPV may be performed at the time of colposcopy if HPV status is unknown. This information can be used to plan follow-up of women with normal cervical, endocervical, or endometrial biopsy results. Figure 34-1 shows the management of women with normal histologic results. Given inherent limitations of colposcopic biopsies and endocervical curettage, continued surveillance is necessary. Women with cervical intraepithelial neoplasia identified on histologic evaluation should follow national guidelines for the management of cervical intraepithelial neoplasia.

Subsequent Management of Women with Atypical Glandular Cells (AGC)

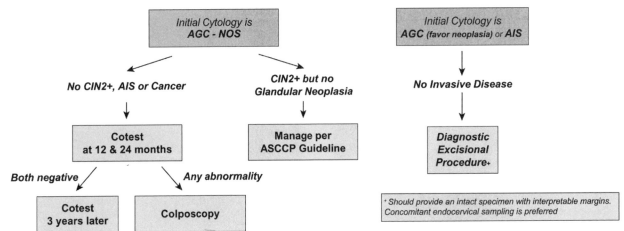

FIG. 34-1. Subsequent management of women with atypical glandular cells. Abbreviations: AGC–NOS indicates atypical glandular cells–not otherwise specified; AIS, adenocarcinoma in-situ; ASCCP, American Society for Colposcopy and Cervical Pathology; CIN, cervical intraepithelial neoplasia. (Massad LS, Einstein MH, Huh WK, Katki HA, Kinney WK, Schiffman M, et al. 2012 updated consensus guidelines for the management of abnormal cervical cancer screening tests and cancer precursors. 2012 ASCCP Consensus Guidelines Conference. J Low Genit Tract Dis 2013;17[5 Suppl1]: S1–S27. Reprinted from *The Journal of Lower Genital Tract Disease* Volume 17, Number 5, with the permission of ASCCP © American Society for Colposcopy and Cervical Pathology 2013. No copies of these ASCCP algorithms may be made without the prior consent of ASCCP.)

In the case of an AGC–favor neoplasia result, colposcopic evaluation with endocervical curettage and endometrial sampling is recommended in all patients. Because of the association of AGC Pap test results and neoplasia and the poor sensitivity of each testing modality, no single test (Pap test, cervical biopsy, endocervical curettage, or endometrial biopsy) is sufficient for evaluation. Therefore, in a woman with a negative biopsy result but a cervical cytology result that indicates AGC–favor neoplasia, a diagnostic excisional procedure is recommended. Cold knife conization or LEEP may be performed. The advantage of cold knife conization is that pathologic specimens will not have cauterized margins.

The advantages of LEEP are the ease of scheduling an in-office procedure and the low risks of bleeding and anesthetic complications. If LEEP is performed for glandular lesions, effort should be made to provide a single surgical specimen with intact pathologic margins to maximize interpretation of glandular disease.

Massad LS, Einstein MH, Huh WK, Katki HA, Kinney WK, Schiffman M, et al. 2012 updated consensus guidelines for the management of abnormal cervical cancer screening tests and cancer precursors. 2012 ASCCP Consensus Guidelines Conference. Obstet Gynecol 2013;121: 829–46.

Miroshnichenko GG, Parva M, Holtz DO, Klemens JA, Dunton CJ. Interpretability of excisional biopsies of the cervix: cone biopsy and loop excision. J Low Genit Tract Dis 2009;13:10–2.

35

Perioperative pulmonary complications

A 60-year-old woman undergoes an uncomplicated bilateral salpingo-oophorectomy for a 20-cm benign mucinous cystadenoma. On postoperative day 1, you are contacted by the nursing staff and informed that the patient has developed a fever of 38.4°C (101°F). The patient states that despite the fever she feels fine. Her oxygen saturation is 92% on room air that improves to 98% with ambulation. Physical examination findings are remarkable for decreased breath and bowel sounds, a clean and intact incision and peripheral intravenous site, and trace bilateral pedal edema with bilateral sequential devices and compression stockings in place. The best next step in management is

*   (A) aggressive pulmonary therapy
        (B) blood and urine cultures
        (C) broad-spectrum antibiotics
        (D) therapeutic anticoagulation
        (E) computed tomography of the chest

Appropriate evaluation of febrile morbidity in the postoperative period is important. A complete history and physical examination may help direct treatment and limit unnecessary laboratory and imaging tests with low yield. Timing of febrile events is important because pulmonary infections will generally precede urinary tract and wound infections. A workup that does not demonstrate any of these three types of infections as possible causes of the fever underscores the potential for thromboembolic events or drug reactions.

Pulmonary issues in the postoperative period include atelectasis, pneumonia, and pulmonary embolus with or without atelectasis. Often, atelectasis is caused by decreased airway space that improves with incentive spirometer use and ambulation. Patients often have a low-grade fever in the postoperative period, as in the described woman who likely has atelectasis. Aggressive pulmonary therapy (removal of excess fluids and mucus) and a chest X-ray to exclude underlying pneumonia constitute reasonable first steps. In cases in which a chest X-ray scan is inconclusive or the patient's clinical condition deteriorates, computed tomography of the chest may be a reasonable step.

A complete blood count, basic metabolic profile, urinalysis, and blood and urine cultures have been demonstrated to have a limited role in the early management of a patient with postoperative fever. However, blood culture is more likely to yield positive results if the patient has a persistent or increased fever, malignancy, bowel resection, and moderately increased white blood cell count. In the absence of these comorbid conditions, further postoperative workup increases cost with low yield. Initiation of broad-spectrum antibiotics on postoperative day 1 is not indicated for the described patient.

A bilateral salpingo-oophorectomy is viewed as a clean procedure and, although a pelvic abscess is a possibility on postoperative day 1, pulmonary complications are likely. Imaging at this time, such as with Doppler ultrasonography, would increase cost without a clear benefit. Thromboembolic events are possible but of decreased likelihood given her appropriate prophylaxis with sequential compression devices and compression stockings along with improvement of the oxygen saturation with ambulation. Further workup for thromboembolic events may be indicated for patients with decreased oxygen saturation and negative chest X-ray results.

de la Torre SH, Mandel L, Goff BA. Evaluation of postoperative fever: usefulness and cost-effectiveness of routine workup. Am J Obstet Gynecol 2003;188:1642–7.

Garibaldi RA, Brodine S, Matsumiya S, Coleman M. Evidence for the non-infectious etiology of early postoperative fever. Infect Control 1985;6:273–7.

Lazenby GB, Soper DE. Prevention, diagnosis, and treatment of gynecologic surgical site infections. Obstet Gynecol Clin North Am 2010;37:379–86.

36

Recurrent bacterial vaginosis

A 33-year-old woman, gravida 2, para 2, comes to your clinic with recurrent malodorous vaginal discharge and vulvar irritation with symptoms every 1–2 months in the past year. She received a diagnosis and was treated for bacterial vaginosis 4 times in the past 5 months. Each time, she had a complete resolution of symptoms followed by recurrence after sexual intercourse. After treatment of her recent infection, the best management plan is

      (A) treat sexual partner(s)
      (B) recommend weekly douching
      (C) postcoital oral clindamycin
  *   (D) metronidazole vaginal gel twice weekly

Vaginal symptoms are common in the general population and are one of the most frequent reasons for patient visits. Vaginitis is defined as the spectrum of conditions that cause vulvovaginal symptoms, such as itching, burning, irritation, and abnormal discharge. Among symptomatic women, the most common causes of infectious vaginitis are bacterial vaginosis (up to 50%), vulvovaginal candidiasis (up to 30%), and trichomoniasis (up to 20%). Up to 22% of women with symptoms of vaginitis may remain without a diagnosis after complete evaluation.

Bacterial vaginosis is associated with complications, including increased risks of sexually transmitted infections, human immunodeficiency virus (HIV), and adverse pregnancy outcomes. The tendency of bacterial vaginosis to recur is frustrating for those affected and can lead to depression or adverse effects on relationships.

Patients with bacterial vaginosis may report an abnormal vaginal discharge and fishy odor. The clinical diagnosis of bacterial vaginosis requires the presence of three out of four Amsel criteria: 1) abnormal gray discharge, 2) pH greater than 4.5, 3) positive amine test (whiff test) result, and 4) greater than 20% clue cells. Amsel criteria have a diagnostic sensitivity of 92% and specificity of 77%. Similar sensitivity and specificity have been demonstrated with the use of any combination of only two clinical criteria.

Bacterial vaginosis can arise and remit spontaneously but often presents as a chronic or recurrent disease. After treatment, bacterial vaginosis is cleared in up to 88% of patients. However, it may recur in up to 30% of women within 3 months. Prevention of recurrences often is difficult. Possible mechanisms for recurrent bacterial vaginosis include persistence of pathogenic bacteria, reinfection from exogenous sources, or failure of the normal lactobacillus-dominant flora to reestablish itself.

Bacterial vaginosis is strongly associated with sexual activity and appears to recur with an increased frequency in HIV-positive women. Additional factors for bacterial vaginosis include douching, use of sex toys, multiple sexual partners, and new sexual partners. Women who have sex with women share similar lactobacillary types and are at increased risk of bacterial vaginosis. However, studies of partner treatment have failed to show a protective effect.

Three antibiotics are approved for the treatment of bacterial vaginosis: 1) metronidazole, 2) tinidazole, and 3) clindamycin. Metronidazole and clindamycin can be applied locally in the vagina or taken orally with similar efficacy. Generally, topical treatment is more expensive than generic oral metronidazole, although the latter may be associated with significant gastrointestinal symptoms. Disulfiram-like reactions may occur with oral and topical azole therapy (metronidazole and tinidazole). Table 36-1 lists treatment options for bacterial vaginosis and other vulvovaginal infections.

Results from randomized studies show that 500-mg oral metronidazole twice daily for 7 days provides the highest cure rates for bacterial vaginosis. After recurrence, a further course of oral metronidazole is recommended followed by twice weekly treatment with 0.75% metronidazole gel for 4–6 months. However, twice weekly treatment may not affect the subsequent recurrence rate after it is stopped. The use of oral clindamycin after sexual intercourse has not been studied for treatment of recurrent bacterial vaginosis.

Hay P. Recurrent bacterial vaginosis. Curr Opin Infect Dis 2009;22: 82–6.

Vaginitis. ACOG Practice Bulletin No. 72. American College of Obstetricians and Gynecologists. Obstet Gynecol 2006;107:1195–206.

Workowski KA, Berman S. Sexually transmitted diseases treatment guidelines, 2010. Centers for Disease Control and Prevention [published erratum appears in MMWR Morb Mortal Wkly Rep 2011;60:18]. MMWR Recomm Rep 2010;59:1–110.

TABLE 36-1. Therapy for Vulvovaginal Infections (Drugs Listed Alphabetically)

Indication	Drug	Formulation	Dosage	Duration
Uncomplicated vulvovaginal candidiasis	Butoconazole	2% sustained-release cream	5 g daily	1 day
	Clotrimazole	1% cream	5 g daily	7 days
		2% cream	5 g daily	3 days
		100-mg vaginal suppository	100 mg daily	7 days
		200-mg vaginal suppository	200 mg daily	3 days
		500-mg vaginal suppository	500 mg daily	1 day
	Fluconazole	150-mg oral tablet	150 mg daily	1 day
	Miconazole	2% cream	5 g daily	7 days
		100-mg vaginal suppository	100 mg daily	7 days
		200-mg vaginal suppository	200 mg daily	3 days
		1,200-mg vaginal suppository	1,200 mg daily	1 day
	Nystatin	100,000-unit vaginal tablets	daily	14 days
	Terconazole	0.4% cream	5 g daily	7 days
		0.8% cream	5 g daily	3 days
	Tioconazole	2% cream	5 g daily	3 days
		6.5% cream	5 g daily	1 day
Bacterial vaginosis	Clindamycin	2% cream	5 g daily	7 days
		2% sustained-release cream	5 g daily	1 day
		100-mg ovules	100 mg daily	3 days
		300-mg oral tablet	300 mg twice daily	7 days
	Metronidazole	0.75% gel	5 g daily	5 days
		500-mg oral tablet	500 mg twice daily	7 days
Trichomoniasis	Metronidazole	500-mg oral tablet	4 tablets as one dose	1 day
			500 mg twice daily	7 days
	Tinidazole	500-mg oral tablet	4 tablets as one dose	1 day

Data from Sexually transmitted diseases treatment guidelines 2002. Centers for Disease Control and Prevention. MMWR Recomm Rep 2002;51(RR-6):1–78; Sobel JD, Faro S, Force RW, Foxman B, Ledger WJ, Nyirjesy P, et al. Vulvovaginal candidiasis: epidemiologic, diagnostic, and therapeutic considerations. Am J Obstet Gynecol 1998;178:203–11; Cohen L. Treatment of vaginal candidosis using clotrimazole vaginal cream: single dose versus 3-day therapy. Curr Med Res Opin 1985;9:520–3; Faro S, Skokos CK. The efficacy and safety of a single dose of Clindesse vaginal cream versus a seven-dose regimen of Cleocin vaginal cream in patients with bacterial vaginosis. Clindesse Investigators Group. Infect Dis Obstet Gynecol 2005;13:155–60; *and* Gabriel G, Robertson E, Thin RN. Single dose treatment of trichomoniasis. J Int Med Res 1982;10:129–30.

Vaginitis. ACOG Practice Bulletin No. 72. American College of Obstetricians and Gynecologists. Obstet Gynecol 2006;107:1195–206.

37

Alternatives to hysterectomy for myomas

A 38-year-old woman, gravida 3, para 3, has a 4-month history of heavy menstrual bleeding. Past surgical history is significant for three cesarean deliveries with the third procedure complicated by a bowel injury. Laboratory evaluation includes a hemoglobin level of 9.2 g/dL. Sonohysterography shows a 3.5-cm pedunculated fundal submucosal myoma with no intramural extension and a uterine sagittal length of 10 cm. Endometrial biopsy reveals disordered, proliferative phase endometrium. The patient desires future fertility. The best approach for management of this patient is

* (A) hysteroscopic myomectomy
 (B) nonresectoscopic endometrial ablation
 (C) magnetic resonance imaging (MRI)-guided focused ultrasound ablation
 (D) uterine artery embolization
 (E) abdominal myomectomy

Myomas, also known as fibroids, are the leading cause of hysterectomy. In the United States annually, approximately 200,000 hysterectomies for myomas are performed. Women with myomas seek medical treatment most commonly for heavy menstrual bleeding and pelvic pressure; heavy menstrual bleeding may lead to iron deficiency anemia. Few comparative studies of myoma treatment strategies exist. Safety, efficacy, and patient autonomy have to be considered when choosing an alternative to hysterectomy.

Submucosal myomas are a cause of heavy menstrual bleeding. Submucosal myomas distort the uterine cavity and can block the cervical canal and tubal ostia, which adversely affects fertility and potentially causes pregnancy complications.

Myomectomy remains the criterion standard in myoma treatment for patients who desire future fertility. The best approach for management of this patient is hysteroscopic myomectomy. Generally, submucosal myomas up to 4–5 cm in diameter can be removed under hysteroscopic direction by experienced surgeons. Larger and multiple myomas are best removed abdominally. Depth of extension into the myometrium and size of myomas, surgeon's skill, instrumentation, and experience of the surgical staff are considerations when planning a hysteroscopic or an abdominal (ie, laparoscopy or laparotomy) procedure.

The most predictive indicator of surgical success at hysteroscopy is the portion of myoma contained within the uterine cavity. A pedunculated myoma is optimal for resection because 100% of such a myoma is contained within the uterine cavity. Appendix E shows a classification system of submucosal myomas based on their depth of penetration into the myometrium. Hysteroscopic myomectomy minimizes operative risks and potential interference with future fertility. Risks of hysteroscopy related to future fertility include incomplete resection necessitating a

second hysteroscopy, intrauterine adhesions, and uterine rupture in pregnancy.

This patient might benefit from a preoperative 3-month course of gonadotropin-releasing hormone agonist. The goals of this therapy are to shrink the myoma, increasing the chance of complete removal, and to reduce menstrual flow, optimizing preoperative hemoglobin level. Reported intraoperative benefits of gonadotropin-releasing hormone agonists include improved visualization and reduced rate of fluid absorption. Potential benefits must be weighed against adverse effects and the cost of the therapy. This patient, who has not had a vaginal delivery, also may benefit from a cervical ripening agent, such as preoperative laminaria or prostaglandins, and an intraoperative intracervical injection of dilute vasopressin to facilitate cervical dilation.

Endometrial ablation is contraindicated in women who desire future childbearing. Endometrial ablation may be effective in select patients with submucosal myomas less than or equal to 3 cm in diameter that extend into the myometrium. Endometrial ablation has decreased efficacy in treating either submucosal myomas greater than 3 cm or pedunculated submucosal myomas.

Hysteroscopic myomectomy is the preferred procedure for the described patient with a type zero submucosal myoma. Advantages include that it is a same-day procedure and has less risk of intraoperative complications, less blood loss, shorter recovery, less pain, faster return to work, and less delay in attempting to conceive than other procedures. The abdominal approach may be desirable in patients who have submucosal myomas that extend to the uterine serosa or other intramural or large subserosal myomas.

Uterine artery embolization has risks of submucosal myoma expulsion, bleeding, and infection. Uterine artery embolization has an age-related risk of diminished ovarian reserve and compromise of endometrial perfusion to the placenta, leading to placentation problems in pregnancy. Additionally, uterine artery embolization in this patient would result in an increased interval of delay in attempt to conceive. Although healthy term pregnancies have been reported, uterine artery embolization should be reserved for women who do not desire future fertility.

The effects of submucosal myoma treatment with MRI-guided focused ultrasound ablation on reproductive outcomes are not well studied. Additionally, the procedure is limited by the high costs of MRI guidance. Thermal injury to the skin has been reported in women with extensive abdominal wall scarring.

AAGL practice report: practice guidelines for the diagnosis and management of submuous myomas. American Association of Gynecologic Laparoscopists (AAGL): Advancing Minimally Invasive Gynecology Worldwide. J Minim Invasive Gynecol 2012;19:152–71.

Alternatives to hysterectomy in the management of myomas. ACOG Practice Bulletin No. 96. American College of Obstetricians and Gynecologists. Obstet Gynecol 2008;112:387–400.

Gambadauro P. Dealing with uterine fibroids in reproductive medicine. J Obstet Gynaecol 2012;32:210–6.

Laughlin SK, Stewart EA. Uterine myomas: individualizing the approach to a heterogeneous condition. Obstet Gynecol 2011;117: 396–403.

Stewart EA. Uterine fibroids and evidence-based medicine—not an oxymoron. N Engl J Med 2012;366:472–3.

38

Perioperative cardiac evaluation

A 63-year-old woman is scheduled to undergo laparoscopic hysterectomy with bilateral salpingo-oophorectomy and pelvic washings along with possible pelvic and paraaortic lymphadenectomy for poorly differentiated endometrial adenocarcinoma. She has a history of morbid obesity with a body mass index (BMI) of 42 (calculated as weight in kilograms divided by height in meters squared) and poorly controlled diabetes mellitus. She has recently developed dyspnea and chest pressure with walking. Her blood pressure is 160 mm Hg systolic, 100 mm Hg diastolic, and her heart rate is 83 beats per minute. A laboratory evaluation reveals a fasting blood sugar level of 120 mg/dL, hemoglobin A_{1c} level of 7.5%, hemoglobin level of 10.5 g/dL, and serum creatinine level of 1.2 mg/dL. The chest X-ray result is normal. She had a normal result on screening colonoscopy 3 years ago. You advise her that it is best to postpone the procedure because of the

      (A) obesity
      (B) hemoglobin A_{1c} level
      (C) blood pressure level
  * (D) dyspnea and chest pressure
      (E) hemoglobin level

The 2007 American College of Cardiology American Heart Association Guidelines on Perioperative Cardiac Evaluation and Care for Noncardiac Surgery constitute the accepted standard for perioperative cardiac evaluation. These guidelines are evidence-based, endorsed by the American Society of Anesthesiologists, and adopted by the Agency for Healthcare Research and Quality.

Clinical risk factors for perioperative cardiac complications include the following:

- History of ischemic heart disease
- History of compensated or prior heart failure
- History of cerebrovascular disease
- Diabetes mellitus
- Renal insufficiency (defined as a preoperative serum creatinine level of more than 2 mg/dL)

Box 38-1 shows the American College of Cardiology and American Heart Association stepwise approach for cardiac evaluation and care for noncardiac surgery. Active cardiac conditions for which patients should undergo treatment before undergoing surgery include the following:

- Unstable coronary syndrome
- Decompensated heart failure
- Significant atrial arrhythmias
- Ventricular arrhythmias
- Severe valvular disease

The goal of the preoperative cardiac evaluation is to identify major risks and optimize perioperative clinical management. Preoperative tests should be ordered only

BOX 38-1

Stepwise Approach to Perioperative Cardiac Assessment

Step 1. The consultant should determine the urgency of noncardiac surgery. In many instances, patient- or surgery-specific factors dictate an obvious strategy (eg, emergent surgery) that may not allow for further cardiac assessment or treatment. In such cases, the consultant may function best by providing recommendations for perioperative medical management and surveillance.

Step 2. Does the patient have one of the active cardiac conditions or clinical risk factors listed? If not, proceed to Step 3. In patients who are being considered for elective noncardiac surgery, the presence of unstable coronary disease, decompensated heart failure, or severe arrhythmia or valvular heart disease usually leads to cancellation or delay of surgery until the cardiac problem has been clarified and treated appropriately.

Step 3. Is the patient undergoing low-risk surgery? In these patients, interventions based on cardiovascular testing in stable patients would rarely result in a change in management, and it would be appropriate to proceed with the planned surgical procedure.

Step 4. Does the patient have good functional capacity without symptoms? In highly functional asymptomatic patients, management will rarely be changed on the basis of results of any further cardiovascular testing. Therefore, it is appropriate to proceed with the planned surgery. In patients with known cardiovascular disease or at least one clinical risk factor, perioperative heart rate control with β-blockers appears appropriate. If the patient has not had a recent exercise test, functional status usually can be estimated from the ability to perform activities of daily living. For this purpose, functional capacity has been classified as excellent (greater than 10 METs [metabolic equivalents of task]), good (7–10 METs), moderate (4–7 METs), poor (less than 4 METs), or unknown.

Step 5. If the patient has poor functional capacity, is symptomatic, or has unknown functional capacity, then the presence of active clinical risk factors will determine the need for further evaluation. If the patient has no clinical risk factors, then it is appropriate to proceed with the planned surgery, and no further change in management is indicated. If the patient has one or two clinical risk factors, then it is reasonable either to proceed with the planned surgery or, if appropriate, with heart rate control with β-blockers, or to consider testing if it will change management. In patients with three or more clinical risk factors, the surgery-specific cardiac risk is important.

Reprinted from the Journal of the American College of Cardiology, Volume 50, Fleisher LA, Beckman JA, Brown KA, Calkins H, Chaikof EL, Fleischmann KE, et al. ACC/AHA 2007 Guidelines on Perioperative Cardiovascular Evaluation and Care for Noncardiac Surgery: Executive Summary: A Report of the American College of Cardiology/American Heart Association Task Force on Practice Guidelines (Writing Committee to Revise the 2002 Guidelines on Perioperative Cardiovascular Evaluation for Noncardiac Surgery) Developed in Collaboration With the American Society of Echocardiography, American Society of Nuclear Cardiology, Heart Rhythm Society, Society of Cardiovascular Anesthesiologists, Society for Cardiovascular Angiography and Interventions, Society for Vascular Medicine and Biology, and Society for Vascular Surgery, pages 1707–32, copyright 2007, with permission from the American College of Cardiology.

if results are likely to affect perioperative care. Box 38-2 lists possible interventions that may be implemented as a result of test outcomes.

The patient's new onset dyspnea and chest pressure on exertion reflect a decompensation in functional capacity possibly caused by unstable coronary syndrome. These are active cardiac issues that need to be evaluated before surgery. The patient should have a stress test (dobutamine echo, exercise, or nuclear imaging) before surgery.

Perioperative β-blocker use is recommended for patients already taking β-blockers. Routine administration of perioperative β-blockers, especially in high doses, is no longer recommended. Preoperative β-blocker therapy should be individualized based on the patient's clinical and surgical risks. Identification of preoperative active cardiac conditions may require intensive management and a delay or cancellation of a nonemergent surgery.

Morbid obesity, diabetes mellitus, and hypertension are chronic diseases and risk factors for surgery, but they are not contraindications to surgery. The blood glucose

BOX 38-2

Potential Interventions That May Result From Knowledge Gained Through Testing

- Delaying the operation because of unstable symptoms
- Coronary revascularization
- Attempting medical optimization before surgery
- Involving additional specialists or providers in the patient's perioperative care
- Modification of intraoperative monitoring
- Modification of postoperative monitoring
- Modification of the surgical location, particularly when the procedure is scheduled for an ambulatory surgical center

Reprinted with permission from Fleisher LA. Cardiac risk stratification for noncardiac surgery: update from the American College of Cardiology/American Heart Association 2007 guidelines. American College of Cardiology/American Heart Association. Cleve Clin J Med 2009;76(Suppl 4):S9–15. Copyright © 2009 Cleveland Clinic Foundation. All rights reserved.

levels and blood pressure can be medically managed perioperatively. The anemia in this patient may be contributing to the dyspnea on exertion and chest pressure, and a perioperative blood transfusion may improve these symptoms. Most importantly, she should be evaluated for coronary heart disease.

Perioperative tests and treatments improve outcomes only when targeted to specific subsets of patients. Evidence-based perioperative evaluation optimizes patient care and reduces health care-related costs.

Chopra V, Flanders SA, Froehlich JB, Lau WC, Eagle KA. Perioperative practice: time to throttle back. Ann Intern Med 2010;152:47–51.

Fleischmann KE, Beckman JA, Buller CE, Calkins H, Fleisher LA, Freeman WK, et al. 2009 ACCF/AHA focused update on perioperative beta blockade: a report of the American college of cardiology foundation/American heart association task force on practice guidelines. Circulation 2009;120:2123–51.

Fleisher LA. Cardiac risk stratification for noncardiac surgery: update from the American College of Cardiology/American Heart Association 2007 guidelines. American College of Cardiology/American Heart Association. Cleve Clin J Med 2009;76(Suppl 4):S9–15.

Fleisher LA, Beckman JA, Brown KA, Calkins H, Chaikof E, Fleischmann KE, et al. ACC/AHA 2007 guidelines on perioperative cardiovascular evaluation and care for noncardiac surgery: executive summary: a report of the American College of Cardiology/American Heart Association Task Force on Practice Guidelines (Writing Committee to Revise the 2002 Guidelines on Perioperative Cardiovascular Evaluation for Noncardiac Surgery). American College of Cardiology/American Heart Association Task Force on Practice Guidelines (Writing Committee to Revise the 2002 Guidelines on Perioperative Cardiovascular Evaluation for Noncardiac Surgery), American Society of Echocardiography, American Society of Nuclear Cardiology, Heart Rhythm Society, Society of Cardiovascular Anesthesiologists, Society for Cardiovascular Angiography and Interventions, and Society for Vascular Medicine and Biology; Society for Vascular Surgery. Anesth Analg 2008;106:685–712.

Vigoda MM, Sweitzer B, Miljkovic N, Arheart KL, Messinger S, Candiotti K, et al. 2007 American College of Cardiology/American Heart Association (ACC/AHA) Guidelines on perioperative cardiac evaluation are usually incorrectly applied by anesthesiology residents evaluating simulated patients. Anesth Analg 2011;112:940–9.

39

Lynch II syndrome

A 35-year-old woman, gravida 2, para 2, comes to your office for her annual examination. Recently, she received the diagnosis of Lynch II syndrome. Her mother had uterine cancer at age 52 years, her maternal uncle had colon cancer at age 47 years, and her older sister had ovarian cancer at age 46 years. The best strategy to decrease the patient's risk of gastrointestinal and gynecologic cancer over the next 5 years is

      (A) annual computed tomography examination of abdomen and pelvis
      (B) annual colonoscopy and transvaginal ultrasonography with endometrial biopsy
      (C) prophylactic colectomy with annual transvaginal ultrasonography
*   (D) prophylactic hysterectomy and bilateral salpingo-oophorectomy with annual colonoscopy

Lynch II syndrome, also known as hereditary nonpolyposis colorectal cancer, is associated with an increased risk of cancer of the colon, endometrium, small bowel, and renal area of the pelvis. Patients without a cancer diagnosis but with a new diagnosis of Lynch II syndrome should receive gastrointestinal and gynecologic surveillance. Patients with Lynch II syndrome have been identified to possess the four most commonly mutated DNA mismatch repair genes, ie, *MLH1, MSH2, MSH6,* and *PMS2.* Such patients have a lifetime risk for endometrial cancer of up to 60% and for colon cancer of up to 70%.

Patients with Lynch II syndrome need to be directly involved in decision-making because of their genetic risk for gynecologic cancer. Patients should consider prophylactic surgery after childbearing is complete, particularly from age 30–40 years onward. Annual colonoscopy and prophylactic gynecologic surgery constitute the only intervention with data that support a decrease in cancer risk.

Annual colonoscopy with transvaginal ultrasonography and endometrial biopsy provide reasonable options for women who wish to maintain fertility. However, available data are limited in regard to any benefit of serial ultrasonography and endometrial biopsy. Prophylactic colectomy is not indicated without a diagnosis of malignancy, and the increased risk of morbidity with this type of surgery must be considered. Annual transvaginal ultrasonography is limited by lack of data to support this modality alone; to date, it has not been demonstrated to reduce the risk of gynecologic cancer. Similarly, it has not been demonstrated that computed tomography reduces the risk of such cancer.

Lancaster JM, Powell CB, Kauff ND, Cass I, Chen LM, Lu KH, et al. Society of Gynecologic Oncologists Education Committee statement on risk assessment for inherited gynecologic cancer predispositions. Society of Gynecologic Oncologists Education Committee. Gynecol Oncol 2007;107:159–62.

Lindor NM, Petersen GM, Hadley DW, Kinney AY, Miesfeldt S, Lu KH, et al. Recommendations for the care of individuals with an inherited predisposition to Lynch syndrome: a systematic review. JAMA 2006;296:1507–17.

Lu KH. Hereditary gynecologic cancers: differential diagnosis, surveillance, management and surgical prophylaxis. Fam Cancer 2008;7:53–8.

Schmeler KM, Lynch HT, Chen LM, Munsell MF, Soliman PT, Clark MB, et al. Prophylactic surgery to reduce the risk of gynecologic cancers in the Lynch syndrome. N Engl J Med 2006;354:261–9.

Smith RA, Cokkinides V, Brooks D, Saslow D, Brawley OW. Cancer screening in the United States, 2010: a review of current American Cancer Society guidelines and issues in cancer screening. CA Cancer J Clin 2010;60:99–119.

40

Abnormal uterine bleeding in a reproductive-aged woman

A 38-year-old woman, gravida 4, para 4, comes to your office and requests contraception. She has a 4-month history of irregular bleeding that lasts up to 17 days per month. Her past medical history is significant for poorly controlled hypertension. On physical examination, her blood pressure (BP) is 160 mm Hg systolic, 110 mm Hg diastolic and her body mass index (BMI) is 32 (calculated as weight in kilograms divided by height in meters squared). A urine pregnancy test result is negative. Other laboratory values are normal except for a hemoglobin level of 11.3 g/dL. Endometrial biopsy reveals a disordered, proliferative phase endometrium. The best contraceptive choice for this patient is

      (A) depot medroxyprogesterone acetate
      (B) contraceptive vaginal ring
      (C) combined oral contraceptives
*   (D) levonorgestrel IUD
      (E) copper IUD

Abnormal uterine bleeding in nonpregnant women can be categorized as chronic, acute, and intermittent. *Chronic abnormal uterine bleeding* can be defined as bleeding from the uterine endometrium that is abnormal in volume, regularity, or timing, and has been present for most of the past 6 months.

The most common form of noncyclic uterine bleeding, *anovulatory bleeding,* is defined as noncyclic menstrual blood flow that may range in volume from spotty to excessive. It originates from the uterine endometrium, is not attributed to an anatomic lesion, and is caused by anovulatory sex steroid production. Box 40-1 lists causes of anovulation.

In anovulation, a corpus luteum is not formed, serum progesterone production remains low, and estrogen production persists. Estrogen stimulates endometrial proliferation and, without adequate progesterone levels, leads to unpredictable, desynchronized sloughing of the endometrial lining.

The described patient has abnormal uterine bleeding that is most likely anovulatory in nature. Laboratory evaluation should include a pregnancy test and serum thyroid-stimulating hormone level measurement. Endometrial assessment should be performed as a first-line test in

---

BOX 40-1

Causes of Anovulation

Physiologic
- Adolescence
- Perimenopause
- Lactation
- Pregnancy

Pathologic
- Hyperandrogenic anovulation (eg, polycystic ovary syndrome, congenital adrenal hyperplasia, and androgen-producing tumors)
- Hypothalamic dysfunction (eg, secondary to anorexia nervosa)
- Hyperprolactinemia
- Hypothyroidism
- Primary pituitary disease
- Ovarian insufficiency
- Iatrogenic (eg, secondary to radiation or chemotherapy)

American College of Obstetricians and Gynecologists. Management of anovulatory bleeding. ACOG Practice Bulletin 14. Washington, DC: ACOG; 2000.

patients older than 45 years with abnormal uterine bleeding. Endometrial sampling also is recommended for patients younger than 45 years with a history of unopposed estrogen exposure, such as obese women or women with polycystic ovary syndrome, patients with failed medical management, and those with persistent abnormal uterine bleeding. In deciding the most appropriate medical therapy for an individual patient, consideration should be given to the patient's comorbidities. Clinicians should refer to the World Health Organization's Medical Eligibility Criteria (Appendix B) to determine the safest options.

The treatment of choice for anovulatory uterine bleeding is medical therapy. Estrogen-containing contraceptives, such as the contraceptive vaginal ring and combined oral contraceptives, are contraindicated in women with a history of uncontrolled hypertension. Women younger than 35 years with adequately controlled and monitored hypertension are candidates for combined hormonal contraceptives.

In patients with systolic BP greater than or equal to 160 mm Hg and diastolic BP greater than or equal to 90 mm Hg, combined hormonal contraceptives are considered Category 4. In this hypertensive subgroup, depot medroxyprogesterone acetate is a Category 3 progestin-only contraceptive. Limited evidence suggests that among women with elevated BP (systolic BP greater than or equal to 160 mm Hg or diastolic BP greater than 90 mm Hg), women who used progestin-only oral contraceptives or progestin-only injectables had a small increased risk of cardiovascular events compared with women who did not use these methods. In this subgroup, the levonorgestrel IUD and the copper IUD are Category 2 and Category 1 contraceptives, respectively. However, the copper IUD would be ineffective in treating anovulatory bleeding and anemia in this patient. Therefore, the levonorgestrel IUD is the best choice for the described patient.

American College of Obstetricians and Gynecologists. Management of anovulatory bleeding. ACOG Practice Bulletin 14. Washington, DC: ACOG; 2000.

Diagnosis of abnormal uterine bleeding in reproductive-aged women. Practice Bulletin No. 128. American College of Obstetricians and Gynecologists. Obstet Gynecol 2012;120:197–206.

Munro MG, Critchley HO, Broder MS, Fraser IS. FIGO classification system (PALM-COEIN) for causes of abnormal uterine bleeding in nongravid women of reproductive age. FIGO Working Group on Menstrual Disorders. Int J Gynaecol Obstet 2011;113:3–13.

U.S. Medical Eligibility Criteria for Contraceptive Use, 2010. Centers for Disease Control and Prevention. MMWR Recomm Rep 2010; 59:1–86.

41

Pelvic floor anatomy

A 48-year-old woman undergoes a total laparoscopic hysterectomy and bilateral salpingo-oophorectomy for abnormal uterine bleeding. The uterus is noted to be homogeneously enlarged at 10-week-of-gestation size with grossly normal appearing ovaries. The procedure is uncomplicated with the exception of some bleeding at the vaginal cuff that is cauterized. On postoperative day 2, the patient has right flank pain and intravenous pyelography reveals a dilated and obstructed distal right ureter. The most likely surgical step that led to the ureteral injury in this patient is

     (A) ligation of the infundibulopelvic ligament
     (B) opening the broad ligament
  * (C) coagulation of the uterine vessels
     (D) transection of the uterosacral ligament
     (E) incision for colpotomy

In the United States, approximately 530,000–600,000 hysterectomies are performed each year. Complications of hysterectomy include urinary tract injuries and bowel injuries, infection, hemorrhage, thromboembolism, and death.

The ureters measure 25–30 cm in length from the kidney to the bladder (Fig. 41-1; see color plate). They are located in the retroperitoneum over the psoas muscle and posterior to the ovarian vessels. At the level of the pelvic brim, the ureters traverse over the bifurcation of the common iliac vessels to enter the pelvis and remain medial to the internal iliac artery. They then pass under the uterine vessels at approximately 15-mm distance from the uterus and into the paracervical tissue (ureteral tunnel). Once they pass the paracervical tissue, the ureters travel in an anteromedial direction to the trigone of the bladder.

The detection of urinary tract injuries during laparoscopic hysterectomy has been noted to be fivefold higher when routine intraoperative cystoscopy was performed compared with when it was not performed. Routine intraoperative cystoscopy detected 89% of ureteral injuries and 95% of bladder injuries intraoperatively. The route of hysterectomy plays a role in the rate of ureteric injury. Vaginal surgery presents the lowest risk of ureteral injury at 0.2 per 1,000 surgical procedures compared with abdominal surgery at 1.3 per 1,000 surgical procedures and laparoscopic surgery at 7.8 per 1,000 surgical procedures.

The most common site of injury during total laparoscopic hysterectomy and bilateral salpingo-oophorectomy is at the coagulation and ligation of the uterine vessels. Other sites of possible injury include the infundibulopelvic ligament, the tunnel of Wertheim, the intramural portion of the ureters, and the lateral pelvic sidewall above the uterosacral ligament. Damage to the ureters during gynecologic surgery caused by thermal spread must be considered during minimally invasive hysterectomy. This type of injury usually will present 2–5 days after the procedure. Improvements in energy modalities have decreased collateral damage to approximately 2–3 mm from the point of contact. Other types of injuries, such as

transection, incision, or ligation also can occur and may be recognized intraoperatively or postoperatively.

In an open abdominal hysterectomy, the most common site of injury of the ureters is at the clamping and ligation of the infundibulopelvic ligament, especially when bleeding is encountered.

In the described patient, the most likely cause of ureteral injury is coagulation of the uterine vessels. Ligation of the infundibulopelvic ligament would be correct if the patient underwent abdominal hysterectomy. Opening the broad ligament and transection of the uterosacral ligament are less often associated with ureteral injury than coagulation of the uterine vessels. Colpotomy is unlikely to be a cause of ureteral injury.

Gilmour DT, Das S, Flowerdew G. Rates of urinary tract injury from gynecologic surgery and the role of intraoperative cystoscopy. Obstet Gynecol 2006;107:1366–72.

Underwood P Jr. Operative injuries to the ureter. In: Rock JA, Jones HW 3rd, editors. Te Linde's operative gynecology. 10th ed. Philadelphia (PA): Wolters Kluwer/Lippincott Williams & Wilkins; 2011. p. 960–72.

42

Bradycardia during minor gynecologic surgery

A healthy 33-year-old woman is having a laparoscopic ovarian cystectomy for a symptomatic dermoid cyst. A pneumoperitoneum is created under pressure less than 8 mm Hg and is increased for trocar insertion. During insertion of the umbilical trocar, the anesthesiologist informs you that the patient's blood pressure has decreased suddenly to 70 mm Hg systolic, 30 mm Hg diastolic. The patient's pulse is 32 beats per minute and oxygen saturation is 90%. The most appropriate next step in management is to

      (A) continue laparoscopic procedure
      (B) perform immediate laparotomy
      (C) terminate procedure
*   (D) desufflate the abdomen

Many common gynecologic procedures are now being performed with minimally invasive techniques. Laparoscopic surgery decreases infection rates and hospital stay and also shortens the time to regain normal function. The carbon dioxide (CO_2) pneumoperitoneum used during laparoscopic surgery causes potentially significant hemodynamic, pulmonary, renal, splanchnic, and endocrine physiologic changes. Tachycardia and bradycardia have been observed in 14–27% of patients during laparoscopy. The risk of arrhythmia is increased with CO_2 pneumoperitoneum over nitrous oxide insufflation.

Cardiovascular and hemodynamic changes are caused by hypercarbia and increased intraabdominal pressure. Carbon dioxide is highly soluble and is absorbed readily

into the circulation. Hypercarbia develops as a result of increased peritoneal absorption of CO_2 and insufficient excretion of CO_2 by ventilation. Ventilation is reduced in patients with compromised cardiopulmonary function, in steep Trendelenburg position, with prolonged operative time, or with high intraabdominal pressure. The main cause for hypercarbia is prolonged elevated intraabdominal pressure.

Increased intraabdominal pressure from a pneumoperitoneum also triggers the sympathetic stress response, which includes the vagal reflex. The increased intraabdominal pressure impairs venous return and reduces cardiac output. Arrhythmias during laparoscopy include tachycardia and extrasystoles from catecholamine release or bradycardia from a vagal-mediated reflex triggered by rapid stretching of the peritoneum. Most patients with arrhythmias respond to a reduction in intraabdominal pressure and 100% oxygen hyperventilation. A report in the urologic literature suggests that bradycardia can be prevented by pretreatment with atropine 3–5 minutes before induction of anesthesia.

Cardiac arrhythmia may occur during gynecologic laparoscopic surgery, although most cases are transient and without significant sequelae. Even in a healthy patient, a profound bradycardia and asystole can occur. Arrhythmia with minimally invasive surgery has been reported in 14–27% of patients during laparoscopic procedures. Tachycardia usually is related to catecholamine release and generally is self-limiting. Bradycardia can be life threatening. The operating gynecologist should understand the mechanism of this arrhythmia in order to intervene appropriately. The described patient is healthy, with no predisposing risk for cardiac arrhythmia. She

demonstrates a vagal reaction with hypotension and bradycardia in response to intraabdominal insufflation. The most appropriate next step is to desufflate the abdomen to reduce peritoneal stretch and to improve venous return. Once the patient has returned to her baseline vital signs and received atropine, a gentle reinsufflation can begin with a lower sustained intraabdominal pressure. To not release the pneumoperitoneum or to proceed with trocar insertion potentially puts the patient at risk for further deterioration. Laparotomy is not indicated because this is not a surgical emergency. The cardiac arrhythmia is likely to be transient and, thus, the procedure does not need to be terminated.

Aghamohammadi H, Mehrabi S, Mohammad Ali Beigi F. Prevention of bradycardia by atropine sulfate during urological laparoscopic surgery: a randomized controlled trial. Urol J 2009;6:92–5.

Gutt CN, Oniu T, Mehrabi A, Schemmer P, Kashfi A, Kraus T, et al. Circulatory and respiratory complications of carbon dioxide insufflation. Dig Surg 2004;21:95–105.

43

Metformin hydrochloride and polycystic ovary syndrome

A 20-year-old woman visits your office for infertility. She and her partner have been unsuccessful in attempting conception for 13 months. She has a history of Class III obesity with a body mass index of 36 (calculated as weight in kilograms divided by height in meters squared) and polycystic ovary syndrome (PCOS). She previously used oral contraceptives for birth control. After discontinuing the oral contraceptives, she had four menstrual periods over the past 14 months. A 2-hour plasma glucose level after ingestion of a 75-g glucose load was 160 mg/dL. The best first step in the management of her infertility is

     (A) metformin hydrochloride
     (B) rosiglitazone
*   (C) weight loss
     (D) clomiphene citrate
     (E) exogenous gonadotropins

Polycystic ovary syndrome is characterized by anovulation, hyperandrogenism, and polycystic ovaries, but no universally accepted definition of PCOS has been established. The 2003 Rotterdam criteria for PCOS are listed in Box 43-1. Women with PCOS, especially women who are obese, have impaired insulin sensitivity. They are at an increased risk of insulin resistance and type 2 diabetes mellitus, cardiovascular disease, hypertriglyceridemia, and endometrial cancer. Obesity is associated with pregnancy loss, preeclampsia, gestational diabetes mellitus, preterm labor, and failure or delayed response to ovulation induction agents, such as clomiphene citrate and gonadotropin. Hyperinsulinemia affects granulosa

cell function and theca cell function, which causes amplification of luteinizing hormone action, contributing to the arrest of follicle growth (leading to anovulation) and excessive androgen production by theca cells.

Weight loss and exercise are the treatments of choice in the management of reproductive and metabolic sequelae in obese women with PCOS who seek fertility. Weight loss of 5% has been shown to improve metabolic abnormalities and fertility. This also may improve the efficacy of ovulation induction agents.

Metformin hydrochloride is considered an insulin-sensitizing agent but its primary mechanism of action is probably reduction of hepatic glucose output. It has been

BOX 43-1

Rotterdam Criteria for Polycystic Ovary Syndrome*

Revised diagnostic criteria of PCOS (2 out of 3)

- Oligo- and/or anovulation
- Clinical and/or biochemical signs of hyper-androgenism
- Polycystic ovaries

and exclusion of other etiologies (congenital adrenal hyperplasias, androgen-secreting tumors, Cushing's syndrome).
Thorough documentation of applied diagnostic criteria should be done (and described in research papers) for future evaluation.

*The 2003 Rotterdam criteria for polycystic ovary syndrome listed here supplanted the 1990 National Institutes of Health diagnostic criteria.

Revised 2003 consensus on diagnostic criteria and long-term health risks related to polycystic ovary syndrome (PCOS). Rotterdam ESHRE/ASRM-Sponsored PCOS consensus workshop group. Hum Reprod 2004;19:41–7, by permission of Oxford University Press.

shown to increase ovulation rates in women with PCOS, but this may be confounded by concomitant weight loss. Use of metformin alone does not improve fertility rates. When metformin is used in combination with clomiphene citrate, pregnancy rates are slightly increased, but live birth rates are unchanged. Metformin use in women with PCOS should be limited to treatment of glucose intolerance.

Rosiglitazone is an insulin-sensitizing agent in the category of drugs called thiazolidinediones (glitazones). It increases ovulation, but adverse effects of hepatotoxicity and cardiovascular morbidity have been reported. It has been classified by the U.S. Food and Drug Administration as pregnancy category C. Insulin-sensitizing agents should not be used as first-line therapy for ovulation induction.

Some women who have difficulty achieving weight loss may reject weight loss as first-line therapy in the management of obesity, PCOS, and infertility and choose to initiate drug therapy instead. Clomiphene citrate, an antiestrogen drug, is the recommended first-line treatment for ovulation induction. Its mechanism of action involves the blockade of negative feedback that leads to increased secretion of follicle-stimulating hormone. Approximately 75–80% of women with PCOS will ovulate with clomiphene citrate therapy with pregnancy rates of 22% per cycle, multiple gestation pregnancy rates of 5–7% per cycle, and a cumulative live birth rate of 50–60% for up to six cycles.

Recommended second-line treatment for ovulation induction when clomiphene citrate therapy failed is exogenous gonadotropin therapy. The goal in the use of exogenous gonadotropin is to generate a limited number of developing follicles to optimize live singleton birth rates and minimize the risks of multiple gestations and ovarian hyperstimulation syndrome. Authors of a study using low-dose regimens (ie, gonadotropin, 37.5–75 international units per day) reported monofollicular ovulation rate of 70%, pregnancy rate of 20%, live birth rate of 5.7% with multiple pregnancies less than 6%, and ovarian hyperstimulation syndrome less than 1%.

Consensus on infertility treatment related to polycystic ovary syndrome. Thessaloniki ESHRE/ASRM-Sponsored PCOS Consensus Workshop Group [published erratum appears in Hum Reprod 2008;23:1474]. Hum Reprod 2008;23:462–77.

Franks S. When should an insulin sensitizing agent be used in the treatment of polycystic ovary syndrome? Clin Endocrinol (Oxf) 2011;74:148–51.

Polycystic ovary syndrome. ACOG Practice Bulletin No. 108. American College of Obstetricians and Gynecologists. Obstet Gynecol 2009;114:936–49.

Revised 2003 consensus on diagnostic criteria and long-term health risks related to polycystic ovary syndrome (PCOS). Rotterdam ESHRE/ASRM-Sponsored PCOS consensus workshop group. Hum Reprod 2004;19:41–7.

44

Ectopic pregnancy

A 24-year-old woman presents to the emergency department with vaginal bleeding and pelvic pain for 2 days. Her menses are irregular and she thinks her last menstrual period was 12 weeks ago. She was treated for chlamydial infection 8 months ago. The examination is unremarkable except for tenderness in the right lower abdominal quadrant. Laboratory values are as follows: blood type, A+; hemoglobin level, 12.4 g/dL; hematocrit, 35%; white blood cell count, 13,000 cells per microliter; platelet count, 86×10^3 per microliter; quantitative serum β-hCG level, 3,600 mIU/mL; aspartate aminotransferase level, 60 units/L; alanine aminotransferase level, 52 units/L; and serum creatinine level, 1.4 mg/dL. Pelvic ultrasonography reveals a 2.8-cm cystic mass with a yolk sac within the right adnexa and no intrauterine pregnancy. No free fluid is observed. The most appropriate management is

*   (A) laparoscopic salpingostomy
    (B) methotrexate
    (C) repeat β-hCG level measurement in 48 hours
    (D) laparotomy with salpingostomy

Methotrexate medical therapy for ectopic pregnancy was introduced in the 1980s. It is an acceptable treatment modality for properly selected patients. Methotrexate is a folic acid antagonist used to treat some types of cancer, severe psoriasis, and rheumatoid arthritis. It is relatively safe in the low doses used for treatment of ectopic pregnancy, but it is associated with a slight risk of renal, hepatic, hematologic, or pulmonary toxicity. At least 35% of patients with ectopic pregnancy are candidates for medical therapy. Ideal candidates for medical treatment with methotrexate for ectopic pregnancy are women who are hemodynamically stable, able to adhere to posttreatment evaluations, have β-hCG levels less than 5,000 mIU/mL, and exhibit no fetal cardiac activity.

The described patient has an ectopic pregnancy. A delay of treatment to obtain another β-hCG measurement in 48 hours would not be appropriate. Based on her laboratory studies, methotrexate is contraindicated. The generally accepted contraindications to methotrexate treatment are shown in Box 44-1. The increased levels in aminotransferases, low platelet count, and an increased creatinine level suggest increased risk of complications with methotrexate. It is important that clinicians remember to obtain complete blood count, renal function test results, and liver function test results before administering methotrexate to a patient for ectopic pregnancy.

Given that methotrexate is contraindicated in this patient, she should undergo surgery. Laparoscopic surgery is preferable to laparotomy in almost all cases of ectopic pregnancy, but especially in a patient who is hemodynamically stable, as in this case. Randomized clinical trials show that laparoscopy results in shorter operative time, less perioperative blood loss, shorter hospital stay, and faster postoperative recovery than other

---

BOX 44-1

Common Contraindications to Methotrexate Treatment

- Hemodynamic instability or signs of ongoing rupture (more than 300 mL of blood or fluid in the peritoneal cavity)
- Abnormalities of baseline renal, hepatic, or hematologic laboratory test values
- Immunodeficiency
- Acute pulmonary disease
- Peptic ulcer
- Coexistent intrauterine pregnancy
- Breastfeeding
- Inability to monitor the patient after treatment
- Hypersensitivity to methotrexate

---

modalities. In cases where equipment or a trained surgeon may not be available, the best option would be laparotomy. The decision to perform a salpingostomy versus salpingectomy is not clear. Salpingostomy has a higher risk of persistent trophoblastic tissue than salpingectomy; therefore, follow-up β-hCG level measurement is mandatory with salpingostomy. Subsequent pregnancy rates do not appear to be different with salpingostomy versus salpingectomy.

American College of Obstetricians and Gynecologists. ACOG Practice Bulletin No. 94: Medical management of ectopic pregnancy. Obstet Gynecol 2008;111:1479–85.

Hajenius PJ, Mol F, Mol Ben WJ, Bossuyt PMM, Ankum WM, Van der Veen F. Interventions for tubal ectopic pregnancy. Cochrane Database of Systematic Reviews 2007, Issue 1. Art. No.: CD000324. DOI: 10.1002/14651858.CD000324.pub2.

45

Clinical depression

A 43-year-old woman, gravida 2, para 2, comes to your office for follow-up of depression. Two months ago, you prescribed a selective serotonin reuptake inhibitor (SSRI) for symptoms of depression, and her mood has now improved. She notes a decrease in orgasmic response; however, she feels comfortable with the decreased response because her husband is currently deployed with the military. She asks how long she will need to take the SSRI. The minimum suggested duration to take the SSRI is

    (A) 3 months
*   (B) 6 months
    (C) 15 months
    (D) 21 months
    (E) indefinitely

Nearly one in five women will have depression during their lifetime compared with one in ten men. Depression is a common illness that is often undiagnosed, untreated, or undertreated. Depression may be triggered by serious physical illness, psychosocial stress, loss of a support system, or other situational events. Obstetrician–gynecologists should be aware of the factors that contribute to depression and of the manifestations and treatment of depression to optimize their patients' global well-being.

The diagnosis of major depression is based on standard clinical criteria, such as those published by the American Psychiatric Association (Box 45-1). Numerous screening tools are available to assess depression. However, simply asking a patient if they are feeling depressed may be all that is required to prompt evaluation and therapeutic intervention.

Various treatment approaches can be used to manage depression, such as pharmacotherapy, psychotherapy, and cognitive behavioral therapy. In patients with mild to moderate depression, psychosocial therapies may be used alone or in conjunction with antidepressant medication. Clinical trials have shown little difference in effectiveness among the various available SSRIs and between SSRIs and other classes of antidepressants. Regardless of the modality of treatment selected for initial therapy, the goal should be symptom resolution.

Antidepressant medication generally should be taken for a minimum of 6–9 months with the initial diagnosis of depression. The goal of treatment is elimination of residual symptoms, restoration to the prior level of functioning, and prevention of recurrent symptoms, including early relapse. Patients who have depression in the setting of known precipitants, such as psychologic stress or personal loss, should continue drug therapy until a significant change in adaptation to those factors has been accomplished and for at least 6 months. Patients should be counseled that medication leads to a genuine change in underlying neurochemistry. Patients may take several weeks to adjust to initiation of medication and to its discontinuation to minimize symptoms associated with abrupt cessation of therapy.

If the event of recurrence or relapse during therapy, gradual discontinuation of drug therapy may be planned for most patients after at least 6 months of treatment. Tapering of medication over several weeks permits detection of recurrent symptoms that require reinstitution of dosing for another 3–6 months. Long-term treatment should be undertaken in patients with recurrent episodes of depression.

Bhatia SC, Bhatia SK. Depression in women: diagnostic and treatment considerations. Am Fam Physician 1999;60:225–34, 239–40.

Mann JJ. The medical management of depression. N Engl J Med 2005;353:1819–34.

Qaseem A, Snow V, Denberg TD, Forciea MA, Owens DK. Using second-generation antidepressants to treat depressive disorders: a clinical practice guideline from the American College of Physicians. Clinical Efficacy Assessment Subcommittee of American College of Physicians [published erratum appears in Ann Intern Med 2009;150:148]. Ann Intern Med 2008;149:725–33.

BOX 45-1

Major Depressive Disorder Diagnostic Criteria

A. Five (or more) of the following symptoms have been present during the same 2-week period and represent a change from previous functioning; at least one of the symptoms is either (1) depressed mood or (2) loss of interest or pleasure.

Note: Do not include symptoms that are clearly attributable to another medical condition.

1. Depressed mood most of the day, nearly every day, as indicated by either subjective report (eg, feels sad, empty, or hopeless) or observation made by others (eg, appears tearful). (Note: In children and adolescents, can be irritable mood.)

2. Markedly diminished interest or pleasure in all or almost all activities most of the day, nearly every day (as indicated by either subjective account or observation).

3. Significant weight loss when not dieting or weight gain (eg, a change of more than 5% of body weight in a month) or decrease or increase in appetite nearly every day. (Note: In children, consider failure to make expected weight gain.)

4. Insomnia or hypersomnia nearly every day.

5. Psychomotor agitation or retardation nearly every day (observable by others, not merely subjective feelings of restlessness or being slowed down).

6. Fatigue or loss of energy nearly every day.

7. Feelings of worthlessness or excessive or inappropriate guilt (which may be delusional) nearly every day (not merely self-reproach or guilt about being sick).

8. Diminished ability to think or concentrate or indecisiveness nearly every day (either by subjective account or as observed by others).

9. Recurrent thoughts of death (not just fear of dying), recurrent suicidal ideation without a specific plan, or a suicide attempt or a specific plan for committing suicide.

B. The symptoms cause clinically significant stress or impairment in social, occupational, or other important areas of functioning.

C. The episode is not attributable to the physiologic effects of a substance or to another medical condition.

Note: Criteria A–C represent a major depressive episode.

Note: Responses to a significant loss (eg, bereavement, financial ruin, losses from a natural disaster, a serious medical illness, or disability) may include the feelings of intense sadness, rumination about loss, insomnia, poor appetite, and weight loss noted in Criterion A, which may resemble a depressive episode. Although such symptoms may be understandable or considered appropriate to the loss, the presence of a major depressive episode in addition to the normal response to a significant loss also should be carefully considered. This decision inevitably requires the exercise of clinical judgment based on the individual's history and cultural norms for the expression of distress in the context of loss.

D. The occurrence of the major depressive episode is not better explained by schizoaffective disorder, schizophrenia, schizophreniform disorder, delusional disorder, or other specified and unspecified schizophrenia spectrum and other psychotic disorders.

E. There has never been a manic episode or a hypomanic episode.

Note: This exclusion does not apply if all of the manic-like or hypomanic-like episodes are substance-induced or are attributable to the physiologic effects of another medical condition.

American Psychiatric Association. Diagnostic and statistical manual of mental disorders: DSM-5. 5th ed. Washington, DC: American Psychiatric Publishing, 2013. p. 160–1. Reprinted with permission from the Diagnostic and Statistical Manual of Mental Disorders, Fifth Edition, (Copyright © 2013). American Psychiatric Association. All Rights Reserved.

46

Severe dyspareunia

A 62-year-old woman comes to your clinic with a 1-year history of severe dyspareunia and inability to tolerate vaginal penetration for the past several months. Your examination reveals the vulvar and oral findings shown in Fig. 46-1 (see color plate) and Fig. 46-2 (see color plate), respectively. Test results are negative for *Candida* species. The most likely diagnosis is

* (A) erosive lichen planus
  (B) lichen sclerosus
  (C) atrophic vaginitis
  (D) desquamative inflammatory vaginitis
  (E) Behçet disease

Symptoms of vulvovaginal disorders are common and account for approximately one in 10 office visits to obstetrician–gynecologists. Despite the frequency with which women present with their concerns, chronic or recurrent forms of vulvovaginal disease can be difficult to diagnose. Obtaining a patient's history, including symptom onset, duration, location, and precipitating factors, in combination with the physical examination, including vaginal microscopy, will help to guide the use of subsequent diagnostic tests.

Lichen planus is an inflammatory disorder most likely related to cell-mediated immunity. The disorder exhibits a wide range of morphologies. Erosive lichen planus is the most common form, and it affects multiple mucocutaneous tissues, most commonly the oral cavity and vulva. Symptoms include pruritus, burning, bleeding, vaginal discharge, and dyspareunia. The classic presentation of erosive lichen planus is sharply demarcated erosive changes with Wickham striae—a white reticulate, lacy pattern. The vestibule and vaginal epithelium can become erythematous, eroded, and denuded. Over time, the eroded surfaces may adhere, resulting in anatomic changes, scarring, and synechiae. Biopsy of the affected area is important to secure the diagnosis. The described patient has erosive lichen planus.

Lichen sclerosus is a chronic disorder most likely related to an autoimmune process of unclear etiology. Most commonly it affects genital skin, with extragenital lesions reported in up to 13% of women. The most common symptom reported is pruritus, followed by irritation, burning, dyspareunia, and tearing. On examination, the skin appears thinned, whitened, and parchment-like, often with areas of ecchymoses. As with erosive lichen planus, anatomic changes, including introital narrowing, fusion of the labia minora, and phimosis of the clitoral hood, are commonly noted. Biopsy of the affected area may be considered to confirm the diagnosis.

Atrophic changes are associated with menopause and the loss of estrogen. At least 50% of postmenopausal women experience vulvovaginal irritation, dryness, dyspareunia, and lower urinary tract problems. Unlike other menopausal symptoms (eg, hot flushes), vulvovaginal symptoms do not resolve. Rather, vulvovaginal symptoms often manifest in late menopause. On examination, the tissue appears thin, pale, smooth, and dry. When present, discharge may be clear to yellow. The diagnosis of atrophic vaginitis is based on the clinical setting, examination findings, elevated vaginal pH, and the presence of parabasal or intermediate cells on microscopy.

Desquamative inflammatory vaginitis is an inflammatory vaginal condition of unknown etiology. The typical symptom is a persistent, copious, purulent discharge. Additional vulvovaginal symptoms include dyspareunia, pain, pruritus, and irritation. On examination, glazed erythema of the vulva and vagina and presence of purulent discharge are noted. The diagnosis of desquamative inflammatory vaginitis is based on clinical history and examination, including discharge findings (ie, increased vaginal pH, negative amine [whiff] test, a marked increase in inflammatory cells and immature squamous cells [basal and parabasal cells], and absence of lactobacilli, yeast, and trichomonas).

Behçet disease is a rare disorder first described as a triad of oral aphthous ulcers, genital aphthous ulcers, and uveitis. It is now considered a multisystem disease. Patients present with painful ulcers (oral or genital). Diagnosis often requires a multidisciplinary approach to differentiate Behçet disease from complex aphthosis.

Diagnosis and management of vulvar skin disorders. ACOG Practice Bulletin No. 93. American College of Obstetricians and Gynecologists. Obstet Gynecol 2008;111:1243–53.

Edwards L, Lynch PJ. Genital dermatology atlas. First edition. Philadelphia (PA): Lippincott Williams & Wilkins; 2004.

Farage MA, Miller KW, Ledger WJ. Determining the cause of vulvovaginal symptoms. Obstet Gynecol Surv 2008;63:445–64.

Kennedy CM, Galask RP. Erosive vulvar lichen planus: retrospective review of characteristics and outcomes in 113 patients seen in a vulvar specialty clinic. J Reprod Med 2007;52:43–7.

47

Postoperative intestinal obstruction

A 32-year-old woman comes to the emergency department with abdominal distension, abdominal pain, and bilious vomiting at day 4 from after a laparoscopic ovarian cystectomy for a 14-cm mature teratoma. Her temperature is 38.7°C (101.7°F). Her heart rate is 115 beats per minute. Her blood pressure is 98 mm Hg systolic, 54 mm Hg diastolic. On examination, the abdomen is distended and soft but diffusely tender with maximal tenderness over the umbilical port site. The umbilical port site appears erythematous. Bowel sounds are hypoactive. Her total white cell count is 22,000 cells per microliter with 12% neutrophils. Based on computed tomography (CT) of the abdomen (Fig. 47-1), the best management course is

*   (A) surgery
      (B) bowel rest with nasogastric suction
      (C) small-bowel series
      (D) ultrasonography
      (E) intravenous antibiotic administration and observation

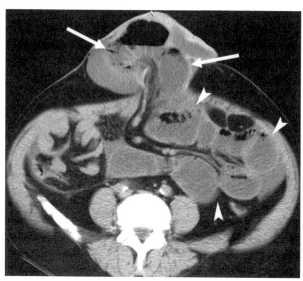

FIG. 47-1

Computed tomography shows a strangulated umbilical hernia (see arrows) causing small bowel obstruction (see arrowheads). Hernias at the port site are an uncommon complication of laparoscopic surgery with an estimated incidence of 0.8–1.2%. Most of these hernias occur within 10 days of surgery. Hernias at the port site necessitate a second surgery and may lead to considerable morbidity caused by bowel strangulation or incarceration.

Hernias at the port site can be classified into three different categories based on the timing of presentation and the defect involved:

1. Early-onset hernias present immediately postoperatively and indicate dehiscence of the anterior and posterior fascia and peritoneum.

2. Special hernias usually present in the immediate postoperative period and refer to complete dehiscence of the anterior abdominal wall with evisceration of peritoneal contents externally often without a hernia sac. Early-onset and special hernias present surgical emergencies.

3. Late-onset hernias present several months to years after surgery and involve dehiscence of the anterior and posterior fascial layers alone. They can be repaired electively because strangulation is unlikely.

Nutritional status, chronic obstructive pulmonary disease, postoperative chest infection, diabetes mellitus, connective tissue disorders, and prior abdominal surgery have been postulated as risk factors for hernias at the port site. However, they have not been convincingly shown to be risk factors in large studies.

Hernias at the port site more commonly occur with ports of 10 mm or more than smaller ports, although hernias with 3- and 5-mm ports have been reported. The umbilical port is a common site for hernias to occur. This may be caused by a single fascial layer at the linea alba and more contact with the small bowel compared with lateral ports. Hernias can occur with any port site and are related to diameter of the trocar-cannula, specimen retrieval through this port, design of the trocar-cannula tip, and preexisting hernia.

This patient has a small bowel obstruction with strangulation as a result of port site hernia. She requires immediate surgery because of increased morbidity and mortality. Diagnosis is confirmed with the clinical presentation and CT findings. Therefore, no additional imaging studies are required. Bowel rest with nasogastric suction is reserved for a patient with a postoperative ileus where high-grade small bowel obstruction is not present. Intravenous antibiotic administration is reasonable. However, the option of antibiotic administration plus observation constitutes inappropriate management for a patient with peritonitis and high-grade bowel obstruction. Small bowel series may be used for an indeterminant CT result to diagnose a low-grade or partial bowel obstruction. Ultrasonography may be comparable with plain-film imaging for the diagnosis of strangulated bowel.

Aguirre DA, Santosa AC, Casola G, Sirlin CB. Abdominal wall hernias: imaging features, complications, and diagnostic pitfalls at multi-detector row CT. Radiographics 2005;25:1501–20.

Diaz JJ Jr, Bokhari F, Mowery NT, Acosta JA, Block EF, Bromberg WJ, et al. Guidelines for management of small bowel obstruction. J Trauma 2008;64:1651–64.

Moreaux G, Estrade-Huchon S, Bader G, Guyot B, Heitz D, Fauconnier A, et al. Five-millimeter trocar site small bowel eviscerations after gynecologic laparoscopic surgery. J Minim Invasive Gynecol 2009; 16:643–5.

Owens M, Barry M, Janjua AZ, Winter DC. A systematic review of laparoscopic port site hernias in gastrointestinal surgery. Surgeon 2011;9:218–24.

48

Hormone therapy after hysterectomy

A 50-year-old woman comes to your office to discuss hormone therapy (HT). Two months ago, she underwent hysterectomy with bilateral salpingo-oophorectomy and appendectomy for bilateral adnexal masses with a pathologic diagnosis of mucinous cystadenomas. She has no menopausal symptoms but has heard about the "critical timing hypothesis" and is interested in beginning HT. You explain to her that the reasons for initiating systemic HT should be limited to

    (A) prevention of coronary heart disease
    (B) treatment of osteoporosis
*   (C) treatment of menopausal symptoms
    (D) prevention of dementia
    (E) treatment of urinary incontinence

Current guidelines recommend that menopausal HT be limited to the treatment of menopausal vasomotor symptoms with the lowest effective dose for the shortest amount of time possible. Hormone therapy should be individualized, and continued use should be reevaluated on a periodic basis. In 2012, the North American Menopause Society stated that recent data support the initiation of HT primarily around the time of menopause to treat menopause-related symptoms and also to prevent osteoporosis in women at high risk of fracture. The increased breast cancer risk in women who take combination HT precludes a recommendation for use beyond 3–5 years. Estrogen therapy may be used for a more extended period.

Several determinants and interactions that predict health and wellness and disease risk in middle-aged women have been proposed. Major factors that affect disease risk include race, ethnicity, socioeconomic status, adverse life events, and high body mass index, especially metabolically unhealthy obesity. Late perimenopause (3 months of amenorrhea) appears to be the timeframe that coincides most strongly with symptoms and measurable physiologic changes in bone, cardiovascular, and psychosocial health; alterations in hemostasis; and sleep difficulty. Continued attention and individualized counseling based on these factors that affect disease risk should be readdressed across the patient's lifespan.

The critical timing hypothesis refers to a hypothetic age-related "window of opportunity" for exogenous menopause hormone treatment to preserve cognitive function and reduce the risk of atherosclerosis in women when initiated early (up to 10 years) in menopause. Large, observational studies showed a protective benefit from exogenous estrogen-only therapy and estrogen plus progestin therapy against coronary heart disease. By contrast, results from large-scale, randomized controlled trials have shown no cardioprotective effect. An increase was observed in coronary heart disease events, strokes, venous thromboemboli, and pulmonary emboli in patients in the combined estrogen plus progestin groups and a decrease in strokes and venous thromboemboli in patients in the estrogen-only groups. However, no difference was observed in coronary heart disease events in the estrogen-only groups. Current guidelines recommend that menopausal HT should not be used for the prevention of primary or secondary coronary heart disease events.

Osteoporosis is a systemic skeletal disease that involves deterioration of bone microarchitecture. The World Health Organization defines osteoporosis based on the total bone density of the hip. Osteoporosis increases the risk of fractures even in the absence of trauma. Multiple studies show a beneficial effect of systemic estrogen therapy with or without progestin on decreasing fracture risk. Use of HT for the prevention of osteoporosis should be individualized and take into account the patient's history and vasomotor symptoms. First-line pharmacologic options determined by the U.S. Food and Drug Administration to be safe and effective for treatment of osteoporosis include bisphosphonates and selective estrogen receptor modulators.

Older, prospective epidemiologic studies reported a decreased risk for dementia among women who took menopausal HT. A number of prospective observational studies found no protective effect of estrogen on either prevention of dementia or cognitive functioning. A more recent large, randomized controlled study concluded that conjugated equine estrogen with or without depot medroxyprogesterone acetate increased the risk of dementia and global cognitive decline.

Topical local estrogen therapy may improve or cure urinary incontinence. However, data are limited concerning long-term effects of therapy and rates of urinary incontinence after discontinuation of therapy. Systemic estrogen therapy with conjugated equine estrogens may worsen incontinence. Insufficient evidence exists to support the long-term use of HT to improve cardiovascular health, cognition, and memory.

Cody JD, Jacobs ML, Richardson K, Moehrer B, Hextall A. Oestrogen therapy for urinary incontinence in post-menopausal women. Cochrane Database of Systematic Reviews 2012, Issue 10. Art. No.: CD001405. DOI: 10.1002/14651858.CD001405.pub3.

Coker LH, Espeland MA, Rapp SR, Legault C, Resnick SM, Hogan P, et al. Postmenopausal hormone therapy and cognitive outcomes: the Women's Health Initiative Memory Study (WHIMS). J Steroid Biochem Mol Biol 2010;118:304–10.

Hormone therapy and heart disease. Committee Opinion No. 565. American College of Obstetricians and Gynecologists. Obstet Gynecol 2013;121:1407–10.

Osteoporosis. Practice Bulletin No. 129. American College of Obstetricians and Gynecologists. Obstet Gynecol 2012;120:718–34.

Santoro N, Sutton-Tyrrell K. The SWAN song: Study of Women's Health Across the Nation's recurring themes. Obstet Gynecol Clin North Am 2011;38:417–23.

Schmidt P. The 2012 hormone therapy position statement of The North American Menopause Society. Menopause 2012;19:257–71.

49

Oliguria in the elderly patient

You evaluate a 73-year-old woman, gravida 2, para 2, for low urine output that occurs 90 minutes after total vaginal hysterectomy. The surgery was uneventful, with an estimated blood loss of 300 mL. She received 2,000 mL of isotonic crystalloid fluid during and after surgery. Before surgery, she followed *nil per os* (NPO) instructions. Bladder volume was 70 mL when the Foley catheter was placed at the conclusion of the surgery. Her past medical history is significant for hypertension, well controlled with lisinopril, and diet-controlled type 2 diabetes mellitus. On examination, the patient has a temperature of 36.8°C (98.2°F), pulse of 100 beats per minute, respiratory rate of 18 breaths per minute, and blood pressure of 136 mm Hg systolic, 82 mm Hg diastolic. Her abdomen is soft and tender to palpation. No drainage or discharge from the vagina is present. The Foley catheter is in place with 7 mL of yellow urine in the bag. You irrigate the catheter with return of an equal amount of fluid. The next step in management is

(A) diagnostic laparoscopy
(B) cystoscopy
(C) computed tomography of abdomen and pelvis
(D) intravenous furosemide
* (E) fractional excretion of sodium (FE_{Na})

This patient has oliguria. Oliguria is defined as urine excretion of less than 400 mL in 24 hours or urine output of less than 0.5 mL/kg/hr. The causes of oliguria are separated into three categories: 1) prerenal injury, 2) postrenal injury, and 3) intrinsic renal injury. Prerenal causes are related to a decrease in renal perfusion because of hypovolemia, cardiac failure, systemic vasodilation, or renal artery occlusion. Postrenal causes are caused by outflow obstruction of either the ureter or urethra. Intrinsic renal causes include acute tubular necrosis, glomerulonephritis, or vasculitis.

Based on the described patient's evaluation in the recovery room, you are concerned about bilateral ureteral ligation or injury. Most ureteral injuries are not recognized until postoperative sequelae occur. The most important principle of postoperative diagnosis of urinary tract injury is to have a high index of suspicion, because early symptoms and signs often are subtle, and delay in diagnosis may result in renal failure and permanent loss of renal function. Complete ureteral obstruction may present with ipsilateral flank pain and transient elevation in serum creatinine within 24 hours after surgery. Partial ureteral obstruction may progress over time to complete obstruction. Patients with undiagnosed ureteral injuries may experience flank pain, fever, ureterovaginal fistulas, ileus, and urine peritonitis with or without pyelonephritis. However, many patients may be asymptomatic or may present with diffuse discomfort (masked by postoperative analgesics). Renal failure can result from unrecognized ureteral injury and delays in diagnosis, with a permanent loss of renal function.

The next step in the evaluation of this patient is laboratory evaluation, including measurements of FE_{Na}, serum electrolytes, blood urea nitrogen, and creatine. To differentiate between a prerenal cause of oliguria and acute tubular necrosis, FE_{Na} measurement is the most accurate screening test and measures the percent of filtered sodium that is excreted in the urine. A value of less than 1% suggests a prerenal cause, and a value greater than 2% usually indicates acute tubular necrosis. The formula for calculation of FE_{Na} is shown in Box 49-1.

If the FE_{Na} level suggests a prerenal cause, fluid bolus with normal saline solution would be appropriate. Beyond the immediate postoperative period, a diuretic challenge may be indicated in patients who are diuretic dependent, especially in those who have underlying medical conditions, including cardiopulmonary dysfunction or renal disease.

Alternatively, if the FE_{Na} level is indeterminate or suggests acute tubular necrosis, immediate evaluation for urinary tract injury should be initiated. Traditionally, intravenous pyelography was the initial imaging study

---

BOX 49-1

Calculation of Fractional Excretion of Sodium

$$*FE_{Na} = ([U_{Na} \times P_{Cr}]/[P_{Na} \times U_{Cr}]) \times 100$$

*Abbreviations: FE_{Na} indicates fractional excretion of sodium; P_{Cr}, plasma creatinine; P_{Na}, plasma sodium; U_{Cr}, urine creatinine; U_{Na}, urine sodium.

to evaluate for a ureteral injury. However, computed tomography is commonly employed as the initial imaging study because the anatomy of the surrounding structures is assessed in addition to the renal collecting system. Cystoscopy is performed to assess for bladder injury and evaluate ureteral patency. Although further surgery may be warranted, diagnostic laparoscopy is not typically employed in the evaluation of a potential ureteral injury.

Lameire N, Van Biesen W, Vanholder R. Acute renal failure. Lancet 2005;365:417–30.

Underwood P Jr. Operative injuries to the ureter. In: Rock JA, Jones HW 3rd, editors. Te Linde's operative gynecology. 10th ed. Philadelphia (PA): Wolters Kluwer/Lippincott Williams & Wilkins; 2011. p. 960–72.

Wu HH, Yang PY, Yeh GP, Chou PH, Hsu JC, Lin KC. The detection of ureteral injuries after hysterectomy. J Minim Invasive Gynecol 2006;13:403–8.

50

Squamous dysplasia of the cervix

A 27-year-old primiparous woman consults you regarding management of the abnormal cervical cytology result. She had normal Pap test results until 12 months ago when a Pap test showed that she had a low-grade squamous intraepithelial lesion (LSIL). A colposcopic biopsy showed cervical intraepithelial neoplasia (CIN) 1. Twelve months later, she received a positive human papillomavirus (HPV) test result. The next step in the management of this patient is

(A) cryotherapy
(B) loop electrosurgical excision procedure
(C) testing for HPV in 1 year
(D) Pap test in 6 months
* (E) colposcopy

Low-grade squamous intraepithelial lesion cytologic results are consistent with HPV infection and mild dysplasia or CIN 1. Observation of the natural history of HPV infection and dysplasia indicates that most CIN 1 lesions will regress within 1–2 years. Prior research indicates that no useful triage strategy exists to determine histologic correlation of LSIL; therefore, immediate colposcopy is recommended.

If diagnosis of CIN 1 or normal pathology is confirmed, women may be monitored with Pap tests in 6 months and 12 months or HPV testing in 12 months. If any of these tests yield abnormal results, as in this patient, colposcopy should be performed.

Normal results of 6-month and 12-month Pap tests or negative result of HPV testing at 12 months should be followed by routine screening. Treatment procedures, such as laser, cryotherapy, loop electrosurgical excision procedure, or cold knife cone biopsy may be considered after 2 years of persistent mild dysplasia. The risks of excisional procedures include bleeding and pain. Conflicting evidence indicates possible risk of preterm delivery in a subsequent pregnancy. Therefore, excisional procedures should be limited to women with appropriate indications or risk factors. In this patient with CIN 1 and then subsequent positive result of HPV testing 12 months later, the appropriate management is colposcopic evaluation.

A randomized trial on the management of low-grade squamous intraepithelial lesion cytology interpretations. ASCUS-LSIL Triage Study (ALTS) Group. Am J Obstet Gynecol 2003;188:1393–400.

Massad LS, Einstein MH, Huh WK, Katki HA, Kinney WK, Schiffman M, et al. 2012 updated consensus guidelines for the management of abnormal cervical cancer screening tests and cancer precursors. 2012 ASCCP Consensus Guidelines Conference. Obstet Gynecol 2013;121:829–46.

51

Ethical management of unexpected surgical findings

A 41-year-old woman with abnormal uterine bleeding comes to you for a hysterectomy. Before the surgery, you review the consent form with her. You advise her of the risks and benefits of the procedure, discuss the alternatives to the surgical procedure, and answer her questions. The procedure listed on the surgical consent is "Laparoscopic Total Hysterectomy." During the surgery, a trocar injures the internal iliac artery. You request a scalpel and ask the circulator to set up for an open procedure. The circulator states that the patient has not consented to laparotomy. In reference to the concerns regarding the consent form, you inform the circulator that

* (A) the medical emergency justifies the change
  (B) the patient's family in the waiting room should be asked for consent
  (C) the risk management personnel should be contacted for guidance
  (D) another gynecologic surgeon agreeable to the change should be called

Informed consent is an ethical and legal concept that is integral to routine medical practice. Obtaining informed consent for medical treatment, medical research, or participation in teaching exercises that involve students and resident physicians is an ethical requirement. Seeking informed consent expresses respect for the patient as a person and her individual autonomy. It protects the patient from unwanted medical treatment and allows her to be actively involved in her medical care. Informed consent is a process that requires two-way communication and exploration of a patient's values and concerns. See Box 51-1 for the American College of Obstetricians and Gynecologists' statement regarding the ethical importance of informed consent.

When informed consent is not possible, a surrogate decision maker, such as the patient's spouse, family member, or legal guardian, should be identified to represent the patient's wishes or best interests. In the case of an emergency, medical professionals may act according to their perceptions of the best interests of the patient. In rare circumstances, informed consent can be overridden in the case of a significant ethical obligation, such as protecting the public health. Physicians should be aware of federal and state legal requirements and institutional policies for informed consent.

In the described scenario, an informed consent discussion should have reviewed risks of the procedure, includ-

ing bleeding, infection, and injury to other organs during the procedure. Because this was a laparoscopic procedure, the surgeon also should have discussed the possibility of laparotomy if the procedure could not be completed laparoscopically. Additionally, surgical consent may have included review of risks of blood transfusion and whether the patient had an Advanced Directive order.

Although this patient's consent form did not explicitly list laparotomy as the planned procedure, injury to the internal iliac artery is a life-threatening condition; immediate control of bleeding and repair of vascular injury is necessary. For a nonemergent condition, in a situation where a patient cannot give informed consent it is helpful to determine the course of action that the patient would likely have chosen by consulting with family, consider legal implications through discussion with risk management personnel, or obtain consultative advice from other medical practitioners. However, this scenario is considered a medical emergency; therefore, the change in treatment plan and decision for laparotomy by the patient's surgeon is justified.

Informed consent. ACOG Committee Opinion No. 439. American College of Obstetricians and Gynecologists. Obstet Gynecol 2009; 114:401–8.

Surgery and patient choice. ACOG Committee Opinion No. 395. American College of Obstetricians and Gynecologists. Obstet Gynecol 2008;111:243–7.

BOX 51-1

American College of Obstetricians and Gynecologists statement on the Ethical Importance of Informed Consent

1. Obtaining informed consent for medical treatment, for participation in medical research, and for participation in teaching exercises involving students and residents is an ethical requirement that is partially reflected in legal doctrines and requirements.

2. Seeking informed consent expresses respect for the patient as a person; it particularly respects a patient's moral right to bodily integrity, to self-determination regarding sexuality and reproductive capacities, and to support of the patient's freedom to make decisions within caring relationships.

3. Informed consent not only ensures the protection of the patient against unwanted medical treatment, but it also makes possible the patient's active involvement in her medical planning and care.

4. Communication is necessary if informed consent is to be realized, and physicians can and should help to find ways to facilitate communication not only in individual relations with patients but also in the structured context of medical care institutions.

5. Informed consent should be looked on as a process rather than a signature on a form. This process includes a mutual sharing of information over time between the clinician and the patient to facilitate the patient's autonomy in the process of making ongoing choices.

6. The ethical requirement to seek informed consent need not conflict with physicians' overall ethical obligation of beneficence; that is, physicians should make every effort to incorporate a commitment to informed consent within a commitment to provide medical benefit to patients and, thus, to respect them as whole and embodied persons.

7. When informed consent by the patient is impossible, a surrogate decision maker should be identified to represent the patient's wishes or best interests. In emergency situations, medical professionals may have to act according to their perceptions of the best interests of the patient; in rare instances, they may have to forgo obtaining consent because of some other overriding ethical obligation, such as protecting the public health.

8. Because ethical requirements and legal requirements cannot be equated, physicians also should acquaint themselves with federal and state legal requirements for informed consent. Physicians also should be aware of the policies within their own practices because these may vary from institution to institution.

Informed consent. ACOG Committee Opinion No. 439. American College of Obstetricians and Gynecologists. Obstet Gynecol 2009;114:401–8.

52

Prevention of human papillomavirus transmission

A 17-year-old patient comes to your office for the annual school physical examination. On reviewing her immunization record, you realize that she received two doses of the bivalent human papillomavirus (HPV) vaccine last year but missed her appointment for the third dose. The patient informs you that she has been sexually active with two prior partners. Regarding HPV vaccination, you counsel her that the most appropriate next step is to

       (A) restart the vaccination series
       (B) do nothing because she has likely been exposed to HPV
*   (C) administer one more dose of the bivalent vaccine
       (D) administer the quadrivalent vaccine
       (E) perform HPV testing before further vaccination

Human papillomavirus infection has been identified in 96–98% of cervical cancer cases, and HPV genotypes 16 and 18 account for more than 70% of cervical cancer cases. Although routine cervical screening has been shown to decrease the incidence of cervical cancer, the prevalence of HPV infection in adolescents and young adults continues to be significant. It is estimated that over 20 million Americans are infected with HPV and that individuals who have been sexually active have a 50–90% lifetime risk of HPV infection. In most immunocompetent individuals, HPV infection typically is transient and resolves within 6–24 months; however, in a small percentage of individuals, it can lead to cervical dysplasia and even cervical carcinoma. Vaccination has been shown to decrease HPV infections. The Centers for Disease Control and Prevention (CDC) recommends routine vaccination of males and females as early as age 9 years and up to age 26 years.

Currently, the vaccine is offered in a quadrivalent form (HPV genotypes 6, 11, 16, and 18) and a bivalent form (HPV genotypes 16 and 18). Both vaccines are administered as a three-part series at baseline, 1–2 months, and 6 months. In case of an interruption in the schedule of administration, the series should not be restarted. Instead, subsequent vaccine should be administered as soon as possible. The minimal time interval between the first and second dose is 4 weeks whereas the third dose should be given no sooner than 12 weeks after the second dose.

For maximum effectiveness, the vaccine should be administered before the onset of sexual activity. In females who are HPV naïve, studies have shown that the vaccine is effective in preventing more than 98% of cases of moderate to severe dysplasia associated with HPV genotypes 16 and 18. Patients who are already sexually active are candidates for vaccination although the efficacy rates are lower because the vaccine will not protect them from strains to which they have already been exposed. The CDC and the American College of Obstetricians and Gynecologists recommend that individuals receive the same vaccine for all three parts of the series. Because the CDC does not recommend switching vaccine types, the described patient should receive one more dose of the bivalent vaccine and not the quadrivalent vaccine. Human papillomavirus testing is not recommended before administration of the vaccine regardless of the patient's history of sexual activity. Also, patients should be counseled that limiting the number of sexual partners, avoiding tobacco smoking, and consistent condom use can decrease their risk of HPV infection. Regardless of sexual history, cervical cancer screening should not be initiated until age 21 years.

Human papillomavirus vaccination. Committee Opinion No. 467. American College of Obstetricians and Gynecologists. Obstet Gynecol 2010;116:800–3.

Muñoz N, Bosch FX, de Sanjosé S, Herrero R, Castellsagué X, Shah KV, et al. Epidemiologic classification of human papillomavirus types associated with cervical cancer. International Agency for Research on Cancer Multicenter Cervical Cancer Study Group. N Engl J Med 2003;348:518–27.

53

Recurrent yeast infections

A 32-year-old woman comes to your office with recurrent yeast infections that began 14 months ago and increased in frequency in the past 4 months. The patient notes that the use of over-the-counter antifungals initially provided benefit. However, recently, their use has worsened the itching and discomfort. Her main concern is intractable itching that wakes her up at night. Her husband has not been affected. Examination of the vulva reveals the findings shown in Fig. 53-1 (see color plate). Microscopy and cultures yield negative results for bacterial vaginosis and *Candida*. The most likely diagnosis is

*   (A) lichen simplex chronicus
      (B) lichen sclerosus
      (C) vulvar intraepithelial neoplasia (VIN)
      (D) inverse psoriasis
      (E) Paget disease

Vulvar pruritus can be caused by a wide range of infectious and noninfectious etiologies, most commonly including candidiasis, contact dermatitis, lichen simplex chronicus, and lichen sclerosus. Patients who have pruritus should be carefully evaluated to exclude infectious etiologies.

Vulvar lichen simplex chronicus is a chronic eczematous disease characterized by intense and unrelenting itching ("scratch-itch-scratch cycle") that may result in sleep disruption. It represents an end-stage response to a wide variety of possible initiating processes, including environmental factors (restrictive clothing, sweat, heat, and contact irritants) and dermatologic disease. It is more common in women with a history of atopic disease than in other populations. Findings are similar to all eczematous diseases and include erythema, swelling, skin thickening, and excoriations (from scratching). Scaling (lichenification) may be obscured by the warm moist environment. Although the diagnosis is clinical, a biopsy should be performed if the practitioner is uncertain. Based on the observed clinical presentation, the described patient has vulvar lichen simplex chronicus.

Lichen sclerosus is a chronic disorder most likely related to an autoimmune process of unclear etiology. Most commonly it affects genital skin, with extragenital lesions reported in up to 13% of women. The most common symptom reported is pruritus, followed by irritation, burning, dyspareunia, and tearing. On examination, the skin appears thinned, whitened, and parchment-like, often with areas of ecchymoses. Unlike lichen simplex chronicus, anatomic changes, including introital narrowing, fusion of the labia minora, and phimosis of the clitoral hood, are commonly noted. Biopsy of the affected area may be considered to confirm the diagnosis.

Vulvar intraepithelial neoplasia associated with genital human papillomavirus can present as white, red, dark, raised, or eroded lesions. Women may note the presence of a lesion or vulvar irritation, pruritus, or pain or they may be asymptomatic. Distinguishing VIN from genital warts on the basis of appearance alone is not always possible. Thus, a biopsy is necessary for diagnosis of any worrisome vulvar lesion or genital wart that does not respond to treatment. Because multicentric disease is commonly encountered, a complete examination should include the cervix, vagina, and perianal area.

Patients who have "inverse" or vulvar psoriasis usually have other manifestations. As with lichen simplex chronicus, vulvar psoriasis typically does not present with scaling because the vulva is more hydrated than is exposed skin. Rather, well-demarcated salmon pink plaques are noted on the vulvar skin and intertriginous areas. The vagina and vestibule are not involved. Biopsy may be considered for diagnosis but is not necessary when cutaneous psoriasis is present elsewhere.

Paget disease of the vulva is a rare form of intraepithelial neoplasia characterized by adenocarcinomatous cells. As with VIN, patients may present with severe vulvar symptoms or may be asymptomatic. Examination typically reveals multiple bright red, scaly, eczematoid plaques. Biopsy is necessary for diagnosis and underscores the importance of biopsying any lesion that does not respond to treatment. When Paget disease is confirmed, evaluation of the breasts, genitourinary tract, and gastrointestinal tract may be needed.

Diagnosis and management of vulvar skin disorders. ACOG Practice Bulletin No. 93. American College of Obstetricians and Gynecologists. Obstet Gynecol 2008;11:1243–53.

Edwards L. Genital dermatology atlas. First edition. Philadelphia (PA): Lippincott Williams & Wilkins; 2004.

Farage MA, Miller KW, Ledger WJ. Determining the cause of vulvovaginal symptoms. Obstet Gynecol Surv 2008;63:445–64.

Stewart KM. Clinical care of vulvar pruritus, with emphasis on one common cause, lichen simplex chronicus. Dermatol Clin 2010;28:669–80.

54

Molar pregnancy

A 24-year-old woman comes to the emergency department with vaginal bleeding. She had a suction curettage for a complete molar pregnancy 11 weeks ago. The preevacuation serum β-hCG level was 285,000 mIU/mL. On physical examination, she is hemodynamically stable, and a small amount of clotting blood is seen in the vagina. Her quantitative β-hCG level last week was 2,485 mIU/mL and is found to be 2,450 mIU/mL today. The most appropriate management is

   (A) methotrexate therapy
   (B) combination chemotherapy
 * (C) quantitative β-hCG measurement in 1 week
   (D) suction curettage
   (E) transvaginal pelvic ultrasonography

Gestational trophoblastic neoplasia (GTN) is the term used to describe a group of tumors that arise from abnormal proliferation of placental trophoblasts. The group of tumors include partial and complete hydatidiform mole, choriocarcinoma, placental site trophoblastic tumor, and epithelioid trophoblastic tumor. Such tumors can arise after any gestation, including spontaneous abortion.

Most cases of persistent GTN are diagnosed after a molar pregnancy. In the United States, approximately 1 in 6,000 therapeutic abortions and 1 in 1,000–2,000 pregnancies are found to be molar gestations. After evacuation of a molar pregnancy, careful weekly follow-up of serum β-hCG is necessary until the level is zero. Once β-hCG is undetectable, continued follow-up is required biweekly or monthly for 6 months. During the follow-up, use of highly effective contraception is important to avoid confusion of a new pregnancy with persistent GTN. The risk of developing persistent GTN after a complete hydatidiform mole is approximately 15–20%. The risk might be 40–50% if the patient presents with uterine size substantially greater than the appropriate size for gestation and a β-hCG level greater than 100,000 mIU/mL. The risk for partial hydatidiform mole to develop into persistent GTN is approximately 1–4%.

The International Federation of Gynecology and Obstetrics (FIGO) criteria for diagnosis of GTN are as follows:

1. Four or more values indicative of β-hCG plateau over at least 3 weeks (on day 1, day 7, day 14, and day 21);

2. An increase in β-hCG levels of 10% or greater for three or more values over at least 3 weeks (on day 1, day 7, and day 14);

3. The presence of histologic choriocarcinoma

4. The persistence of β-hCG 6 months after molar evacuation

Patients with persistent GTN by FIGO criteria will require an evaluation to determine the extent of disease, including medical history and physical examination, quantitative β-hCG level, complete blood count, liver and renal function tests, and computed tomography of the chest, abdomen, and pelvis. With the use of these data, the FIGO stage and the World Health Organization prognostic score can be calculated (Table 54-1 and Table 54-2). Appropriate therapy can then be determined based on presence or absence of metastases and prognostic score.

Because the described patient had an initial level of β-hCG greater than 100,000 mIU/mL, she is at an increased risk of developing persistent GTN, but two increased β-hCG levels 1 week apart do not meet the FIGO criteria for persistent GTN. Because she does not have a diagnosis of persistent GTN, single agent or combination chemotherapy is not indicated at this time. The patient should have repeat serum β-hCG measurement in 1 week. If she has a plateau or increase that is sustained for 3 weeks, and the diagnosis of persistent GTN is established, imaging should be ordered. With the diagnosis of persistent GTN, computed tomography of the

TABLE 54-1. Staging for Gestational Trophoblastic Neoplasia

Stage	Description
I	Disease confined to uterus
II	Disease extends outside uterus but is limited to genital structures (adnexa, vagina, and broad ligament)
III	Disease extends to lungs with or without genital tract involvement
IV	Disease involves other metastatic sites

Reprinted from American Journal of Obstetrics and Gynecology, Volume 204, Lurain JR, Gestational trophoblastic disease II: classification and management of gestational trophoblastic neoplasia, pages 11–8, copyright 2011, with permission from Elsevier.

TABLE 54-2. Scoring System for Gestational Trophoblastic Neoplasia

Risk Factor	Score			
	0	1	2	4
Age (years)	39 or less	More than 39	Not applicable	Not applicable
Antecedent pregnancy	Mole	Abortion	Term	Not applicable
Period from pregnancy event to treatment (months)	Less than 4	4–6	7–12	12 or more
Pretreatment human chorionic gonadotropin level (mIU/mL)	Less than 103	103–104	104–105	Greater than 105
Largest tumor mass, including uterus (cm)	Less than 3	3–4	5 or more	Not applicable
Site of metastases	Not applicable	Spleen or kidney	Gastrointestinal tract	Brain or liver
Number of metastases	Not applicable	1–4	5–8	Greater than 8
Type of previous failed chemotherapy	Not applicable	Not applicable	Single drug	Two or more drugs

Total score for patient is obtained by adding individual scores for each prognostic risk factor: low risk, less than 7; high risk, greater than 7.

Reprinted from American Journal of Obstetrics and Gynecology, Volume 204, Lurain JR, Gestational trophoblastic disease II: classification and management of gestational trophoblastic neoplasia, pages 11–8, copyright 2011, with permission from Elsevier.

chest, abdomen, and pelvis will determine stage and help define the World Health Organization prognostic score. Pelvic ultrasonography can be helpful to identify patients who might benefit from hysterectomy to reduce tumor burden, but repeat suction curettage is not indicated. Pelvic ultrasonography will likely not lead to a change in management. In the case of persistent GTN, repeat suction curettage does not decrease the need for adjuvant chemotherapy but might increase the risk of uterine bleeding and infection.

Goldstein DP, Berkowitz RS. Current management of gestational trophoblastic neoplasia. Hematol Oncol Clin North Am 2012;26:111–31.

Lurain JR. Gestational trophoblastic disease II: classification and management of gestational trophoblastic neoplasia. Am J Obstet Gynecol 2011;204:11–8.

May T, Goldstein DP, Berkowitz RS. Current chemotherapeutic management of patients with gestational trophoblastic neoplasia. Chemother Res Pract 2011;2011:1–12.

55

Complications of embolization

A 42-year-old woman comes to your office with heavy menstrual bleeding for the past 9 months despite treatment with combination oral contraceptives. Recent ultrasonography revealed an intramural anterior fundal myoma that measured 7.5 cm × 8.1 cm. She recently read about uterine artery embolization as a treatment option. You counsel her that the most common complication associated with uterine artery embolization is

      (A) readmission
*   (B) postembolization syndrome
      (C) sepsis
      (D) unsuccessful bilateral embolization
      (E) prolonged hospital stay

Symptomatic uterine myomas affect approximately 20–40% of women of childbearing age. They account for 30–40% or 150,000–200,000 of all hysterectomies performed in the United States. The two most common symptoms for which women seek treatment of uterine myomas are abnormal uterine bleeding and pelvic pressure. Uterine artery embolization is one of the minimally invasive alternative options for the management of symptomatic uterine myomas. Success of the procedure is defined by the complete occlusion of bilateral feeding vessels with resultant necrosis and shrinkage of the myoma.

The procedure is performed primarily by interventional radiologists. The femoral artery is catheterized and the catheter is advanced over the aortic bifurcation to the internal iliac arteries. Each uterine artery is then identified and an embolic compound (most commonly polyvinyl alcohol particles) is injected into the vessel. This is followed by injection of contrast dye to ensure occlusion of the vessels. Studies have shown a favorable outcome by 3 months with a 42% reduction rate in the volume of the dominant myoma. Most patients are discharged from the hospital within 1–2 days after the procedure.

Hospital readmissions are encountered in 11% of patients, most within the first week after the procedure. Reasons for readmission include pain, fever, or a combination of both. Occasionally, a prolonged initial hospital stay may be encountered for the same reasons.

Postembolization syndrome is a common complication of uterine artery embolization and consists of a constellation of symptoms that include nausea, fever, pelvic pain, and malaise. The syndrome is encountered in 40% of cases and, generally, is self-limited. Most of these patients will experience one or more of these symptoms. Up to one third of these patients will report a febrile

illness. It occurs after the iatrogenic infarction of a solid tumor; in this case, a myoma. The procedural protocol includes a variety of medications, such as antibiotics, nonsteroidal antiinflammatory drugs, antiemetics, and occasional narcotic analgesics, to counter this common complication.

Sepsis after uterine artery embolization is rare and limited to case reports. However, uterine and pelvic organ infections are common. These infections are characterized by delayed fever and purulent discharge. An infected uterus is an indication for admission and may require hysterectomy, which occurs in 1 in 200 patients who underwent uterine artery embolization. The presence of a submucosal myoma may increase the likelihood of this complication.

Procedural difficulties are encountered in 11% of patients and include anatomic variations, vessel spasm, and technical difficulties. Vessel spasm can be overcome by waiting, or with the use of spasmolytics. Unsuccessful bilateral catheterization of the uterine vessels and uterine artery embolization occurs in 4.9% of procedures.

Al-Fozan H, Tulandi T. Factors affecting early surgical intervention after uterine artery embolization. Obstet Gynecol Surv 2002;57:810–5.

Alternatives to hysterectomy in the management of myomas. ACOG Practice Bulletin No. 96. American College of Obstetricians and Gynecologists. Obstet Gynecol 2008;112:387–400.

Gupta Janesh K, Sinha A, Lumsden MA, Hickey M. Uterine artery embolization for symptomatic uterine fibroids. Cochrane Database of Systematic Reviews 2012, Issue 5. Art. No.: CD005073. DOI: 10.1002/14651858.CD005073.pub3.

Hehenkamp WJ, Volkers NA, Donderwinkel PF, de Blok S, Birnie E, Ankum WM, et al. Uterine artery embolization versus hysterectomy in the treatment of symptomatic uterine fibroids (EMMY trial): peri- and postprocedural results from a randomized controlled trial. Am J Obstet Gynecol 2005;193:1618–29.

56

Risk of acquiring human immunodeficiency virus after sexual assault

A 28-year-old woman comes to the emergency department at your hospital 12 hours after being sexually assaulted. She reports vaginal and anal penetration, and physical examination identifies numerous lacerations. The sexual assault involved one unknown perpetrator. The patient's immunization record is unavailable. When counseling the patient about emergency contraception and prophylaxis against sexually transmitted infections (STIs), you advise her against routine prophylaxis for

       (A) pregnancy
       (B) emotional trauma
  * (C) human immunodeficiency virus (HIV)
       (D) hepatitis B virus

Approximately 13–39% of all women will experience sexual assault in their lifetime. Survivors of such attacks are at risk of acute traumatic injury, unwanted pregnancy, acquisition of STIs, and emotional trauma.

The risk of acquiring HIV from a sexual assault is low; however cases of such transmission have been reported in the literature. The incidence of HIV transmission after isolated sexual contact with an HIV-positive person is unknown, but is estimated to be approximately 1–2 per 1,000 cases after vaginal penetration and 1–3 per 100 cases after anal penetration. The risk increases in proportion with a stage of HIV disease and a viral load in the assailant. The presence of genital trauma, genital ulcers, or coinfection in the victim increases the risk of transmission. Although the HIV status of the assailant typically is not known, 1% of prisoners incarcerated for sexual assault are HIV positive. At this prevalence, the estimated risk of transmission of HIV after a sexual assault is 1–2 per 100,000 for vaginal penetration and 20–30 per 100,000 for anal penetration. Trauma that occurs during the assault may increase these estimations.

Postexposure HIV prophylaxis may be offered if the patient presents within 72 hours of exposure, but its use is controversial. The Centers for Disease Control and Prevention (CDC) does not have guidelines for HIV prophylaxis in cases of sexual assault when the HIV status of the assailant is unknown. As a result, decisions should be made on a case-by case basis with consideration given to the estimated risk of infection in the perpetrator, the nature of the assault, and the desire of the patient. The U.S. Department of Health and Human Services recommends that an individual who seeks care within 72 hours after exposure to an individual known to have HIV receive a 28-day course of highly active antiretroviral

therapy, initiated as soon as possible after exposure. A number of regimens have been recommended. If the assailant's HIV status is unknown, clinicians should evaluate the risks and benefits of prophylaxis on an individual basis.

Only 17–43% of women present for medical evaluation after sexual assault. Survivors should be evaluated for acute, physical injury, which occurs in approximately one half of all cases. General body trauma is more common than genital trauma. Injuries may include blunt traumatic injuries to the head, face, torso, or limbs, and penetrating injuries. Defensive injuries, including abrasions, lacerations, and bruising typically are found on the hands, arms, and medial thighs. Injuries should be treated by standard trauma protocols.

The risk of pregnancy after sexual assault is approximately 5%. Progestin-only emergency contraception (1.5 mg oral levonorgestrel, one time) should be given as soon as possible and up to 120 hours after the assault. This regimen is 98.5% effective in preventing pregnancy and is more effective when given earlier after the exposure.

Patients should be given prophylaxis against STIs, including gonorrhea, chlamydial infection, bacterial vaginosis, and hepatitis B. The current CDC guidelines recommend postexposure hepatitis B vaccination for survivors without history of vaccination in addition to the following antibiotic regimen: ceftriaxone, 250 mg intramuscularly as a single dose, plus metronidazole, 2 g orally as a single dose, plus azithromycin, 1 g orally as a single dose, or doxycycline, 100 mg orally twice daily for 7 days. Figure 56-1 shows an algorithm for postexposure prophylaxis against HIV after sexual assault.

Patients also need emotional support acutely when they seek health care. Such patients will benefit from the

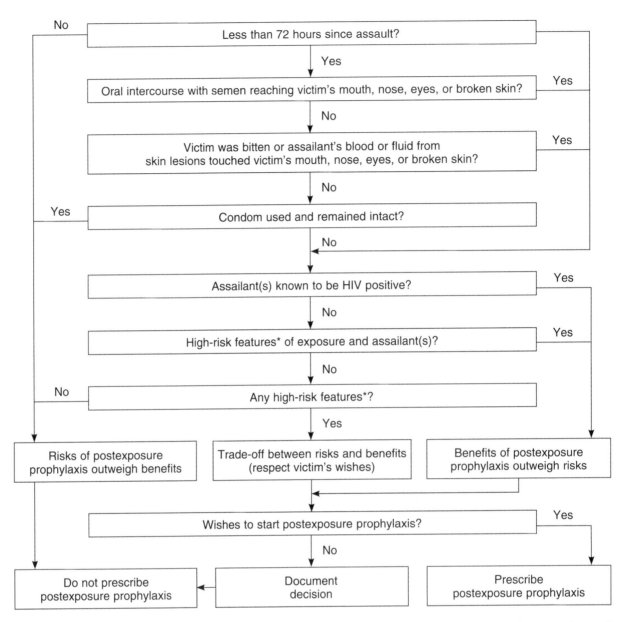

FIG. 56-1. Algorithm for postexposure prophylaxis against human immunodeficiency virus (HIV) after sexual assault. *Exposure high-risk features include defloration, other trauma to penetration site, known current sexually transmitted infection, anal intercourse, multiple assailants, repeated intercourse, survivor bitten by an assailant, and assailant bitten by survivor. Assailant high-risk features include being a man who has sex with men, injection drug use, and being male from high prevalence area. (Adapted by permission from BMJ Publishing Group Limited. BMJ, Welch J, Mason F, Volume 334, pages 1154–8, copyright 2007 and Martin Wiese, Consultant Emergency Physician, Leicester Royal Infirmary, Leicester, UK.)

involvement of a sexual assault crisis counselor or social worker. Long-term mental health assessment and care also should be initiated.

Linden JA. Clinical practice. Care of the adult patient after sexual assault. N Engl J Med 2011;365:834–41.

Sexual assault. Committee Opinion No. 499. American College of Obstetricians and Gynecologists. Obstet Gynecol 2011;118:396–9.

Smith DK, Grohskopf LA, Black RJ, Auerbach JD, Veronese F, Struble KA, et al. Antiretroviral postexposure prophylaxis after sexual, injection-drug use, or other nonoccupational exposure to HIV in the United States: recommendations from the U.S. Department of Health and Human Services. U.S. Department of Health and Human Services. MMWR Recomm Rep 2005;54:1–20.

Welch J, Mason F. Rape and sexual assault. BMJ 2007;334:1154–8.

57

Peer review of operative complications

You participate in a departmental Quality Assurance and Improvement Committee meeting at your hospital. One of the cases involves a ureteral injury during a surgical procedure carried out by a urogynecologist. The division director of urogynecology, who is not a member of the committee, sees you in the cafeteria and asks you about the discussion of this case. You inform her that you

        (A) will forward her the minutes from the meeting

*   (B) cannot discuss the meeting with her

        (C) can tell her about the discussion in a private place

        (D) can relate the outcome of the meeting but no other details

Peer review is an important component of the quality assurance and improvement programs at most institutions. Each department within a hospital will have a quality assurance and improvement committee that has the responsibility for peer review as one of its functions. The primary goal of peer review is to improve the overall quality of patient care. Because of the importance of this function, almost all states have made peer review processes within hospitals confidential and legally non-discoverable. Because the findings of a peer review committee can, in some cases, lead to disciplinary actions, it is important that all members of such committees maintain confidentiality to ensure due process is followed in all cases. All hospitals should have a specific protocol by which disciplinary action must progress to protect the interests of the hospital and the medical practitioner. Discussions outside of this mandated process have the potential to create unwanted repercussions for the hospital or the practitioner.

Because of the principle of peer review protection, it is not appropriate to discuss the confidential information or conclusions of the peer review committee outside of the committee meetings. It is also not appropriate to share the minutes of the meeting. For this reason, you must tell division director that you cannot discuss the meeting or forward the minutes.

American College of Obstetricians and Gynecologists. Guidelines for women's health care: a resource manual. 3rd ed. Washington, DC: ACOG; 2007.

American College of Obstetricians and Gynecologists. Quality and safety in women's health care. 2nd ed. Washington, DC: American College of Obstetricians and Gynecologists; 2010.

Berlin L. Performance improvement and peer-review activities: are they immune from legal discovery? AJR Am J Roentgenol 2003;181: 649–53.

Meyer DJ, Price M. Peer review committees and state licensing boards: responding to allegations of physician misconduct. J Am Acad Psychiatry Law 2012;40:193–201.

58
Sexual dysfunction

A 48-year-old perimenopausal woman, gravida 2, para 2, comes to your clinic for follow-up of decreased libido and hypoactive sexual disorder. She has no medical problems and takes no medications; her examination yields normal results. She notes no improvement after four sessions of couple's counseling and reports a good relationship with her husband. She would like to initiate medical therapy to see if she can improve her sex drive while she continues counseling. The best recommendation to improve her libido is

    (A) phosphodiesterase inhibitor
    (B) selective serotonin reuptake inhibitor
    (C) psychotropic agent
    (D) estrogen therapy
*   (E) testosterone therapy

Hypoactive sexual disorder is the most common female sexual dysfunction with a peak incidence between ages 40 years and 60 years. Often, the condition is untreated because women feel embarrassed to bring up the topic, and many health care providers are unaware of treatment strategies. Female sexual dysfunction is multifactorial and may be exacerbated by situational circumstances, such as relationship issues, depression, dyspareunia, alcohol use, or medications. Thus, a complete evaluation for sexual issues, including physical and psychologic factors that may contribute to the diminished desire, is essential. Medications, particularly selective serotonin reuptake inhibitors and oral contraceptives, can be associated with hypoactive sexual disorder. Psychotropic medications also have been associated with sexual dysfunction. Diagnostic criteria for sexual interest and arousal disorder are listed in Box 58-1.

Treatment for low desire consists primarily of patient counseling and education and treatment of identified underlying comorbid conditions. Currently, no medications are approved by the U.S. Food and Drug Administration (FDA) for the treatment of female sexual dysfunction other than estrogen for vaginal atrophy symptoms, including vaginal dryness and dyspareunia. Other medications evaluated for a possible effect on female sexual dysfunction, including phosphodiesterase inhibitors (used to treat male erectile dysfunction), have not been proved to be effective in women.

Androgen levels decrease in reproductive aged women until menopause and then remain stable. Although no population-based studies have identified a clear association between androgen levels and satisfactory sexual function, women who had a hysterectomy with bilateral oophorectomy reported significantly decreased libido compared with women who retained their ovaries. Several studies have demonstrated a positive effect on female sexual

---

BOX 58-1

Criteria for Sexual Interest and Arousal Disorder

A. Lack of sexual interest/arousal, of at least 6 months' duration, as manifested by at least three of the following criteria:
  1. Absent or reduced interest in sexual activity
  2. Absent or reduced sexual or erotic thoughts or fantasies
  3. No initiation of sexual activity and is not receptive to a partner's attempts to initiate
  4. Absent or reduced sexual excitement or pleasure during sexual activity (in 75% or more of sexual encounters)
  5. Absent or reduced genital, nongenital, or both physical changes during sexual activity (in 75% or more of sexual encounters)

B. The disturbance causes clinically significant distress or impairment, characterized by the following:
  1. Lifelong or acquired distress or impairment
  2. Generalized or situational distress or impairment
  3. Partner factors (eg, partner's sexual problems or partner's health status)
  4. Relationship factors (eg, poor communication, relationship discord, or discrepancies in desire for sexual activity)
  5. Individual vulnerability factors (eg, depression or anxiety, poor body image, or history of abuse)
  6. Cultural or religious factors (eg, inhibitions related to prohibitions against sexual activity)
  7. Medical factors (eg, illness or medication)

With kind permission from Springer Science+Business Media: Arch Sex Behav, The DSM diagnostic criteria for female sexual arousal disorder, Graham CA, volume 39, year 2010, pages 240–55.

dysfunction (improved libido) with the short-term use of androgen therapy (oral, topical, or injectable). Pooled data from trials in surgically and naturally menopausal women found that women who were treated with testosterone reported an increase in sexually satisfying events per 4 weeks (1.9 events versus 0.9 events over a baseline of approximately 3 events) compared with women who received placebo. In the 1990s and 2000s, manufacturers sought approval of androgen therapy for female hypoactive sexual dysfunction by the FDA. However, lack of evidence supported by long-term studies and safety concerns with extended use precluded FDA approval. Generally, use of androgen therapy should be limited to short-term treatment in carefully selected women who are willing to accept the risks of adverse effects of androgen

replacement therapy (eg, hirsutism, acne, virilization, and cardiovascular complications). The use of a compounding pharmacy is recommended to avoid commercially available high-dose formulations that are used in men when prescribing androgen therapy for female sexual dysfunction.

Female sexual dysfunction. Practice Bulletin No. 119. American College of Obstetricians and Gynecologists. Obstet Gynecol 2011;117:996–1007.

Graham CA. The DSM diagnostic criteria for female sexual arousal disorder. Arch Sex Behav 2010;39:240–55.

Shifren JL. The role of androgens in female sexual dysfunction. Mayo Clin Proc 2004;79:S19–S24.

Woodis CB, McLendon AN, Muzyk AJ. Testosterone supplementation for hypoactive sexual desire disorder in women. Pharmacotherapy 2012;32:38–53.

59

Ovarian cancer screening

A 45-year-old woman comes to your office for her annual gynecologic examination. She reports that her mother died of ovarian cancer at age 55 years. No other breast, ovarian, endometrial, or colon cancer occurred in her family. When discussing with her the pros and cons of screening for ovarian cancer, you advise her that the screening test that might have the most clinical benefit for her is

   (A) annual CA 125 testing
   (B) ovarian cancer blood test
 * (C) transvaginal ultrasonography
   (D) inhibin test
   (E) pelvic magnetic resonance imaging

The World Health Organization recommends consideration of screening for a disease in the following circumstances:

- The condition that is screened for should be a major cause of death and have a substantial prevalence in the population being screened.

- The natural history of the disease is well known.

- Effective treatment exists for those with overt disease, and treating early stage disease will improve outcome.

- The test should be acceptable to the population and cost effective.

- The test should have a high positive predictive value, negative predictive value, sensitivity, and specificity.

For a cancer screening test to be helpful, the disease in question should have a long prodromal or in situ phase during which time intervention will be curable, and the

cancer is sufficiently common that the positive predictive values (PPVs) and negative predictive values will inform clinical decisions regarding intervention.

The paradigm for screening tests in gynecology is the Pap test. This simple, accessible, and inexpensive test has decreased the incidence of cervical cancer in the United States by approximately 75% since its adoption in 1947. Cervical cancer has a long precancerous phase during which treatment will prevent progression to cancer.

Epithelial ovarian cancer is the fifth leading cause of cancer death in U.S. women, occurring in nearly 24,000 women annually and accounting for 15,000 deaths annually. Because ovarian cancer often presents at an advanced stage, long-term disease-free survival is uncommon, and 5-year survival is 30–40%. In contrast, ovarian cancer that is diagnosed when confined to the ovary has a 5-year survival of more than 90%. It is essential that any ovarian cancer screening test reliably detect stage I disease and that it have a sensitivity of at least 75%, a specificity of 99.6%, and a PPV of at least 10%. To date, no screening test satisfies the World Health Organization criteria as an adequate screening test for ovarian cancer in the general population. To make the available screening tests more useful by increasing the PPV of the test individualized assessment of a patient's risk of ovarian cancer is necessary.

A strong predictor of ovarian cancer risk is family history. A woman with a single first-degree relative with ovarian cancer is considered at moderate risk of ovarian cancer. The Society of Gynecologic Oncologists (SGO) consensus statement recommends that such a patient undergo annual transvaginal ultrasonography and consideration of annual CA 125 testing. The National Comprehensive Cancer Network recommends screening of women with a family history of ovarian or breast cancer with transvaginal ultrasonography and CA 125 measurements every 6 months. The U.S. Preventive Services Task Force does not recommend routine screening of women without known genetic mutations that increase risk. The American Cancer Society recommends possible screening for women with a family history of ovarian cancer with the caveat that it is not known whether screening such women will improve survival.

Serum CA 125 measurements have been used in combination with transvaginal ultrasonography in several prospective evaluations for the early detection of ovarian cancer. Annual CA 125 testing has not been shown to be useful in screening the general population because more than 50% of stage I ovarian cancer patients will have normal CA 125 values, and in premenopausal women, the specificity of the test is less than 95% because of frequent false-positive results. Serial CA 125 measurements might improve the accuracy of this screening test for the general population and the population at moderate and high risk, and trials are ongoing. Inhibin is a marker for granulosa cell tumors of the ovary, and is not useful for epithelial ovarian cancer screening.

An ovarian cancer blood test that has been approved by the U.S. Food and Drug Administration, is a serum test intended to aid in the management or triage of a complex adnexal mass detected by ultrasonography. The test provides an assessment of the level of six tumor markers that is interpreted by a proprietary algorithm to provide a result of low risk or high risk of ovarian cancer. It is not approved as a screening test.

Prospective studies that have used ultrasonographic screening have shown a PPV ranging from 1.5% to 27%. This wide range is generally attributed to the overall risk of the women included in each study; women of average risk had a PPV of less than 3%. Women at moderate risk in these studies fared better. In a prospective study conducted at the University of Kentucky, 25,327 women older than 50 years or older than 25 years with a family history of ovarian cancer were screened with annual ultrasonography. Strict ultrasonographic criteria were used to triage women. Oophorectomy was performed in 364 women, of whom 29 were found to have invasive ovarian cancer; 14 of 29 women had stage I disease. Overall 5-year survival was 77%, and for stage I patients survival was greater than 90%, which suggests a benefit with ultrasonographic screening. The PPV for ultrasonography in this population was 27%, and sensitivity was 85%. Although this still does not meet the strict World Health Organization criteria, the described patient fulfills these eligibility criteria. She should be counseled regarding the limitations and effectiveness of ultrasonographic screening. No data exist to support the use of pelvic magnetic resonance imaging or computed tomography as screening tests for epithelial ovarian cancer.

Buys SS, Partridge E, Black A, Johnson CC, Lamerato L, Isaacs C, et al. Effect of screening on ovarian cancer mortality: the Prostate, Lung, Colorectal and Ovarian (PLCO) Cancer Screening Randomized Controlled Trial. PLCO Project Team. JAMA 2011;305:2295–303.

Clarke-Pearson DL. Clinical practice. Screening for ovarian cancer. N Engl J Med 2009;361:170–7.

Society of Gynecologic Oncologists. Statement on use of CA 125 for monitoring for ovarian cancer. Chicago (IL): SGO; 2009. Available at:https://www.sgo.org/wp-content/uploads/2012/09/SGO-CA-125-statement.pdf. Retrieved June 6, 2013.

van Nagell JR Jr, Pavlik EJ. Ovarian cancer screening. Clin Obstet Gynecol 2012;55:43–51.

60

Hysteroscopic sterilization

A 23-year-old woman, gravida 4, para 4, comes to your office at 6 weeks postpartum for hysteroscopic sterilization with a metallic microinsert. During the review of her medical records, you notice that her history is complicated by sensitivity to nickel and that she had a finding of atypical squamous cells of undetermined significance (ASC-US) on a recent Pap test. She also reports that when she underwent intravenous pyelography after a complicated cesarean delivery, she developed chest tightness and a rash. The contraindication to metallic microinsert hysteroscopic sterilization in this patient is

(A) her age
* (B) allergy to contrast dye
(C) nickel sensitivity
(D) finding of ASC-US on Pap test
(E) number of weeks postpartum

Approximately 700,000 tubal sterilizations are performed in the United States annually. The methods used to achieve tubal sterilization include laparoscopy, minilaparotomy, and hysteroscopy. Hysteroscopic tubal sterilization offers women a permanent sterilization procedure that does not involve entry into the peritoneal cavity and that should avoid the need for general anesthesia. It is approved to be performed at least 6 weeks after a delivery or pregnancy loss. The procedure involves the deployment of a metallic microinsert, which consists of stainless steel covered by a polyethylene inner coil and an outer nickel-titanium coil into each tubal ostium. The tubal occlusion occurs from a combination of the microinsert's outer coil filling the fallopian tube lumen and the fibers of the inner coil inducing a fibrotic response. Over time, this will lead to tissue ingrowth and fibrosis. Because the occlusion is not immediate, women must use back up contraception for 3 months after device placement to allow time for tubal occlusion to occur. The U.S. Food and Drug Administration currently requires that hysterosalpingography be performed 3 months after sterilization to confirm satisfactory placement of the devices and ensure tubal occlusion. The fact that this patient has an allergy to contrast dye precludes the 3-month confirmatory hysterosalpingography. Therefore, the inability to perform hysterosalpingography is a contraindication.

The contraindications to microinsert hysteroscopic sterilization are shown in Box 60-1. Although the described patient's age places her at risk for regret, her age is not a contraindication to the procedure. The risk of poststerilization regret ranges from 0.9% to 26%. Data from the U.S. Collaborative Review of Sterilization Study found that the cumulative risk of regret over 14 years of follow-up was 12.7%. However, the risk can reach 20.3% for women aged 30 years or younger at the

> **BOX 60-1**
>
> **Contraindications to Microinsert Hysteroscopic Sterilization**
>
> - Patient is uncertain about ending fertility.
> - Patient can have only one insert placed (including contralateral proximal tubal occlusion or suspected unicornuate uterus).
> - Patient has previously undergone a tubal ligation.
> - Patient is pregnant or has a suspected pregnancy.
> - Patient gave birth or terminated a pregnancy less than 6 weeks before the procedure.
> - Patient has an active or recent upper or lower pelvic infection.
> - Patient has a known allergy to contrast media.
>
> Sakhel K. Transcervical sterilization. In: Sakhel K, Lukban JC, Abuhamad AZ, editors. Practical guide to office procedures in gynecology and urogynecology. London: Jaypee Brothers; 2012. p. 97–110. With kind permission of Dr. Sakhel.

time of sterilization, compared with 5.9% for women older than 30 years. Given the significant risk of regret, women should receive adequate counseling. Components of counseling for microinsert hysteroscopic sterilization are listed in Box 60-2.

Nickel hypersensitivity as confirmed by a skin test is no longer a contraindication to the nickel-containing metallic microinsert sterilization. The U.S. Food and Drug Administration has recently approved the removal of this contraindication from the labeling of the product. However, patients with metal allergy should be counseled about the possibility of developing an allergic reaction.

BOX 60-2

Counseling for Sterilization

- Permanent nature of the procedure
- Alternative methods available, including male sterilization
- Reasons for choosing sterilization
- Screening for risk indicators for regret
- Details of the procedure, including risks and benefits of anesthesia
- The possibility of failure, including ectopic pregnancy
- The need to use condoms for protection against sexually transmitted diseases, including human immunodeficiency virus infection
- Completion of informed consent process
- Local regulations regarding interval from time of consent to procedure

Benefits and risks of sterilization. Practice Bulletin No. 133. American College of Obstetricians and Gynecologists. Obstet Gynecol 2013;121:392–404.

An abnormal Pap test result may be an indication for further evaluation; however, it is not a contraindication to metallic microinsert hysteroscopic sterilization. The patient is at 6 weeks postpartum and, therefore, is eligible to undergo the procedure.

Benefits and risks of sterilization. Practice Bulletin No. 133. American College of Obstetricians and Gynecologists. Obstet Gynecol 2013; 121:392–404.

Hysterosalpingography after tubal sterilization. Committee Opinion No. 458. American College of Obstetricians and Gynecologists. Obstet Gynecol 2010;115:1343–5.

61

Adverse effects of pharmacologic therapy for overactive bladder

A 67-year-old woman comes to your office for evaluation of urinary incontinence. She reports no symptoms associated with cough or Valsalva maneuvers, but has repeated episodes of urgency before leakage. Her physical and pelvic examination results are within normal limits. Review of symptoms reveals recent blurring of vision and eye pain, which the patient attributes to stress. You obtain a urine culture, which reveals no growth. Before initiation of a trial of anticholinergic therapy, the most appropriate next step is

*   (A) ophthalmologic evaluation
      (B) hemoglobin A_{1c} test
      (C) Kegel exercises
      (D) urodynamics

Anticholinergic medications represent the criterion standard in the treatment of overactive bladder syndrome. To understand their mechanism of action, it is necessary to review the signaling conduction pathway of micturition. Figure 61-1 (see color plate) shows the neurologic control of voiding and the involved receptors and their ligands. As shown in Figure 61-1, acetylcholine is responsible for the stimulation of the M_3 receptors within the detrusor muscle and the nicotinic receptors in the external urethral sphincter. Thus, blockage of its release has a predominantly inhibitory effect on spontaneous contractions of the detrusor muscle.

Given the widespread use of anticholinergics in the treatment of overactive bladder, it is necessary for the health care practitioner to be aware of the common adverse effects and contraindications, including the following:

• Dry mouth
• Dry eyes
• Constipation
• Increased body temperature and cessation of perspiration
• Increased intraocular pressure and blurred vision

Possible increased intraocular pressure is of particular concern for patients who are affected by angle closure glaucoma. Therefore, it is necessary to rule out this diagnosis before initiation of anticholinergic therapy. Although the closed angle form of glaucoma may occur gradually, angle closure glaucoma is an acute process which, if not diagnosed and treated promptly, can result in blindness.

This patient's chief concern is most consistent with overactive bladder syndrome and, therefore, use of anticholinergic medication is appropriate. The use of screening questions for the following symptoms will help to identify patients with acute angle-closure glaucoma:

• Acute blurred vision
• Eye pain
• Nausea and vomiting associated with eye pain
• A rainbow halo observed around lights

Given this patient's uncertain history and lack of regular health maintenance visits, screening for diabetes mellitus with a hemoglobin A_{1c} test may be a reasonable option. However, with a normal urinalysis result, it is unlikely that this would account for her visual symptoms; nor is diabetes mellitus a contraindication to initiating anticholinergic therapy.

Kegel exercises are useful in a number of urogynecologic conditions; however, they are not likely to be of value in this patient. Similarly, although urodynamics may be a useful adjunct in the diagnostic evaluation of this patient, such testing is unnecessary before starting anticholinergic therapy.

Geoffrion R. Treatments for overactive bladder: focus on pharmacotherapy. J Obstet Gynaecol Can 2012;34:1092–101.

Madhuvrata P, Cody JD, Ellis G, Herbison GP, Hay-Smith EJ. Which anticholinergic drug for overactive bladder symptoms in adults. Cochrane Database of Systematic Reviews 2012, Issue 1. Art. No.: CD005429. DOI: 10.1002/14651858.CD005429.pub2.

Shamliyan T, Wyman JF, Ramakrishnan R, Sainfort F, Kane RL. Benefits and harms of pharmacologic treatment for urinary incontinence in women: a systematic review. Ann Intern Med 2012;156: 861–74, W301–10.

62

Heavy menstrual bleeding in a patient with a low platelet count

You are consulted about an 11-year-old patient who was admitted to the hospital for an inability to tolerate solids or liquids, a 3-day history of acute and severe menstrual bleeding at menarche, and newly diagnosed immune thrombocytopenic purpura (ITP). The girl has never been sexually active nor has she had a pelvic examination. She is currently undergoing a transfusion of packed red blood cells and platelets and is receiving intravenous (IV) fluids, immunoglobulin, and corticosteroids. She is hemodynamically stable with splenomegaly. The physical examination revealed normal external genitalia with a virginal introitus and approximately 500 mL of bright red blood on a pad. Transabdominal pelvic ultrasonography yields normal results. A urine pregnancy test result is negative. Hemoglobin level is 6 g/dL and platelet count is 12×10^3 per microliter. The best next step in management is

* (A) depot medroxyprogesterone acetate
* (B) IV conjugated equine estrogens
* (C) combined oral contraceptives
* (D) oral progestin
* (E) levonorgestrel IUD

Heavy menstrual bleeding is defined as excessive vaginal bleeding that occurs in a woman of childbearing age. Anovulatory bleeding and undiagnosed bleeding disorders are common in adolescents. Bleeding disorders associated with adolescents with heavy menstrual bleeding include von Willebrand disease, platelet dysfunction, clotting factor deficiency, and thrombocytopenia. Von Willebrand disease is one of the most common bleeding disorders associated with chronic heavy menstrual bleeding, with an overall prevalence of 13%.

Few studies have evaluated the incidence of severe heavy menstrual bleeding in women with thrombocytopenia. Immune thrombocytopenic purpura is one of the most common causes of acute heavy menstrual bleeding in adolescents. Optimal management in an adolescent with a bleeding disorder includes a multidisciplinary approach that involves a hematologist, pediatrician, and gynecologist. The goals are the diagnosis and treatment of the underlying blood disorder and gynecologic condition with preservation of fertility.

Although the described patient has heavy menstrual bleeding, she has an normal gynecologic examination and transabdominal pelvic ultrasonography results. The most likely diagnosis is anovulatory bleeding with newly diagnosed ITP. High-dose estrogen therapy is an appropriate initial hormonal therapy for adolescents with acute and severe heavy menstrual bleeding and no contraindication to estrogen therapy. The exact mechanism of action is unknown. The best next step would be to administer IV conjugated equine estrogens. Oral conjugated equine estrogens can be substituted for IV conjugated equine estrogens in patients who can tolerate oral medications.

Combined oral contraceptives and progestins are not appropriate for this patient who cannot tolerate oral medications. An intramuscular injection of depot medroxyprogesterone acetate may cause a hematoma in a severely thrombocytopenic patient. The levonorgestrel IUD has not been studied as a treatment for acute heavy menstrual bleeding in thrombocytopenic patients. Additionally, insertion of the levonorgestrel IUD would most likely require that the patient be transferred to a surgical suite for sedation and monitoring.

This patient with ITP should be transitioned to long-term, combination hormonal contraceptives to stabilize her endometrium and prevent ovulation. Progestin-only pills also should act to reduce endometrial proliferation and thereby reduce menstrual blood loss. A progestin implant is not an appropriate option for a severely thrombocytopenic patient. Currently, no data are available regarding treatment of heavy menstrual bleeding in women with bleeding disorders with other combination hormonal contraceptives, such as transdermal patches or rings, although theoretically they should be effective.

Ahuja SP, Hertweck SP. Overview of bleeding disorders in adolescent females with menorrhagia. J Pediatr Adolesc Gynecol 2010;23:S15–S21.

American College of Obstetricians and Gynecologists. Management of anovulatory bleeding. ACOG Practice Bulletin 14. Washington, DC: ACOG; 2000.

James AH, Kouides PA, Abdul-Kadir R, Dietrich JE, Edlund M, Federici AB, et al. Evaluation and management of acute menorrhagia in women with and without underlying bleeding disorders: consensus from an international expert panel. Eur J Obstet Gynecol Reprod Biol 2011;158:124–34.

Levens ED, Scheinberg P, DeCherney AH. Severe menorrhagia associated with thrombocytopenia. Obstet Gynecol 2007;110:913–7.

63

Perioperative anticoagulants

A 50-year-old woman is scheduled for a total laparoscopic hysterectomy and bilateral salpingo-oophorectomy for simple endometrial hyperplasia. Her medical history is significant for a 20-pack-year smoking history and a body mass index of 40 (calculated as weight in kilograms divided by height in meters squared). Her obstetric history is remarkable for two vaginal births and one cesarean delivery for a breech presentation. The best option to minimize her risk for a perioperative thromboembolic event is

      (A) smoking cessation
      (B) prophylactic warfarin sodium
  * (C) unfractionated heparin
      (D) change from surgery to laparotomy

The incidence of postoperative venous thromboembolic events is approximately 2% in women who undergo gynecologic surgery. Table 63-1 shows risk classification for venous thromboembolism in patients who undergo surgery without prophylaxis. Other risk factors for thromboembolic events include smoking history, hormone therapy, and obesity (Appendix F).

The described patient is aged 50 years. Major surgery will place her at high risk of a venous thromboembolic event. Although she should be counseled to quit smoking, smoking cessation immediately before surgery will not reduce her current venous thromboembolic risk.

Perioperative unfractionated heparin has been studied extensively and is the best option for her. Subcutaneous heparin in the perioperative period can reduce thromboembolic events and may be extended in the postoperative period in high-risk patients for up to 4 weeks. Warfarin sodium is not indicated in the perioperative period and may increase her risk of venous thromboembolic events because protein C and protein S may be affected before factor X, factor IX, factor VII, or factor II.

Postoperative venous thromboembolic events have been studied mostly in patients undergoing open surgery. In the described patient, changing from a minimally invasive surgery to an open procedure would not reduce her risk of a venous thromboembolic event. Research on minimally invasive surgery in gynecologic and gynecologic oncology patients demonstrated that venous thromboembolism was diagnosed in approximately 0.5% of patients who underwent intermediate complexity procedures and 2.8% of patients who underwent high complexity procedures. In this study, intermediate complexity procedures included hysterectomy, removal of ovaries, and bilateral tubal ligation. High complexity procedures included bowel surgery, lymph node dissection, and splenectomy. Recommendations regarding continuation of anticoagulation prophylaxis for up to 4 weeks in the postoperative period are important to consider in high-risk gynecologic patients who undergo surgery. However, definitive data regarding outcomes are lacking.

Agnelli G, Bolis G, Capussotti L, Scarpa RM, Tonelli F, Bonizzoni E, et al. A clinical outcome-based prospective study on venous thromboembolism after cancer surgery: the @RISTOS project. Ann Surg 2006;243:89–95.

Geerts WH, Bergqvist D, Pineo GF, Heit JA, Samama CM, Lassen MR, et al. Prevention of venous thromboembolism: American College of Chest Physicians Evidence-Based Clinical Practice Guidelines (8th Edition). American College of Chest Physicians. Chest 2008; 133:381S–453S.

Nick AM, Schmeler KM, Frumovitz MM, Soliman PT, Spannuth WA, Burzawa JK, et al. Risk of thromboembolic disease in patients undergoing laparoscopic gynecologic surgery. Obstet Gynecol 2010;116: 956–61.

Prevention of deep vein thrombosis and pulmonary embolism. ACOG Practice Bulletin No. 84. American College of Obstetricians and Gynecologists. Obstet Gynecol 2007;110:429–40.

TABLE 63-1. Levels of Thromboembolism Risk and Recommended Thromboprophylaxis in Hospital Patients*

Levels of Risk	Approximate Deep Vein Thrombosis Risk Without Thromboprophylaxis†	Suggested Thromboprophylaxis Options	Other Recommended Management
Low risk (Mobile patients undergoing minor surgery and patients who use medical therapy and are fully mobile)	Less than 10%	No specific thromboprophylaxis	Early and aggressive ambulation
Moderate risk (Most general type of risk—open gynecologic or urologic surgery patients, and medical patients who are on bed rest or sick)	10–40%	Low molecular weight heparin at recommended doses, low-dose unfractionated heparin two or three times a day, and fondaparinux	None
Moderate risk of venous thromboembolism plus high risk of bleeding	Not applicable	Mechanical thromboprophylaxis‡	None
High risk (Patients with hip or knee arthroplasty, hip fracture surgery, major trauma, and spinal cord injury)	40–80%	Low molecular weight heparin (at recommended doses), fondaparinux, and oral vitamin K antagonist (international normalized ratio 2–3)	None
High risk of venous thromboembolism plus high risk of bleeding	Not applicable	Mechanical thromboprophylaxis‡	None

*The descriptive terms are purposely left undefined to allow individual clinician interpretation.

†Rates are based on objective diagnostic screening for asymptomatic deep vein thrombosis in patients not receiving thromboprophylaxis.

‡Mechanical thromboprophylaxis includes intermittent pneumatic compression or venous foot pumps with or without graduated compression stockings; consider switching to anticoagulant thromboprophylaxis when high bleeding risk decreases.

Geerts WH, Bergqvist D, Pineo GF, Heit JA, Samama CM, Lassen MR, et al. Prevention of venous thromboembolism: American College of Chest Physicians Evidence-Based Clinical Practice Guidelines (8th Edition). American College of Chest Physicians. Chest 2008;133:381S–453S. Reproduced with permission from the American College of Chest Physicians.

64

Ovarian remnant syndrome

A 45-year-old woman has been referred to you for a complex left adnexal mass, left lower quadrant and flank pain, hematuria, rectal bleeding, and anemia. Two years ago, she had a total laparoscopic hysterectomy with bilateral salpingo-oophorectomy for stage IV endometriosis. She is otherwise healthy. A left pararectal mass is palpated on examination. Computed tomography (CT)–intravenous pyelography reveals extrinsic compression of the left ureter with severe left hydronephrosis and a 6-cm complex left pelvic mass. Laboratory evaluation shows a hemoglobin level of 10.7 g/dL. Her urologist places a retrograde stent into the left ureter. Cystoscopy yields normal results. The remainder of her medical history is unremarkable. The next step in the management of this patient is

      (A) surgical excision of the pelvic mass
      (B) retrograde pyelography
      (C) nephrostomy
*   (D) colonoscopy

Common symptoms and signs in patients with colorectal cancer, inflammatory bowel disease, and bowel endometriosis include abdominal pain or cramping, change in bowel habits (constipation, diarrhea, and narrowing of stool), rectal bleeding, and hematochezia. Patients with colorectal cancer are more likely to have weakness or fatigue, weight loss, and anemia than patients with bowel endometriosis. Endometriotic lesions rarely cause bowel obstruction.

The described patient needs a colonoscopy because her history of rectal bleeding and anemia are concerning for colorectal cancer. In addition, colonoscopy will assist with preoperative diagnosis and planning for the appropriate surgery. Differentiating between intestinal cancer and endometriosis can be difficult even with diagnostic and imaging studies, such as colonoscopy and CT with barium enema. This is especially true in patients with lesions that involve the mucosal surface of the intestine. After colonoscopy with biopsy, surgical excision of the left adnexal mass should be performed to pathologically confirm the diagnosis and appropriately treat the patient, while preserving the function of her left kidney.

The patient most likely has ovarian remnant syndrome with an endometriotic cyst within an ovarian remnant. This is a surgical diagnosis. *Ovarian remnant syndrome* is defined as pelvic pain in the presence of histologically proved ovarian tissue after salpingo-oophorectomy. Usually, an ovary is incompletely resected because it was densely adherent to the pelvic sidewall due to endometriosis, adhesions, or pelvic inflammatory disease. The residual ovarian tissue continues to have cyclic activity and cystic changes that can cause pain by exerting pressure on the adjacent adherent posterior vagina, rectum, bladder, and ureter. A serum follicle-stimulating hormone level in the premenopausal range supports the

diagnosis in patients suspected of having ovarian remnant syndrome.

Confirmation of ovarian remnant syndrome in a patient who has a negative radiologic imaging study results may be improved by ovarian stimulation with clomiphene citrate followed by reimaging 10 days later. Ovarian stimulation also may facilitate intraoperative identification and removal of the ovarian remnant.

In ovarian remnant syndrome, dense adhesions usually involve the ovarian remnant, bowel, omentum, bladder, and ureters. Surgical management requires meticulous dissection of the retroperitoneum beginning at the pelvic brim and the pelvic sidewall with the goal of complete excision of the diseased tissue. Ovarian remnant excision should be performed by a surgeon with the requisite skill to perform this technically challenging procedure. Advocates for surgical treatment of ovarian remnant syndrome point out risks that cancer may be found in ovarian remnant tissue.

The patient has already undergone CT–intravenous pyelography. Retrograde pyelography would not add any additional information. A nephrostomy would have been necessary if her retrograde stent placement had been unsuccessful.

Kho RM, Magrina JF, Magtibay PM. Pathologic findings and outcomes of a minimally invasive approach to ovarian remnant syndrome. Fertil Steril 2007;87:1005–9.

Nezhat CH, Seidman DS, Nezhat FR, Mirmalek SA, Nezhat CR. Ovarian remnant syndrome after laparoscopic oophorectomy. Fertil Steril 2000;74:1024–8.

Slaughter K, Gala RB. Endometriosis for the colorectal surgeon. Clin Colon Rectal Surg 2010;23:72–9.

Yoshida M, Watanabe Y, Horiuchi A, Yamamoto Y, Sugishita H, Kawachi K. Sigmoid colon endometriosis treated with laparoscopy-assisted sigmoidectomy: significance of preoperative diagnosis. World J Gastroenterol 2007;13:5400–2.

65

Office hysteroscopy

A 34-year-old woman, gravida 1, para 1, comes to your office with irregular bleeding that began 3 months ago. Physical and pelvic examinations yield normal results. The urine pregnancy test result is negative. Sonohysterography shows a 1-cm intrauterine cavitary mass with a feeding vessel through its stalk. You recommend office hysteroscopy with polypectomy preceded by a prostaglandin cervical ripening agent administration. During insertion of the hysteroscope, the patient becomes hypotensive and bradycardic. She maintains her oxygen saturation. She reports no chest pain or shortness of breath, just cramping. Figure 65-1 (see color plate) shows the image you see on the video monitor. Immediate fluid deficit of 500 mL of normal saline solution occurs. Blood pressure and heart rate normalize with removal of the hysteroscope. The best next step in management is

   (A) completion of the procedure
   (B) ventilation–perfusion lung imaging
 * (C) observation
   (D) chest computed tomography angiography
   (E) diagnostic laparoscopy

Invasive gynecologic procedures are increasingly being performed in the office. It is the responsibility of obstetrician–gynecologists to practice patient safety in an office's daily operations. Health care providers should seek the help of all stakeholders to assist in establishing a safe, transparent environment for the delivery of health care.

Uterine perforation occurs in an estimated 1–1.5% of hysteroscopic procedures. Risk factors include cervical stenosis and intrauterine scar tissue. Patients at greatest risk are those who have not had a vaginal delivery, those who have had prior cervical surgery, and postmenopausal women. Many uterine perforations occur during forceful dilation of the cervical canal with a blunt-tipped dilator. Most of these perforations are fundal in location.

The most common signs of uterine perforation are the inability to obtain or maintain uterine distention and rapid fluid loss. Less commonly, hemorrhage occurs. To minimize this type of mechanical injury, preprocedure cervical ripening agents may be administered, such as intravaginal or oral prostaglandin (off-label use) or laminaria.

A preoperative pelvic examination to determine position and flexion of the uterus is essential. If the cervix is stenotic at the time of surgery, the surgeon can choose a smaller hysteroscope, if available. A second option is to intracervically inject diluted vasopressin. This softens the cervix and facilitates cervical dilation without excessive force. As a last resort, the cervical canal and the endocervix can be opened by a loop electrosurgical excision procedure, although this should be performed only if other methods fail.

Care should be taken not to create a false passage during cervical dilation and insertion of the hysteroscope. The hysteroscope can be used for cervical dilation under direct visualization. Hysteroscopy requires a thorough understanding of the relationship between the angle of the lens and the patient's uterine position and flexion. Concurrent abdominal ultrasonography can be used to help guide the hysteroscope in difficult cases.

Management of a uterine perforation is dependent on the location of the injury and the equipment used. If a fundal uterine perforation occurs with blunt trauma, such as from a cervical dilator, the patient can be managed expectantly. If it occurs anteriorly, posteriorly, or laterally, one should consider a cystoscopy, sigmoidoscopy, or laparoscopy to assess for injury to the bladder, rectum, or vessels in the broad ligament, respectively. If a uterine perforation occurs with an energy source, such as a monopolar or bipolar loop, laparoscopy or laparotomy is required to assess for a visceral thermal injury. If bowel or bladder injury is suspected, cystoscopy or sigmoidoscopy may be indicated. Thermal injury may not be recognized for up to 3–7 days postoperatively. Therefore, patients need to be counseled regarding symptoms of a thermal bowel injury, which include fever, elevated heart rate, nausea, vomiting, absence of passage of flatus or stool, abdominal pain and distension, and diminished urine output.

This patient has a uterine perforation and a transient vasovagal episode upon insertion of the hysteroscope. Observation of the patient that includes evaluation of her symptoms, vital signs, heart, lung, abdominal, and pelvic examination is the most appropriate next step. Observation of the patient allows time to confirm that she is stable and does not have a delayed complication, such as bleeding. Completion of the procedure is unwise because of continued rapid fluid absorption, poor visualization, a compromised uterine cavity, and increased risk of visceral injury.

A ventilation–perfusion lung imaging or chest computed tomography angiography to assess for a pulmonary embolism is unnecessary. Gas embolus is a rare complication when using fluid distension media. Although it is possible that this patient had a transient gas embolism, the fact that she had no chest pain, dyspnea, or drop in her oxygen saturation argue against a gas embolus. The rapid absorption of fluid and the image in Figure 65-1 confirm a uterine perforation. The patient had a uterine fundal

perforation with a blunt instrument and is asymptomatic. Therefore, laparoscopy is not indicated at this time and observation is most appropriate.

AAGL practice report: practice guidelines for the diagnosis and management of endometrial polyps. American Association of Gynecologic Laparoscopists. J Minim Invasive Gynecol 2012;19:3–10.

Erickson TB, Kirkpatrick DH, DeFrancesco MS, Lawrence HC 3rd. Executive summary of the American College of Obstetricians and Gynecologists Presidential Task Force on Patient Safety in the Office Setting: reinvigorating safety in office-based gynecologic surgery. Obstet Gynecol 2010;115:147–51.

Hysteroscopy. Technology assessment No. 7. American College of Obstetricians and Gynecologists. Obstet Gynecol 2011;117:1486–91.

Shveiky D, Rojansky N, Revel A, Benshushan A, Laufer N, Shushan A. Complications of hysteroscopic surgery: "Beyond the learning curve." J Minim Invasive Gynecol 2007;14:218–22.

66

Postoperative pelvic abscess

A 55-year-old woman comes to the emergency department 2 weeks after an uncomplicated laparoscopic hysterectomy and bilateral salpingo-oophorectomy. She has been experiencing fever, chills, and pelvic pain but reports normal bowel and bladder functions. Examination is remarkable for an intact vaginal cuff with a 5-cm fluctuant mass noted with mild diffuse abdominal pain. A temperature of 38.4°C (101°F) is noted with otherwise stable vital signs. Laboratory results are remarkable for an elevated white blood cell count. Computerized tomography demonstrates a 10 cm × 10 cm × 10 cm pelvic fluid collection consistent with a postoperative abscess superior to the vaginal cuff. The most important next step in management is

    (A) oral antibiotics
    (B) hospital observation
    (C) intravenous antibiotics
*   (D) drainage of the abscess

Postoperative pelvic abscess is a recognized complication of surgical intervention in the pelvis with a reported incidence of approximately 1%. Early management of postoperative pelvic abscess with broad-spectrum antibiotics can result in clinical improvement in up to 87.5% of patients. Larger abscess volumes (calculated as height × width × length × 0.52) have been found to be statistically associated with higher antibiotic failure rates. Patients who had transvaginal or image-guided drainage showed improvement in clinical outcomes with decreased hospital stays. Therefore, in the case described in this clinical scenario, drainage of the abscess would be the most important next step in management.

To discharge the patient with only oral antibiotics is not indicated and could lead to worsening systemic illness.

Hospital admission without initiation of broad-spectrum antibiotics plus drainage of the abscess also is not reasonable. Interventional radiology consultation is a reasonable option for placement of drains while minimizing the risk of surgery; however, many hospitals do not have access to interventional radiology.

Goharkhay N, Verma U, Maggiorotto F. Comparison of CT- or ultrasound-guided drainage with concomitant intravenous antibiotics vs. intravenous antibiotics alone in the management of tubo-ovarian abscesses. Ultrasound Obstet Gynecol 2007;29:65–9.

McNeeley SG, Hendrix SL, Mazzoni MM, Kmak DC, Ransom SB. Medically sound, cost-effective treatment for pelvic inflammatory disease and tuboovarian abscess. Am J Am J Obstet Gynecol 1998;178:1272–8.

67

Use of prophylactic antibiotics in surgery for patients allergic to penicillin

A 47-year-old woman, gravida 2, para 2, is scheduled for laparoscopy-assisted vaginal hysterectomy for abnormal uterine bleeding. During her recent office visit, she told you she had an allergic reaction to penicillin with a mild body rash that resolved with over-the-counter diphenhydramine. The best step in management to reduce perioperative infection risk is to administer

    (A) clindamycin
    (B) metronidazole and a fluoroquinolone
    (C) vancomycin
*   (D) cefazolin

The decision and timing of antibiotic administration is one of the most important issues that a gynecologic surgeon must consider in the preoperative period. Appendix G lists considerations for the surgeon to take into account when choosing which antibiotic agents to use in the preoperative period.

Box 67-1 shows recommended antibiotic prophylactic regimens for hysterectomy within 1 hour of incision. Cephalosporins are the most studied agent in perioperative infection risk reduction for gynecologic surgery and should be used in patients at low risk of severe allergic reactions. For patients with a history of severe penicillin allergy, alternative antibiotic regimens should be discussed in the preoperative period to ensure that the patient and anesthesiologist understand the clinical indications.

Severe reactions are defined as anaphylactic reactions with acute onset shortness of breath, urticaria, and systemic instability. Respiratory compromise is rare and needs to be elucidated so that patients are not stratified to potentially inferior antibiotic regimens. The allergic reaction to penicillin that this patient has described would not be classified as severe.

Cefazolin is a first-generation cephalosporin and is the first-line antibiotic for operative gynecologic procedures because of its broad antimicrobial spectrum and the low incidence of allergic reactions and adverse effects. The long half-life (1.8 hours) and low cost of cefazolin is another reason that it is a first-line agent for antimicrobial prophylaxis in clean–contaminated procedures, such as hysterectomy.

Often, clindamycin is used to treat Gram-positive and anaerobic infections. However, its use is limited for treatment of Gram-negative infections, and alone it would not be the first choice as a preoperative antibiotic agent. Vancomycin often is used to treat complex Gram-positive infections including methicillin-resistant *Staphylococcus aureus*, but its use is limited for the treatment of anaerobic and Gram-negative infections. In patients with a history of severe allergic reactions to penicillin and cephalosporins, metronidazole and fluoroquinolone are reasonable second-line agents with broad-spectrum coverage but should not be chosen in preference to cefazolin.

BOX 67-1

Antibiotic Prophylactic Regimens for Hysterectomy to be Administered Within 1 Hour of Incision

1. Cefazolin, 1 g or 2 g intravenously (2-g dose if patient's weight is greater than 100 kg or body mass index is greater than 35 [calculated as weight in kilograms divided by height in meters squared])

2. Clindamycin, 600 mg intravenously, + gentamicin, 1.5 mg/kg intravenously), or quinolone, 400 mg intravenously, or aztreonam, 1 g intravenously

3. Metronidazole, 500 mg intravenously + gentamicin, 1.5 mg/kg intravenously, or quinolone, 400 mg intravenously

Antibiotic prophylaxis for gynecologic procedures. ACOG Practice Bulletin No. 104. American College of Obstetricians and Gynecologists. Obstet Gynecol 2009;113: 1180–9.

Antibiotic prophylaxis for gynecologic procedures. ACOG Practice Bulletin No. 104. American College of Obstetricians and Gynecologists. Obstet Gynecol 2009;113:1180–9.

Fonacier L, Hirschberg R, Gerson S. Adverse drug reactions to a cephalosporins in hospitalized patients with a history of penicillin allergy. Allergy Asthma Proc 2005;26:135–41.

Goodman EJ, Morgan MJ, Johnson PA, Nichols BA, Denk N, Gold BB. Cephalosporins can be given to penicillin-allergic patients who do not exhibit an anaphylactic response. J Clin Anesth 2001;13:561–4.

Hemsell DL. Gynecologic postoperative infections. In: Pastorek JG 2nd, editor. Obstetric and gynecologic infectious disease. New York (NY): Raven Press; 1994. p. 141–9.

68

Vaginal cancer screening after hysterectomy

A 60-year-old woman, gravida 3, para 3, with a history of abnormal uterine bleeding recently underwent an abdominal hysterectomy and bilateral salpingo-oophorectomy for uterine myomas. Her past medical history is significant for hypertension and recurrent bacterial vaginosis. Her obstetric and gynecologic history is remarkable for three normal spontaneous vaginal births and a lifetime history of normal Pap test results. She inquires about future Pap tests during her annual examinations. In regard to future Pap tests, you advise her that she should

    (A) have annual tests
    (B) have tests every 3 years
*   (C) discontinue tests
    (D) include testing for human papillomavirus (HPV) every 5 years

The American College of Obstetricians and Gynecologists and the American Cancer Society support continued cytology surveillance in low-risk women. Low-risk women are women who have had a total hysterectomy for benign indications with no prior history of high-grade cervical intraepithelial neoplasia (CIN) and women older than age 65 years who have had three or more consecutive negative cytology test results and no abnormal test results in the past 10 years. Women treated in the past for CIN 2, CIN 3, or cancer remain at risk of persistent or recurrent disease after treatment and should continue to have routine screening for at least 20 years. Bacterial vaginosis is not an indication for cervical cancer screening.

Cervical cancer screening should begin at age 21 years to help avoid overtreatment in women at low risk of developing cervical cancer (Appendix H and Appendix I). Cervical cytology screening is recommended every 3 years for women aged 21–29 years. Screening for women aged 30–65 years can include cervical cytology every 3 years or an extended surveillance with combined cervical cytology and HPV testing every 5 years. Patients with a low-risk history who are older than 65 years may not require further cervical cytology screening. Patients with a low-risk history after hysterectomy are at low risk for vaginal cancer. Therefore, the described patient should not need further cytology screening. The American College of Obstetricians and Gynecologists recommends that women who may require more frequent surveillance are those with the following conditions:

- History of CIN 2 or CIN 3
- Human immunodeficiency virus (HIV) infection or immunocompromised medical history
- Diethylstilbestrol in utero exposure

Co-testing for HPV with cervical cytology is reasonable for women older than 30 years but not for the low-risk patient described in this clinical scenario. Women who have received the HPV vaccine should undergo the same screening as women who have not received the HPV vaccine.

Salani R, Backes FJ, Fung MF, Holschneider CH, Parker LP, Bristow RE, et al. Posttreatment surveillance and diagnosis of recurrence in women with gynecologic malignancies: Society of Gynecologic Oncologists recommendations. Am J Obstet Gynecol 2011;204:466–78.

Screening for cervical cancer. Practice Bulletin No. 131. American College of Obstetricians and Gynecologists. Obstet Gynecol 2012; 120:1222–38.

Smith RA, Cokkinides V, Brooks D, Saslow D, Brawley OW. Cancer screening in the United States, 2010: a review of current American Cancer Society guidelines and issues in cancer screening. CA Cancer J Clin 2010;60:99–119.

69

Hormone therapy after hysterectomy for endometriosis

You have just performed a hysterectomy with bilateral salpingo-oophorectomy (BSO) in a 33-year-old woman for treatment of severe pelvic pain associated with stage IV endometriosis because she desired definitive surgery. At the time of surgery, you were able to remove all of the visible endometriosis. In regard to hormone therapy (HT) after the procedure, the most appropriate choice is

      (A) prescribe combined estrogen–progestin postoperatively
      (B) delay estrogen administration for at least 12 months
      (C) administer depot leuprolide injections postoperatively
*   (D) prescribe estrogen postoperatively

Endometriosis is the presence of ectopic endometrium, ie, endometrium outside of the uterus. It is estimated to occur in 7–10% of women. Although often asymptomatic, it may be associated with dysmenorrhea, dyspareunia, chronic pelvic pain, and infertility. Clear evidence exists that conservative laparoscopic treatment of endometriosis-associated pelvic pain is efficacious. However, the risk of recurrence of endometriosis is high with conservative surgery. Reoperation is required in at least 20% of patients within 2 years after conservative surgery compared with 4% of patients after hysterectomy with BSO. As in the described case, if a patient does not desire preservation of fertility, is older than 30 years, has advanced disease, and wants definitive treatment, hysterectomy with BSO is indicated.

Different types of HT used for treatment of endometriosis have not been well studied after hysterectomy with BSO. However, the primary mode of action of depot leuprolide therapy is by suppressing estrogen levels through downregulation of the hypothalamic–pituitary–ovarian axis. Depot leuprolide decreases gonadotropin-releasing hormone levels to induce a hypoestrogenic state. In a patient without ovaries, as in this case, a hypoestrogenic state already exists. Therefore, the administration of depot leuprolide will not have any effect on the efficacy of hysterectomy with BSO, so its use postoperatively is not indicated.

Expert opinion has long held that estrogen HT should not be started for 6–12 months after hysterectomy with BSO to decrease the chance of recurrence of endometriosis or stimulation of residual endometriotic lesions. The reported rate of recurrence with estrogen HT after hysterectomy with BSO is approximately 0.9% or less per year, suggesting that the true risk of estrogen treatment is very low and is outweighed by the benefits of preventing premature menopausal changes, such as hot flushes, vaginal dryness and atrophy, and bone loss. The decision to never use estrogen therapy after BSO in a young woman is not an appropriate clinical decision in an otherwise healthy woman.

Delaying the start of estrogen HT for 6 months results in notable postmenopausal symptoms with no evidence that it changes the risk of recurrence, so it is not recommended. Recurrence or persistence of symptoms with HT after hysterectomy with BSO has been observed in cases in which not all of the endometriosis was removed. Current opinion is that all endometriotic tissue should be removed at the time of hysterectomy with BSO. In this patient, the most appropriate step would be to prescribe estrogen postoperatively. In otherwise healthy women, many practitioners would continue estrogen treatment until approximately age 50 years. Combined HT is not indicated for patients who have undergone hysterectomy with BSO. Theoretic concerns regarding stimulating endometriotic implants or unopposed estrogen stimulating progression to endometrial cancer have not been substantiated.

Abbott J, Hawe J, Hunter D, Holmes M, Finn P, Garry R. Laparoscopic excision of endometriosis: a randomized, placebo-controlled trial. Fertil Steril 2004;82:878–84.

MacDonald SR, Klock SC, Milad MP. Long-term outcome of nonconservative surgery (hysterectomy) for endometriosis-associated pain in women <30 years old. Am J Obstet Gynecol 1999;180:1360–3.

Matorras R, Elorriaga MA, Pijoan JI, Ramon O, Rodriguez-Escudero FJ. Recurrence of endometriosis in women with bilateral adnexectomy (with or without total hysterectomy) who received hormone replacement therapy. Fertil Steril 2002;77:303–8.

Shakiba K, Bena JF, McGill KM, Minger J, Falcone T. Surgical treatment of endometriosis: a 7-year follow-up on the requirement for further surgery [published erratum appears in Obstet Gynecol 2008;112:710]. Obstet Gynecol 2008;111:1285–92.

Sutton CJ, Ewen SP, Whitelaw N, Haines P. Prospective, randomized, double-blind, controlled trial of laser laparoscopy in the treatment of pelvic pain associated with minimal, mild, and moderate endometriosis. Fertil Steril 1994;62:696–700.

70

Pelvic organ prolapse

An 85-year-old woman, gravida 4, para 4, comes to your office for treatment of a bothersome vaginal bulge and accompanying urinary retention. Her medical history is significant for hypertension, coronary artery disease, and emphysema, for which she requires supplemental oxygen at home. Her prior surgical procedures include vaginal hysterectomy at age 45 years and coronary artery bypass grafting 5 years ago. On pelvic examination, she has significant anterior wall and apical prolapse, with minimal posterior wall prolapse. Results of a pelvic organ prolapse quantification examination are consistent with Stage III pelvic organ prolapse. When the anterior prolapse is reduced in the office, she has no incontinence. She desires to retain coital ability. The most appropriate next step in managing this patient is

   (A) observation
* (B) support pessary
   (C) suburethral sling procedure
   (D) anterior repair
   (E) colposacropexy

The Pelvic Organ Prolapse Quantification technique is used to determine prolapse in a patient (Appendix C). In the Pelvic Organ Prolapse Quantification technique, the support defects of the vagina and perineum are systematically measured, including the anterior, posterior, and apical dimensions, together with the genital hiatus and perineal body measurements.

The management options for the patient with pelvic organ prolapse include observation, pessary use, or surgery. In women with few symptoms that do not interfere with quality of life, observation is an excellent option. Usually, these patients present with prolapse that does not extend past the hymen. This patient, however, has significant symptomatic anterior and apical pelvic organ prolapse that extends beyond the hymen, with accompanying urinary retention. The urinary retention puts her at significant risk of urinary tract infections with the potential for developing urosepsis. Therefore, observation would not be the best option for her.

The goals for treatment of the described patient are to alleviate her symptomatic vaginal bulge and discomfort, and to address her urinary retention without causing her significant morbidity. Given her age and medical comorbidities, it would be prudent to first try a nonsurgical option. The risk associated with use of pessaries is minimal compared with surgery, and thus a support pessary would be the best next step in her management.

Figure 70-1 (see color plate) and Figure 70-2 (see color plate) show various types of pessaries. Pessary use before reconstructive surgery in women with urinary retention has been shown to resolve the urinary retention in 75% of patients. Although no clear consensus exists regard-

ing the best type of pessary, indication, or follow-up care, support pessaries are considered first-line therapy when the prolapse is apical or anterior, as seen in this patient. Data on the effectiveness of pessaries are scarce. However, the ring with support (a support pessary) has been found to be equivalent to the Gellhorn pessary (a space-filling pessary) in treating symptoms of protrusion and voiding dysfunction.

The suburethral sling procedure is an excellent option for the patient with stress urinary incontinence. However, it has not been shown to improve symptomatic pelvic organ prolapse nor does it help with urinary retention. In fact, one of the potential postoperative complications of the suburethral sling procedure is urinary retention. Suburethral sling is sometimes necessary for the stress incontinence that may occur after pelvic reconstructive surgery for pelvic organ prolapse. This patient has no evidence of incontinence when her prolapse is reduced; therefore, suburethral sling would not be indicated for her.

The surgical options for treating pelvic organ prolapse include anterior repair (anterior colporrhaphy), colposacropexy, colpocleisis, and vaginal sacrospinous ligament suspension. Anterior colporrhaphy involves centrally plicating the fibromuscular layer of the anterior vaginal wall to repair anterior vaginal prolapse. Success rates of anterior colporrhaphy for reduction of prolapse have been reported to be 40–60% in randomized trials. Colposacropexy involves the use of a graft to suspend the upper vagina from the sacral promontory. Studies have shown that abdominal colposacropexy is associated with lower risk of recurrent prolapse but longer operating time and greater morbidity and cost than sacrospinous ligament suspension. Laparoscopic colposacropexy has success rates comparable with the open technique but is associated with reduced blood loss and need for admission. The introduction of robotic colposacropexy may reduce operative times and postoperative complications without compromising efficacy and thus may become the surgical procedure of choice in pelvic organ prolapse. Colpocleisis, also known as the Lefort procedure, repairs the prolapse by closing the vagina, and thus would not be appropriate for this patient because she wishes to remain sexually active. Given her age and significant comorbidities,

surgical intervention may be considered later in the event of failure of conservative management with a support pessary.

Atnip SD. Pessary use and management for pelvic organ prolapse. Obstet Gynecol Clin North Am 2009;36:541–63.

Bump RC, Mattiasson A, Bø K, Brubaker LP, DeLancey JO, Klarskov P, et al. The standardization of terminology of female pelvic organ prolapse and pelvic floor dysfunction. Am J Obstet Gynecol 1996;175: 10–7.

Jelovsek JE, Maher C, Barber MD. Pelvic organ prolapse. Lancet 2007;369:1027–38.

71

Abnormal cervical cytology results

A 33-year-old woman, gravida 3, para 3, comes to your office for her annual gynecologic examination. She is married and reports being in good health. The patient has normal breast and pelvic examination results. You perform a Pap test and send the specimen for cytology and human papillomavirus (HPV) co-testing. The Pap test result is normal, but the HPV test result is positive. You counsel the patient that the most appropriate next step is to

    (A) repeat the Pap test with HPV cotesting in 3 years

    (B) perform colposcopy

    (C) repeat the Pap test in 1 year

    (D) perform HPV testing in 1 year

*   (E) test for HPV 16 and 18 genotypes

The American Society for Colposcopy and Cervical Pathology in conjunction with the American Cancer Society has released revised cervical cancer screening guidelines. The protocol allows for less frequent screening in an effort to decrease the number of unnecessary procedures. Women aged 21–29 years who have a normal Pap test result are now recommended to undergo repeat screening no more frequently than every 3 years. Co-testing for HPV is not recommended in this age group because HPV infection is highly prevalent and frequently spontaneously resolves. Women aged 30–65 years with a history of normal Pap test results are advised to undergo cytology with HPV co-testing every 5 years. Women with abnormal cervical cytology result and a negative HPV test result have a low risk of severe dysplasia, ie, a 0.16% risk of developing cervical intraepithelial neoplasia 3 in 5 years.

    Women who have abnormal cytology results, such as low-grade squamous intraepithelial lesion or high-grade squamous intraepithelial lesion, are advised to undergo further investigation in accordance with the American Society for Colposcopy and Cervical Pathology guidelines. Women who have a normal cytology result with

a positive high-risk HPV test result are recommended to immediately undergo testing for HPV 16 and HPV 18. The HPV 16 and HPV 18 genotypes are implicated in approximately 68% cases of squamous cell cancer and in 85% cases of adenocarcinoma cervical cancer. A positive result for either HPV 16 or HPV 18 increases the risk of cervical intraepithelial neoplasia 3 from 0.16% to 10% and, therefore, justifies colposcopy. In areas where HPV 16 and HPV 18 testing is not available, the alternative is to repeat cytology and HPV co-testing in 1 year. If the follow-up Pap test result is abnormal or if the HPV cotesting still yields a positive result, the patient should undergo colposcopic examination.

    Repeating the Pap test in 3 years for the described patient would be inappropriate because she has been identified as being at an increased risk of dysplasia. Although progression to cervical cancer tends to be a slow process, women older than 30 years with a positive HPV test result are at an increased risk and should be followed up frequently. Colposcopy is unnecessary at this stage because HPV co-testing can yield positive results for any one of 13 or 14 HPV genotypes. Many of these are unlikely to lead to severe cervical dysplasia.

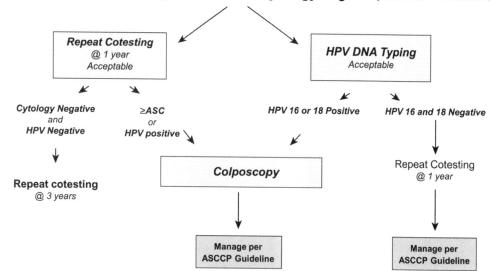

Management of Women ≥ Age 30, who are Cytology Negative, but HPV Positive

FIG. 71-1. Management of women aged 30 years or older who have cervical cytology negative results but human papillomavirus positive results. (Reprinted from *The Journal of Lower Genital Tract Disease* volume 17, Number 5, with the permission of ASCCP © American Society for Colposcopy and Cervical Pathology 2013. No copies of the algorithms may be made without the prior consent of ASCCP. Massad LS, Einstein MH, Huh WK, Katki HA, Kinney WK, Schiffman M, et al. 2012 updated consensus guidelines for the management of abnormal cervical cancer screening tests and cancer precursors. 2012 ASCCP Consensus Guidelines Conference. J Low Genit Tract Dis 2013; 17[5 Suppl 1]:S1–S27.)

Co-testing for high-risk HPV has been shown to have a higher sensitivity and negative predictive value compared with the Pap test or HPV testing alone. Therefore, it is recommended that, when available, cytology and HPV screening should be performed simultaneously to improve detection rates in women older than 30 years. According to the guidelines, the most appropriate next step is to order HPV 16 and HPV 18 genotyping to further assess this patient's risk of cervical dysplasia (Fig. 71-1).

Chelmow D, Waxman A, Cain JM, Lawrence HC 3rd. The evolution of cervical screening and the specialty of obstetrics and gynecology. Obstet Gynecol 2012;119:695–9.

Fontaine PL, Saslow D, King VJ. ACS/ASCCP/ASCP guidelines for the early detection of cervical cancer. Am Fam Physician 2012;86:501, 506–7.

Massad LS, Einstein MH, Huh WK, Katki HA, Kinney WK, Schiffman M, et al. 2012 updated consensus guidelines for the management of abnormal cervical cancer screening tests and cancer precursors. 2012 ASCCP Consensus Guidelines Conference. Obstet Gynecol 2013; 121:829–46.

Screening for cervical cancer. Practice Bulletin No. 131. American College of Obstetricians and Gynecologists. Obstet Gynecol 2012; 120:1222–38.

Smith RA, Cokkinides V, Brawley OW. Cancer screening in the United States, 2012: a review of current American Cancer Society guidelines and current issues in cancer screening. CA Cancer J Clin 2012;62:129–42.

72

Asymptomatic myomas

A 43-year-old multiparous woman comes to your office for her annual gynecologic examination. She reports regular menses that last for 4 days. She has no pelvic pain, pressure, or dyspareunia. She has completed childbearing and her partner has had a vasectomy. On physical examination, she has a palpable abdominal pelvic mass that extends to the midpoint between the umbilicus and the pubic symphysis. Bimanual examination reveals a globally enlarged uterus the size of a 14-week gestation. Ultrasonography confirms multiple myomas and normal-appearing ovaries. The best next step in her management is

* (A) reassurance and follow-up in 1 year
(B) levonorgestrel IUD
(C) myomectomy
(D) endometrial ablation
(E) hysterectomy

Symptomatic uterine myomas are the most common indication for hysterectomy in U.S. women. Urinary frequency, pelvic pain and pressure, dyspareunia, and abnormal uterine bleeding are all common symptoms of uterine myomas. Treatment should focus on the symptom complex that is occurring. Symptoms associated with uterine myomas generally correlate with their location. Subserosal and intramural myomas are most commonly associated with pelvic pressure and urinary or fecal urgency from uterine size. Intramural and submucosal myomas are commonly associated with abnormal uterine bleeding from a poorly supported endometrium or an enlarged endometrial cavity.

The described patient has no symptoms related to the uterine myomas. She reports 4-day menses that are regular. On pelvic examination, the uterus appears to be equivalent in size to a gestation of 14 weeks, and ultrasonography confirmed uterine myomas. Location and number of myomas in addition to overall uterine size can help guide future management should the patient become symptomatic. Pelvic ultrasonography is most useful to distinguish uterine enlargement from an adnexal mass. Before the advent of ultrasonography, removal of an

asymptomatic fibroid uterus was recommended once the uterus was equivalent in size to a gestation of 14 weeks because, at this time, a pelvic examination would no longer adequately assess the ovaries. With ultrasonography, the ovaries can be identified and assessed for size and the presence of an abnormal mass. Medical options for treating abnormal uterine bleeding include the levonorgestrel intrauterine device, monthly progestins, tranexamic acid, gonadotropin-releasing hormone agonists, or combined hormonal contraceptives. Surgical treatment for uterine myomas ranges from endometrial ablation, uterine artery embolization, myomectomy, and hysterectomy. At the present time, no treatment is necessary for the woman described. She should be advised to return in 1 year for her routine well-woman examination.

Alternatives to hysterectomy in the management of myomas. ACOG Practice Bulletin No. 96. American College of Obstetricians and Gynecologists. Obstet Gynecol 2008;112:387–400.

Donnez J, Tatarchuk TF, Bouchard P, Puscasiu L, Zakharenko NF, Ivanova T, et al. Ulipristal acetate versus placebo for fibroid treatment before surgery. PEARL I Study Group. N Engl J Med 2012;366: 409–20.

Parker WH. Uterine myomas: management. Fertil Steril 2007;88: 255–71.

73

Persistent vulvar pain

A 55-year-old woman, gravida 2, para 2, comes to your office with vulvar pain for 8 months. She has been treated repeatedly for yeast infections. She reports a constant raw feeling like sandpaper on the vulva. The pain increases after intercourse. Your evaluation shows no visible abnormalities of the vulva or vagina. Pain is present with separation of the labia minora. No tenderness is reported with a cotton swab palpation of the vulva or vestibule. Pain mapping pelvic examination reveals no areas of palpable tenderness. Microscopic evaluation of the vaginal discharge is unremarkable. She is in good health and has no significant past medical history. The most likely diagnosis is

     (A) chronic fungal infection
     (B) lichen sclerosus
     (C) bilateral pudendal neuralgia
 *   (D) vulvodynia
     (E) provoked vestibulodynia (vulvar vestibulitis)

Vulvar pain is relatively common, with an estimated prevalence of approximately 3–16%. The terminology related to vulvar pain syndromes has been inconsistent, but generally vulvar pain syndromes are classified into two major categories: 1) vulvar pain related to a specific disorder and 2) vulvodynia.

Specific disorders related to vulvar pain may be infectious, inflammatory, neoplastic, or neurologic (Fig. 73-1). Neurologic disorders may include referred pain from musculoskeletal disorders, radicular pain related to spinal disc disorders, multiple sclerosis, neurofibromatosis, pudendal neuralgia caused by injury or entrapment, postherpetic neuralgia, and possibly sacral–meningeal cysts (Tarlov cysts). None of these are consistent with the described case except possibly bilateral pudendal neuralgia. The absence of any vulvar tenderness and any areas of pelvic tenderness makes a diagnosis of bilateral pudendal neuralgia unlikely. Neoplastic conditions include Paget disease, vulvar intraepithelial neoplasia, or carcinoma. The absence of any visual abnormalities makes these conditions unlikely.

Inflammatory disorders include diagnoses, such as lichen sclerosus, lichen simplex chronicus, lichen planus, and atrophic vaginitis. However, the absence of any visible abnormalities and a negative result of microscopic examination of vaginal discharge similarly make such diagnoses unlikely. Infectious disorders may include candidiasis, trichomoniasis, or herpes simplex. Cultures for yeast infection should be performed as part of the diagnostic evaluation. Based on the clinical history and

findings in this case, culture will likely yield negative results and, thus, chronic fungal infection is not the likely diagnosis.

The most likely diagnosis in the described patient is vulvodynia. However, the diagnosis of vulvodynia is largely a diagnosis of exclusion. Vaginal pH, microscopic evaluation, and cultures of vaginal discharge should almost always be obtained. Ulcers or vesicle-like lesions are found, assessment for herpes zoster and herpes simplex is indicated. Vulvar biopsy is warranted if possible neoplastic or inflammatory diagnoses are of concern.

Most often, vulvodynia is classified as provoked or nonprovoked vulvodynia. Provoked vulvodynia usually is localized to the vulvar vestibule and is termed vulvar vestibulitis or provoked vestibulodynia. Marked tenderness to cotton-tip applicator palpation of the vestibule is characteristic in patients with provoked vestibulodynia, a finding not present in this case. Thus, a diagnosis of provoked vestibulodynia (vulvar vestibulitis) is not likely. It is important diagnostically to make this distinction because surgery is not recommended for treatment of provoked vulvodynia in contrast to provoked vestibulodynia (vulvar vestibulitis) for which vestibulectomy often is performed.

Bergeron S, Binik YM, Khalifé S, Pagidas K, Glazer HI, Meana M, et al. A randomized comparison of group cognitive–behavioral therapy, surface electromyographic biofeedback, and vestibulectomy in the treatment of dyspareunia resulting from vulvar vestibulitis. Pain 2001;91:297–306.

Vulvodynia. ACOG Committee Opinion: No. 345. American College of Obstetricians and Gynecologists. Obstet Gynecol 2006;108:1049–52.

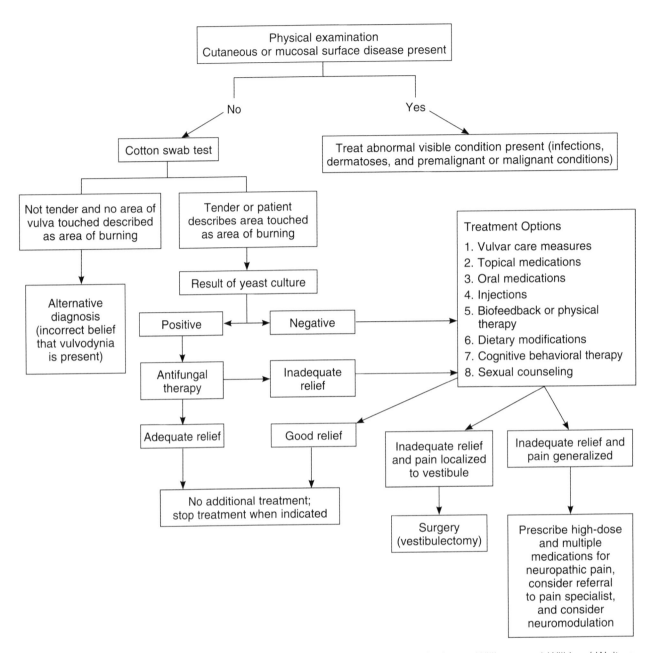

FIG. 73-1. Vulvodynia treatment algorithm. (Adapted with permission from Lippincott Williams and Wilkins / Wolters Kluwer Health: Haefner HK, Collins ME, Davis GD, Edwards L, Foster DEC, Hartmann EH, et al. The vulvodynia guideline. J Low Genit Tract Dis 2005;9:40–51. Copyright 2005.)

74

Appropriate treatment of sexually transmitted diseases

A 16-year-old patient comes to your office with a 1-week history of increased vaginal discharge and lower abdominal cramping. Her last menstrual period was 2 weeks ago. She reports being sexually active, and says that she and her partner do not always use condoms. She has no fever, vomiting, or diarrhea. She reports a possible mild reaction when given penicillin at age 4 years. Pelvic examination reveals mucopurulent discharge and uterine tenderness. Microscopy reveals an abundance of white blood cells, but yields negative results for trichomonas, monilia, and bacterial vaginosis. A urine pregnancy test result is negative. The most appropriate antibiotic treatment for this patient is

   (A) outpatient azithromycin and metronidazole
 * (B) outpatient ceftriaxone and doxycycline
   (C) inpatient clindamycin and gentamicin
   (D) inpatient levofloxacin and doxycycline
   (E) outpatient levofloxacin and metronidazole

In 2010, the Centers for Disease Control and Prevention (CDC) published the most recent guidelines for the diagnosis and management of pelvic inflammatory disease (PID). Women with lower abdominal pain and at least one other contributing symptom, including cervical motion tenderness, uterine tenderness, or adnexal tenderness, should be considered for the treatment of PID. Because the long-term consequences of untreated PID include infertility, pelvic pain, and pelvic adhesions, the threshold to treat patients should be low. Because PID often is a polymicrobial infection, treatment should include broad-spectrum antibiotics with coverage for *Neisseria gonorrhea* and *Chlamydia trachomatis*. The CDC recommends outpatient treatment unless the patient is pregnant, unable to tolerate oral intake, severely ill, or found to have a pelvic abscess or the previous outpatient therapy was ineffective. The preferred outpatient antibiotic regimen includes single-dose intramuscular ceftriaxone and 14 days of oral doxycycline with or without oral metronidazole. The preferred inpatient antibiotic regimen is intravenous cefotetan or cefoxitin with doxycycline (Appendix J).

The combination of azithromycin and metronidazole would provide adequate coverage for *C trachomatis*, but it would not be appropriate coverage for *N gonorrhea*. Although the patient is a minor and previous guidelines recommended inpatient management, no data support improved outcomes. Therefore, the patient qualifies for the outpatient regimen outlined earlier in this section.

Clindamycin and gentamicin can be used for intravenous therapy and are preferred for patients with allergy to cephalosporins. The described patient was reported to have a possible mild allergy to penicillin as a child.

Prior reports of cross-reactivity between cephalosporins and penicillin have been overemphasized. Recent studies show that the risk of allergy to cephalosporins in a patient with a confirmed allergy to penicillin is less than 0.17–2%. The likelihood of a cross-reaction is decreased if the patient's reaction was more than 10 years ago and was considered mild. Therefore, ceftriaxone use is still an appropriate first choice for this patient.

With the widespread emergence of quinolone-resistant gonorrhea, the recommendation for levofloxacin has been removed from the CDC guidelines. Fluoroquinolones should be reserved for use in individuals who are unable to take the preferred antibiotics. If fluoroquinolones are to be used, the CDC recommends sending a gonorrhea culture for sensitivity when starting treatment to confirm quinolone sensitivity. If quinolone resistant, the patient should be treated with parenteral cephalosporins or high-dose azithromycin. Therefore, levofloxacin and doxycycline would not be the best antibiotic regimen for this patient. Similarly, levofloxacin with metronidazole will not provide adequate coverage of gonorrhea or chlamydia. Although metronidazole is recommended if there is evidence of bacterial vaginosis, trichomoniasis, or a pelvic abscess is present, it does not treat chlamydial infections.

Ness RB, Soper DE, Holley RL, Peipert J, Randall H, Sweet RL, et al. Effectiveness of inpatient and outpatient treatment strategies for women with pelvic inflammatory disease: results from the Pelvic Inflammatory Disease Evaluation and Clinical Health (PEACH) Randomized Trial. Am J Obstet Gynecol 2002;186:929–37.

Workowski KA, Berman S. Sexually transmitted diseases treatment guidelines, 2010. Centers for Disease Control and Prevention [published erratum appears in MMWR Morb Mortal Wkly Rep 2011;60:18]. MMWR Recomm Rep 2010;59:1–110.

75

Screening for vaginal intraepithelial neoplasia

A 30-year-old nulligravid woman has a colposcopic evaluation for a high-grade squamous intra-epithelial lesion (HSIL) Pap test result. No ectocervical lesions are observed, and endocervical curettage result is reported as negative. In light of these findings, the lesion that must be excluded is

      (A) vulvar intraepithelial neoplasia 3
      (B) adenocarcinoma in situ of the cervix
*   (C) vaginal intraepithelial neoplasia (VAIN) 3
      (D) endometrial hyperplasia
      (E) chronic cervicitis

The goal of Pap test screening is to detect precancer-ous lesions of the cervix and to prevent morbidity and mortality of cervical cancer. In 2012, new guidelines that incorporated age-specific screening intervals and human papillomavirus (HPV) cotesting were approved by the American Cancer Society, American Society for Colposcopy and Cervical Pathology (ASCCP), and American Society for Clinical Pathology (Appendix H) and further updated in 2013 (Appendix I). Infection with HPV is associated with neoplasia in the cervix, vagina, vulva, anus, and nasopharynx. Vaginal intraepithelial neoplasia is less common than cervical intraepithelial neoplasia, with an incidence of 2–3 per million women. Approximately 50–90% of women with VAIN have or have had intraepithelial neoplasia or cancer of the cervix or vulva. Human papillomavirus serotypes 16 and 18 are the most common serotypes seen with VAIN. The natural history of VAIN is not well characterized, but progres-sion of VAIN 3 to invasive cancer has been reported. As with cervical intraepithelial neoplasia 3, treatment of VAIN 3 is recommended to prevent progression to invasive disease.

The patient described in this clinical scenario has a Pap test–biopsy result discrepancy, and further evaluation of the vagina is indicated. If a patient has no obvious vaginal or cervical dysplasia after thorough colposcopic evalu-ation, the ASCCP guidelines recommend either close follow-up or a conization procedure to identify occult high-grade intraepithelial neoplasia. Complications of conization, whether cold knife conization or loop electro-cautery excision, include infection, hemorrhage, preterm labor, cervical incompetence, and cervical stenosis. In the nulligravid patient who desires future pregnancy, coniza-tion can lead to significant complications. Therefore, attempts should be made to exclude VAIN as a cause for the abnormal Pap test result. Before recommending close follow-up or a conization procedure, this patient should have a thorough colposcopic evaluation of the entire vagina with acetic acid staining and Lugol staining. Most

commonly, VAIN occurs in the upper third of the vagina and shows a raised, white, and granular appearance after acetic acid staining. After application of Lugol solution, the normal vagina will stain dark brown, whereas VAIN will appear a bright mustard yellow. Biopsy can be per-formed with the use of cervical biopsy forceps.

If VAIN 2 or VAIN 3 is identified, several treatment options are available based on the size and location of the lesion—VAIN can be ablated with a carbon dioxide laser, excised with a cold knife or electrosurgical loop, or treated with topical medications, such as imiquimod or 5-fluourouracil. Recurrence rates are 20% with any of these therapies. If VAIN 1 is identified on biopsy, no treatment is necessary. This represents chronic HPV infection and should be managed conservatively with annual Pap test and colposcopic evaluation. Vulvar intraepithelial neoplasia 3 is unlikely to cause an HSIL Pap test result. Endometrial hyperplasia usually occurs in the context of abnormal menstrual bleeding, as a glan-dular change, and should not be confused with HSIL. Cervical adenocarcinoma in situ should be detected on endocervical curettage. Chronic cervicitis can cause an atypical squamous cells of undetermined significance (ASC-US) Pap test result, but is unlikely to be interpreted as HSIL. If no vaginal lesion is identified, this patient should be managed according to ASCCP and American College of Obstetricians and Gynecologists guidelines.

Jakobsson M, Gissler M, Paavonen J, Tapper AM. Loop electrosurgi-cal excision procedure and the risk for preterm birth. Obstet Gynecol 2009;114:504–10.

Massad LS, Einstein MH, Huh WK, Katki HA, Kinney WK, Schiffman M, et al. 2012 updated consensus guidelines for the management of abnormal cervical cancer screening tests and cancer precursors. 2012 ASCCP Consensus Guidelines Conference. Obstet Gynecol 2013;121:829–46.

Saslow D, Solomon D, Lawson HW, Killackey M, Kulasingam SL, Cain J, et al. American Cancer Society, American Society for Colposcopy and Cervical Pathology, and American Society for Clinical Pathology screening guidelines for the prevention and early detection of cervical cancer. ACS-ASCCP-ASCP Cervical Cancer Guideline Committee. CA Cancer J Clin 2012;62:147–72.

Watson M, Saraiya M, Wu X. Update of HPV-associated female genital cancers in the United States, 1999-2004. J Womens Health (Larchmt) 2009;18:1731–8.

Werner CL, Lo JY, Heffernan T, Griffith WF, McIntire DD, Leveno KJ. Loop electrosurgical excision procedure and risk of preterm birth. Obstet Gynecol 2010;115:605–8.

76

Atypical endometrial hyperplasia and endometrial cancer

A 53-year-old woman comes to your office for abnormal uterine bleeding. Her body mass index is 35 (calculated as weight in kilograms divided by height in meters squared). Endometrial biopsy is performed and the pathology report shows complex atypical endometrial hyperplasia and well-differentiated endometrioid adenocarcinoma with squamous differentiation, International Federation of Gynecology and Obstetrics grade 1. During counseling, you explain to the patient that the component of surgical staging for endometrial cancer that remains most controversial in this setting is

      (A) appendectomy
      (B) bilateral salpingo-oophorectomy
*   (C) lymphadenectomy
      (D) omentectomy
      (E) random peritoneal biopsies

Endometrial cancer is the most common type of female genital tract cancer. It occurs in approximately 2.6% of women in the United States during their lifetime. Approximately 72% of cases are diagnosed in stage I; 12% in stage II; 13% in stage III; and 3% in stage IV. Approximately 99% of women with endometrial cancer have symptomatic bleeding or vaginal discharge. Most cases of endometrial cancer occur in postmenopausal women. However, up to 14% of women with endometrial cancer are premenopausal and 4% are younger than 40 years. Younger women are at an increased risk of cancer associated with the Lynch syndrome, also known as hereditary nonpolyposis colorectal cancer, ie, colorectal, small bowel, ovarian, ureteral, or renal pelvic cancer, and synchronous or metachronous ovarian types of cancer other than Lynch syndrome.

Endometrial cancer exists in two forms: 1) type I and 2) type II. The more common form is type I or estrogen-dependent endometrial cancer, which includes endometrioid adenocarcinoma. Excess endogenous estrogen or unopposed exogenous estrogen can predispose women to development of endometrial hyperplasia and, subsequently, endometrial cancer. Table 76-1 lists risk factors for type I endometrial cancer.

In type II endometrial cancer, the background endometrium is atrophic or associated with polyps. There are no known epidemiologic risk factors. Type II endometrial cancer is more aggressive and lethal than the more indo-lent type I endometrial cancer and includes clear-cell and serous carcinomas and uterine carcinosarcomas.

Endometrial cancer should be comprehensively surgically staged based on guidelines of the International Federation of Gynecology and Obstetrics. *Comprehensive surgical staging of endometrial cancer* is defined as removal of the uterus, cervix, adnexa, pelvic and para-aortic lymph node tissues and obtaining pelvic washing samples. Controversy exists about whether to perform pelvic or paraaortic lymphadenectomy in women with early stage disease. Proponents of comprehensive surgical staging point out the benefits of prognosis, diagnosis, and proper triage to help in the decision about adjuvant treatment. Opponents of comprehensive surgical staging cite morbidity associated with lymphadenectomy without a clear 5-year disease-free survival benefit. Complications of paraaortic and pelvic lymphadenectomy include injury to major vessels or nerves, lymphedema, and associated cellulitis. Those who do not advocate comprehensive staging have differing views on degree of lymphadenectomy. Recommendations range from no lymphadenectomy to pelvic lymphadenectomy only, limited intramesenteric paraaortic lymphadenectomy, or sentinel node mapping.

Younger women with early stage endometrial cancer and a desire for childbearing may be treated with progestins and surveillance with endometrial sampling approximately every 3 months. Alternatively, women may have surgical staging without bilateral salpingo-oophorectomy

TABLE 76-1. Risk Factors for Uterine Cancer

Factors Influencing Risk	Estimated Relative Risk*
Older age	2–3
Residency in North America or Northern Europe	3–18
Higher level of education or income	1.5–2
White race	2
Nulliparity	3
History of infertility	2–3
Menstrual irregularities	1.5
Late age at natural menopause	2–3
Early age at menarche	1.5–2
Long-term use of high dosages of menopausal estrogens	10–20
Long-term use of high dosages of combination oral contraceptives	0.3–0.5
High cumulative doses of tamoxifen citrate	3–7
Obesity	2–5
Polycystic ovary syndrome	Less than 5
History of diabetes mellitus, hypertension, gallbladder disease, or thyroid disease	1.3–3
Cigarette smoking	0.5

*Relative risks depend on the study and referent group employed.

Modified from Management of endometrial cancer. ACOG Practice Bulletin No. 65. American College of Obstetricians and Gynecologists. Obstet Gynecol 2005;106:413–25.

to enable possible future oocyte retrieval or to avoid surgical menopause. Careful oncologic, psychotherapeutic, genetic, and reproductive counseling is recommended along with follow-up.

Endometrial cancer spreads through lymphatic and hematogenous dissemination. Omentectomy is included in complete surgical staging for type II endometrial cancer and only for type I disease if the omentum is involved with the tumor. Staging for endometrial cancer does not include either appendectomy or random peritoneal biopsies.

Management of endometrial cancer. ACOG Practice Bulletin No. 65. American College of Obstetricians and Gynecologists. Obstet Gynecol 2005;106:413–25.

Penner KR, Dorigo O, Aoyama C, Ostrzega N, Balzer BL, Rao J, et al. Predictors of resolution of complex atypical hyperplasia or grade 1 endometrial adenocarcinoma in premenopausal women treated with progestin therapy. Gynecol Oncol 2012;124:542–8.

Rungruang B, Olawaiye AB. Comprehensive surgical staging for endometrial cancer. Rev Obstet Gynecol 2012;5:28–34.

Trimble CL, Method M, Leitao M, Lu K, Ioffe O, Hampton M, et al. Management of endometrial precancers. Society of Gynecologic Oncology Clinical Practice Committee. Obstet Gynecol 2012;120:1160–75.

Wright JD, Barrena Medel NI, Sehouli J, Fujiwara K, Herzog TJ. Contemporary management of endometrial cancer. Lancet 2012;379:1352–60.

Zivanovic O, Carter J, Kauff ND, Barakat RR. A review of the challenges faced in the conservative treatment of young women with endometrial carcinoma and risk of ovarian cancer. Gynecol Oncol 2009;115:504–9.

77

Etonogestrel subdermal implants

A 19-year-old woman comes to your office for insertion of an etonogestrel subdermal implant for contraception. She reports that her menstrual cycles are regular and that her last menses were 5 days ago. Her body mass index is 28.4 (calculated as weight in kilograms divided by height in meters squared). During counseling, you tell her that the most common adverse effect of the etonogestrel subdermal implant is

* (A) abnormal uterine bleeding
  (B) headache
  (C) weight gain
  (D) breast pain
  (E) emotional lability

Long-acting reversible contraceptive (LARC) methods, including intrauterine device and the subdermal contraceptive implant, are characterized by high continuation rates and low failure rates. The number of unintended pregnancies in the United States remains high, at approximately 50%. For this reason, the Institute of Medicine has recommended an increase in the long-acting reversible contraceptive use among young women.

The subdermal etonogestrel implant is a 4-cm long single-rod that contains 68 mg of etonogestrel, which is the biologically active metabolite of the progestin desogestrel, embedded in an ethylene vinyl acetate core. The implant releases etonogestrel at a rate of 60–70 micrograms per day in the first few weeks after insertion and then decreases to 25–30 micrograms per day by the end of the third year. The primary mechanism of action of the implant is suppression of ovulation, in addition to thickening of the cervical mucus and thinning of the endometrial lining. It is approved in the United States for up to 3 years of use and is prepackaged in a sterile applicator that is preloaded with the rod. The insertion is subdermal at the medial aspect of the nondominant upper arm. The etonogestrel implant is one of the most effective contraceptive options available, with a risk of pregnancy of approximately 0.05%.

The most common adverse effect is abnormal uterine bleeding. More than 50% of women who use the implant report infrequent vaginal bleeding or amenorrhea. Approximately 25% of these patients report either prolonged bleeding (16.9%) or frequent bleeding (6.1%). Other adverse effects include headache (15.3%), weight gain (11.8%), acne (11.4%), breast pain (10.2%), and emotional lability (5.7%).

Approximately 25% of patients will discontinue the use of the implant prematurely, with abnormal uterine bleeding being the most common reason cited (11.3%). Other reasons for discontinuation include emotional lability (2.3%), weight increase (2.3%), acne (1.3%), headache (1.6%), and depression (1.0%).

Complications related to the insertion procedures are rare (approximately 1%) and include pain, bleeding at the insertion site, hematoma, difficult insertion, and unrecognized noninsertion. Complications related to the removal procedures also are uncommon (approximately 1.7%) and include breakage of the rod and inability to palpate or locate the implant.

Casey PM, Long ME, Marnach ML, Bury JE. Bleeding related to etonogestrel subdermal implant in a US population. Contraception 2011;83:426–30.

Espey E, Ogburn T. Long-acting reversible contraceptives: intrauterine devices and the contraceptive implant. Obstet Gynecol 2011;117:705–19.

Long-acting reversible contraception: implants and intrauterine devices. Practice bulletin No. 121. American College of Obstetricians and Gynecologists. Obstet Gynecol 2011;118:184–96.

Mansour D, Korver T, Marintcheva-Petrova M, Fraser IS. The effects of Implanon on menstrual bleeding patterns. Eur J Contraception Reprod Healthcare 2008;13(Suppl 1):13–28.

78

Recurrent genital herpes

A 33-year-old woman, gravida 2, para 2, comes to your office for routine well-woman care. Her medical history is significant for genital herpes (a genital lesion that was culture-positive for herpes simplex virus type 2 [HSV-2]) diagnosed 3 years ago. Since that time, she has noted recurrent outbreaks every 1–2 months. She uses an oral antiviral drug as needed for outbreaks. Currently she is asymptomatic. Your examination confirms normal vulvar anatomy without lesions. The best management plan for this patient is

      (A) confirmation of diagnosis with type-specific serologic test
      (B) episodic antiviral therapy
      (C) local antiviral therapy
*   (D) suppressive antiviral therapy

Herpes simplex virus type 1 (HSV-1) and HSV-2 can both cause genital herpes. Infection with HSV is chronic. The prevalence of HSV-2 antibody among U.S. women aged 12 years and older is approximately 26%, with more than 910,000 new infections annually. However, most cases of HSV are misdiagnosed by women or their health care providers; it has been estimated that only 10% of cases of HSV-2 infections are actually diagnosed.

Especially among younger women, HSV-1 is becoming a frequent cause of genital herpes. Overall, the seroprevalence of HSV-1 in the United States is 67% (including all sites of infection). Although the initial presentation of genital herpes is the same for HSV-1 and HSV-2, the rate of recurrence of genital HSV is lower for HSV-1 than for HSV-2.

A definitive diagnosis should be confirmed by laboratory testing, even if the infection was established in the past on clinical grounds because the sensitivity and specificity of clinical diagnosis alone are poor. In addition to viral detection methods (culture), type-specific antibodies can help to establish the diagnosis. Antibodies to HSV-2 are detected 2–12 weeks after acquisition of infection and persist indefinitely. The described patient had confirmation of HSV-2 by previous culture of a lesion.

The frequency of clinical and subclinical viral reactivation varies widely and probably depends more on the host than viral factors. Antiviral agents cannot eradicate latent HSV infection and hence do not change the frequency or severity of recurrences once therapy is stopped.

In the absence of antiviral therapy, the median recurrence rate after the first episode of HSV-2 infection is approximately four recurrences per year, with approximately 40% of patients having at least six recurrences and 20% of patients having more than 10 recurrences in the first year. In most patients, disease activity and HSV shedding are highest in the first year after infection, then gradually decrease with time.

Recurrent episodes of genital herpes can be managed effectively with either daily suppressive or episodic antiviral drugs. Management of genital herpes with antiviral drugs aims to abate the signs and symptoms of genital herpes, which results in faster symptom resolution and lesion healing, decreased viral shedding, and prevention of new lesions. Episodic antiviral therapy provides the greatest benefit when patients are educated to recognize prodromal and early symptoms and are able to self-initiate treatment. The greatest chance of resolving a recurrence without development of a lesion occurs when oral treatment is initiated within 24 hours of the first prodromal sign or symptom. Although this may be considered for the described patient, her outbreaks occur quite frequently and they would be better addressed with suppressive therapy (Box 78-1 and Box 78-2).

Suppressive therapy for genital herpes prevents approximately 80% of recurrent HSV episodes. If they do occur, breakthrough recurrences last shorter. In some patients, suppressive therapy may eliminate recurrences for several years. Reduction also has been noted in asymptomatic viral shedding, with an approximately 48% reduction rate in transmission between discordant sexual partners. Although clinicians have traditionally reserved suppressive therapy for patients with frequent recurrences, studies show that patients with low frequency of recurrence may benefit, with reduction or elimination of recurrences. Patients rate their quality of life higher when receiving suppressive therapy compared with episodic therapy.

Topical acyclovir antiviral medication is not effective therapy and does not add to the benefit of oral medication. Penciclovir cream and over-the-counter preparations for oral herpes have not been assessed for effectiveness against genital herpes and are not recommended. The management of genital herpes should be tailored to the individual. It should include counseling regarding the variable natural history, appearance of lesions, educa-

---

BOX 78-1

Suggested Regimens for Suppressive Therapy for Recurrent Genital Herpes

Acyclovir, 400 mg orally, twice a day, or
Famciclovir, 250 mg orally, twice a day, or
Valacyclovir, 500 mg orally, once a day*, or
Valacyclovir, 1 g orally, once a day

*Valacyclovir, 500 mg orally once a day, might be less effective than other valacyclovir or acyclovir dosages in patients who have very frequent recurrences (ie, 10 episodes per year or more).

Workowski KA, Berman S. Sexually transmitted diseases treatment guidelines, 2010. Centers for Disease Control and Prevention [published erratum appears in MMWR Morb Mortal Wkly Rep 2011;60:18]. MMWR Recomm Rep 2010;59:1–110.

---

tion about prevention of transmission, and psychosocial aspects.

Gupta R, Warren T, Wald A. Genital herpes. Lancet 2007;370:2127–37.

Gynecologic herpes simplex virus infections. ACOG Practice Bulletin No. 57. American College of Obstetricians and Gynecologists. Obstet Gynecol 2004;104:1111–8.

Workowski KA, Berman S. Sexually transmitted diseases treatment guidelines, 2010. Centers for Disease Control and Prevention [published erratum appears in MMWR Morb Mortal Wkly Rep 2011;60:18]. MMWR Recomm Rep 2010;59:1–110.

BOX 78-2

Suggested Regimens for Episodic Therapy for Recurrent Genital Herpes

Acyclovir, 400 mg orally, three times a day for 5 days, or
Acyclovir, 800 mg orally, twice a day for 5 days, or
Acyclovir, 800 mg orally, three times a day for 2 days, or
Famciclovir, 125 mg orally, twice a day for 5 days, or
Famciclovir, 1,000 mg orally, twice a day for 1 day, or
Famciclovir, 500 mg orally, once, then 250 mg twice a day for 2 days, or
Valacyclovir, 500 mg orally, twice a day for 3 days, or
Valacyclovir, 1 g orally, once a day for 5 days

Workowski KA, Berman S. Sexually transmitted diseases treatment guidelines, 2010. Centers for Disease Control and Prevention [published erratum appears in MMWR Morb Mortal Wkly Rep 2011;60:18]. MMWR Recomm Rep 2010;59:1–110.

79

Coding for office-based procedures

A 29-year-old woman, gravida 3, para 3, undergoes hysteroscopic sterilization in your office. During the procedure, you perform paracervical block and cervical dilation. The right fallopian tube is successfully occluded; however, the left fallopian tube cannot be cannulated because of spasm despite repeated efforts. You decide to terminate the procedure and advise the patient to return in 2 weeks for hysteroscopic occlusion of the left fallopian tube. When you submit the billing for the initial procedure, in addition to the *Current Procedural Terminology* (CPT) code[1] for hysteroscopic tubal occlusion (58565), you will need to include a code for

     (A) cervical dilation

 *   (B) reduced service modifier

     (C) paracervical block

     (D) diagnostic hysteroscopy

The use of the reduced service code modifier 52 provides the means to report that the performed procedure was altered because of changing circumstances that did not allow the completion of the procedure as planned. Because a unilateral procedure was performed, the billing should include only partial procedure indicated by using modifier, which should also be used when the procedure is repeated for the contralateral fallopian tube. Modifiers also can be used when a service has both components— professional and technical. This reduced service code should not be used when the planned procedure is unsuccessful and a different approach is used during the same surgical session, eg, if hysteroscopy is unsuccessful and laparoscopy is then performed.

The CPT codes 58563 (Hysteroscopy, surgical; with endometrial ablation, eg, endometrial resection, electrosurgical ablation, thermoablation) and 58565 (Hysteroscopy, surgical; with bilateral fallopian tube cannulation to induce occlusion by placement of permanent implants) are bundled to include the hysteroscopy, cervical dilation, and paracervical block. The practice expense that is associated with these codes includes the allowance for the procedure kit that was used so no additional reimbursement can be given for the kit.

For non-Medicare patients, the paracervical block (CPT code 64435) may be reported separately when the procedure is performed with the following hysteroscopy codes:

- 58555 Hysteroscopy, diagnostic (separate procedure)

- 58558 Hysteroscopy, surgical; with sampling (biopsy) of endometrium and/or polypectomy, with or without dilation and curettage

- 58559 Hysteroscopy, surgical; with lysis of intrauterine adhesions (any method)

- 58560 Hysteroscopy, surgical; with division or resection of intrauterine septum (any method)

- 58561 Hysteroscopy, surgical; with removal of myomas

- 58562 Hysteroscopy, surgical; with removal of affected foreign body

For Medicare patients, the paracervical block is bundled into the aforementioned CPT codes. However, it can be reimbursed when performed, and modifier 59 (distinct procedural services) is used.

American Congress of Obstetricians and Gynecologists. 2013 Ob/Gyn coding manual: components of correct procedural coding. Washington, DC: American Congress of Obstetricians and Gynecologists; 2013.

American Medical Association. Current procedural terminology 2013. Chicago (IL): AMA; 2012.

80

Complications of uterine artery embolization

A 38-year-old woman, gravida 2, para 2, comes to the emergency department with vaginal bleeding and severe abdominal cramping. She underwent uterine artery embolization 14 weeks ago. Her temperature is 38.5°C (101.3°F), blood pressure is 100 mm Hg systolic and 80 mm Hg diastolic, and the heart rate is 104 beats per minute. Blood workup is significant for a white blood cell count of 12,800 per microliter and hemoglobin level of 10.2 g/dL, decreased from a preoperative hemoglobin level of 13.5 g/dL. The physician in the emergency department had difficulty performing the speculum examination because of a mass in the vagina. Pelvic examination reveals uterine tenderness but no adnexal tenderness. Gas is not present within the myoma as per the abdominal and pelvic computed tomography (CT) scan. The most likely diagnosis is

    (A) normal findings
    (B) tubo–ovarian abscess
    (C) pyomyoma
 *   (D) prolapsed submucosal myoma
    (E) uterine embolization material

Treatment of abnormal uterine bleeding and bulk-related symptoms associated with myomas has traditionally been by myomectomy or hysterectomy. Since its inception in 1995, uterine artery embolization has developed into another popular treatment modality.

Short-term data that compare hysterectomy and myomectomy with uterine artery embolization suggest that the benefits of uterine artery embolization include a shorter procedure length, less likelihood of a blood transfusion, shorter hospital stay, and reduced time to resumption of routine activities. Major complication rates, quality of life, and patient satisfaction rates are similar among the three procedures. However, uterine artery embolization is associated with higher rates of minor short- and long-term complications, more unscheduled readmissions after discharge, and an increased surgical reintervention rate. Long-term data show a fivefold increased reintervention rate at 5 years. Three studies cited reintervention rates at 5 years in the range of 14–32% in contrast with hysterectomy (4–11%) and myomectomy (4–23%). This may balance out the initial cost advantage of uterine artery embolization. Myomectomy may be associated with better fertility outcomes than uterine artery embolization, but more research is needed.

Absolute contraindications to uterine artery embolization include active infection and viable pregnancy. In patients who desire future fertility, uterine artery embolization is still considered investigational. Live births have been reported after uterine artery embolization. Potential complications after uterine artery embolization are ovarian failure caused by impairment of ovarian blood flow and infection that possibly causes adhesive disease with

subsequent infertility. In one report, uterine rupture at childbirth after uterine artery embolization was noted. In addition, a theoretical risk exists of an adverse effect on placental blood flow after uterine artery embolization. Studies have shown increased risks of preterm labor, intrauterine growth restriction, and postpartum hemorrhage in women who become pregnant after uterine artery embolization.

The goal of uterine artery embolization for treatment of myomas is to totally occlude both of the uterine vessels. Afterwards, the myometrium rapidly establishes a new blood supply through collateral vessels from the ovarian and vaginal circulations. In contrast, blood to myomas appears to be supplied by end arteries without the collateral blood flow. Therefore, they are preferentially affected by the reduction in flow. This results in a decrease in myoma volume with resultant improvement in the woman's symptoms.

The described patient has fever, an elevated white blood cell count, heavy menstrual bleeding, and submucosal myoma expulsion with a closed cervix. She has uterine tenderness but no adnexal tenderness. Gas is not present within the myoma on abdominal and pelvic CT. The most likely diagnosis is prolapsed submucosal myoma. Appropriate management includes antibiotic therapy and analgesics and myomectomy or hysterectomy. Figure 80-1 shows a suggested management algorithm.

Myoma expulsion can occur weeks to years after embolization. Rates of myoma expulsion are in the range of 1.7–50%. Myomas that are expelled are submucosal in location. The entire tumor may be expelled at once

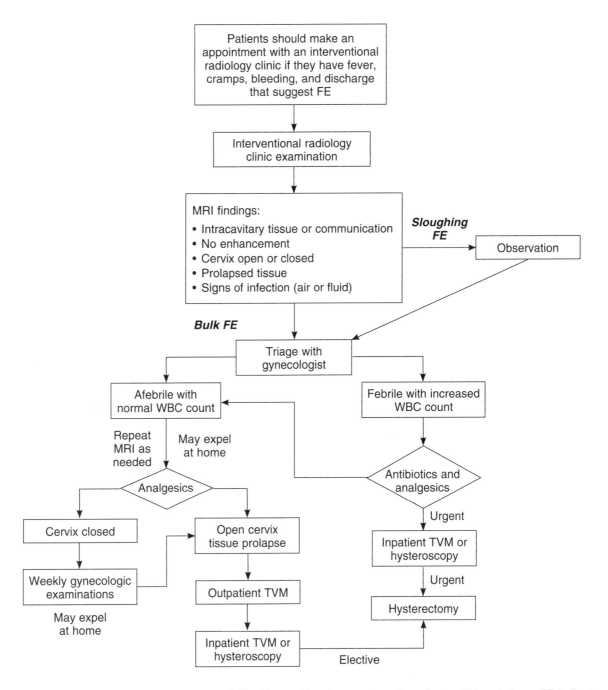

FIG. 80-1. Algorithm for the management of fibroid expulsion in symptomatic patients. Abbreviations: FE indicates fibroid expulsion; MRI, magnetic resonance imaging; TVM, transvaginal myomectomy; WBC, white blood count. (Reprinted from Journal of Vascular and Interventional Radiology, Volume 22, Shlansky-Goldberg RD, Coryell L, Stavropoulos SW, Trerotola SO, Mondschein J, Beshara M, et al. Outcomes following fibroid expulsion after uterine artery embolization, pages 1586–93, Copyright 2011, with permission from Elsevier.)

or it can incrementally slough or fragment over time. Symptoms include vaginal discharge, bleeding, pain, and fever.

Pyomyoma, a suppurative myoma, usually submucosal in location, is a rare complication of uterine artery embo-

lization. The clinical triad of pyomyoma is a fibroid uterus, sepsis, and no other source of infection. The presence of gas within the myoma on CT is pathognomonic of a pyomyoma. Postprocedural imaging, usually magnetic resonance imaging, is employed to assess percentage of infarction of the dominant myoma and the overall myoma infarction compared with baseline. The embolization material cannot be visualized on postprocedural imaging studies.

Burke CT, Funaki BS, Ray CE, Kinney TB, Kostelic JK, Loesberg A, et al. ACR Appropriateness Criteria® on treatment of uterine myomas. J Am Coll Radiol 2011;8:228–34.

Gupta JK, Sinha A, Lumsden MA, Hickey M. Uterine artery embolization for symptomatic uterine fibroids. Cochrane Database of Systematic Reviews 2012, Issue 5. Art. No.: CD005073. DOI: 10.1002/14651858. CD005073.pub3.

Kroencke TJ, Scheurig C, Poellinger A, Gronewold M, Hamm B. Uterine artery embolization for myomas: percentage of infarction predicts clinical outcome. Radiology 2010;255:834–41.

Moss JG, Cooper KG, Khaund A, Murray LS, Murray GD, Wu O, et al. Randomised comparison of uterine artery embolisation (UAE) with surgical treatment in patients with symptomatic uterine fibroids (REST trial): 5-year results. BJOG 2011;118:936–44.

Shlansky-Goldberg RD, Coryell L, Stavropoulos SW, Trerotola SO, Mondschein J, Beshara M, et al. Outcomes following fibroid expulsion after uterine artery embolization. J Vasc Interv Radiol 2011;22:1586–93.

81

Abnormal uterine bleeding in an adolescent patient

A 14-year-old patient, who underwent menarche 15 months ago, has irregular, heavy menses that occur every 2–8 weeks and last up to 14 days. She reports the bleeding to be heavy with clots, and she is having accidents at school and at home. She has been experiencing menstrual cramps, but reports that they are relieved by ibuprofen. Her blood pressure is 110 mm Hg systolic and 80 mm Hg diastolic and the heart rate is 82 beats per minute. Her abdomen is soft and nontender; no masses are noted. The remainder of the physical examination is unremarkable. An office urine pregnancy test yields a negative result. The most likely etiology of her menstrual abnormality is

   (A) chlamydial cervicitis
   (B) hypothyroidism
   (C) bleeding disorder
 * (D) anovulation
   (E) endometriosis

Anovulation is the most common etiology of abnormal uterine bleeding in adolescents. Profuse and prolonged menstruation is one of the most common adolescent gynecologic problems. In most patients, anovulation will be the underlying cause. Up to 85% of cycles in the first gynecologic year are anovulatory. The median age of menarche in the United States has been stable for the past 40–50 years at 12.43 years. By the third gynecologic year, 60–80% of the menstrual cycles will be ovulatory and occur at 21–34-day intervals. Often, it is difficult to assess the amount of flow because young patients are not familiar with what is considered a normal flow, and accidents may occur because of many reasons other than heavy flow, such as restrictions to bathroom access during the school day. Most teenagers will need to change their pads or tampons 3–6 times per day; changing more frequently may suggest a clinical concern. Cases of younger patients who report passing blood clots have been associated with an increased risk of anemia. Anovulatory cycles typically resolve with gynecologic age, but if treatment is indicated, these patients respond well to hormonal therapy.

Bleeding disorders should be considered in young women with heavy menstrual bleeding, but are not the most common cause of abnormal bleeding in patients shortly after menarche. The most common bleeding disorders are von Willebrand disease and platelet function disorders. Patients who report any of the following symptoms should be screened for bleeding disorders:

- Menses that last more than 7 days
- "Gushing blood" or having bleeding heavy enough to limit activity
- History of anemia
- Family history of a bleeding disorder
- Abnormal bleeding after a hemostatic challenge, such as tooth extraction or surgery

Based on her history, this patient would qualify for screening for bleeding disorders, although a bleeding disorder is not the most likely diagnosis. Initial laboratory testing includes complete blood count with differential, platelet count, prothrombin time, activated partial thromboplastic time, and fibrinogen level determination. If any of the initial screening laboratory evaluation yields abnormal results or if a bleeding abnormality is suspected, a workup for von Willebrand disease is indicated, including serum testing for factor VIII coagulant activity, ristocetin cofactor activity, and the concentration of von Willebrand factor antigen.

Adolescents with endometriosis typically have dysmenorrhea refractory to treatment with hormonal contraceptives and nonsteroidal antiinflammatory drugs. Dysmenorrhea in this patient is relieved with ibuprofen, which makes endometriosis unlikely. Chlamydial cervicitis can accompany abnormal vaginal bleeding, but it is not the most likely diagnosis in this case. All sexu-

ally active adolescents should be screened annually for *Chlamydia*. Hypothyroidism may be associated with abnormal bleeding, but it is not the most likely cause of this patient's bleeding pattern.

American College of Obstetricians and Gynecologists. Management of anovulatory bleeding. ACOG Practice Bulletin 14. Washington, DC: ACOG; 2000.

Boswell HB. The adolescent with menorrhagia: why, who, and how to evaluate for a bleeding disorder. J Pediatr Adolesc Gynecol 2011;24: 228–30.

Menstruation in girls and adolescents: using the menstrual cycle as a vital sign. ACOG Committee Opinion No. 349. American College of Obstetricians and Gynecologists. Obstet Gynecol 2006;108:1323–8.

Wilkinson JP, Kadir RA. Management of abnormal uterine bleeding in adolescents. J Pediatr Adolesc Gynecol 2010;23:S22–S30.

82

Hysteroscopic complications

A 37-year-old nulligravid woman is scheduled for an in-office diagnostic hysteroscopy for abnormal uterine bleeding. During the procedure, the cervix is noted to be stenotic and dilation is performed. The hysteroscope is then inserted with some force into the uterine cavity with saline solution for distention. At first, distention is inadequate and the saline bag is raised higher on the intravenous pole. A 2–3-mm defect is immediately noted at the top of the fundus with minimal blood oozing into the cavity. No other endometrial pathology is noted. The procedure is terminated and the fluid deficit is 150 mL. At the end of the procedure, the patient is pain free and her abdomen is soft and nontender. She has a blood pressure of 117 mm Hg systolic and 82 mm Hg diastolic and pulse of 72 beats per minute. The best next step in the management of this patient is

* (A) observation
   (B) immediate laparoscopy
   (C) discharge home
   (D) electrolyte measurement
   (E) ultrasonography of abdomen and pelvis

Diagnostic hysteroscopy is used to visualize the endocervical canal, endometrial cavity, and fallopian tube ostia. Hysteroscopes are available in flexible or rigid configurations. A distention medium is required, and the type of medium chosen depends on the requirements of the procedures, especially if electrosurgery is required. The advantages and disadvantages of different types of distention media are shown in Table 82-1. Contraindications to performing hysteroscopy are known pregnancy, active genital tract infections, and active herpetic infection. The most common perioperative complications associated with operative hysteroscopy are hemorrhage (2.4%), uterine perforation (1.5%), and cervical laceration (1–11%).

Fluid overload is a rare complication in hysteroscopy and is suspected when the amount of distention fluid

used far outweighs the amount retrieved. If the resulting fluid deficit reaches 1,000–1,500 mL of a nonelectrolyte solution or 2,500 mL of an electrolyte solution, further infusion should be stopped, and the procedure should be promptly concluded. Level of electrolytes should be assessed, administration of diuretics considered, and further diagnostic and therapeutic intervention begun as indicated.

Generally, hysteroscopic procedures are considered safe. Such procedures are commonly performed in the office. The rate of uterine perforation has been estimated to be approximately 1.1–1.4%. This figure ranges from 0.13% for diagnostic procedures to 4.5% if the procedure is operative hysteroscopy for adhesiolysis. Risk factors for uterine perforation include nulliparity; endometrial

TABLE 82-1. Advantages and Disadvantages of Distention Media

Type	Advantages	Disadvantages and Safety Precautions
Carbon dioxide gas	Ease of cleaning and maintaining equipment Clear view of cavity	To minimize the risk of gas embolization, the flow of carbon dioxide should be limited to 100 mL/min with intrauterine pressure of less than 100 mm Hg and used with a hysteroscopic insufflator. Insufflators designed for use in laparoscopy must not be used for hysteroscopy.
Electrolyte-poor fluid (eg, glycine, 1.5%; sorbitol, 3%; and mannitol, 5%)	Compatible with radiofrequency energy Monopolar devices require electrolyte-poor fluids.	Excessive absorption of this type of fluids can cause hyponatremia, hyperammonemia, and decreased serum osmolality with the potential for seizures, cerebral edema, and death.
Electrolyte-containing fluid	Readily available Isotonic Media of choice during diagnostic hysteroscopy and in operative cases where mechanical, laser, or bipolar energy is used	Although the risk of hyponatremia and decreased serum osmolality can be reduced by using these media, pulmonary edema and congestive heart failure can still occur. Careful attention should be paid to fluid input and output, with particular attention to the fluid deficit.

Hysteroscopy. Technology Assessment No. 7. American College of Obstetricians and Gynecologists. Obstet Gynecol 2011;117:1486–91.

or myometrial thinning as in menopause; gonadotropin-releasing hormone agonist use; distortion of the endocervical canal from prior surgery, such as cone biopsy; markedly retroverted uterus, and the excessive use of force. It is estimated that more than one half of the perforations occur at the time of entry through the cervical canal. Therefore, if cervical stenosis is suspected, preoperative placement of laminaria or osmotic dilators or pretreatment with misoprostol may be recommended.

In the described patient, a uterine perforation was noted during the procedure. Because most diagnostic hysteroscopy equipment uses an outer sheath that is 5 mm or less in diameter, the resulting uterine perforation is small. This patient was noted to be stable hemodynamically, pain free, with no evidence of heavy bleeding, either vaginally or intraabdominally. Therefore, immediate laparoscopy is not indicated. Because a uterine perforation was encountered, immediate discharge is not appropriate before evaluating the patient for hemodynamic stability, bleeding, and pain.

Because suspicion for intraabdominal bleeding is low, ultrasonography of the abdomen and pelvis may reveal a small amount of distention fluid; however, this will not alter this patient's management. In addition, a small fluid deficit was noted and hence checking electrolytes is not indicated. Given that the patient has had a surgical complication, immediate discharge is not appropriate and the best course of management is observation.

Aydeniz B, Gruber IV, Schauf B, Kurek R, Meyer A, Wallwiener D. A multicenter survey of complications associated with 21,676 operative hysteroscopies. Eur J Obstet Gynecol Reprod Biol 2002;104:160–4.

Bradley LD. Complications in hysteroscopy: prevention, treatment and legal risk. Curr Opin Obstet Gynecol 2002;14:409–15.

Hysteroscopy. Technology Assessment No. 7. American College of Obstetricians and Gynecologists. Obstet Gynecol 2011;117:1486–91.

Jansen FW, Vredevoogd CB, van Ulzen K, Hermans J, Trimbos JB, Trimbos-Kemper TC. Complications of hysteroscopy: a prospective, multicenter study. Obstet Gynecol 2000;96:266–70.

83

Use of the levonorgestrel intrauterine device for heavy menstrual bleeding

A 32-year-old woman, gravida 3, para 3, who does not desire future fertility, has been experiencing heavy menstrual bleeding. Her past medical history is significant for asthma; she is otherwise healthy. The workup includes pelvic ultrasonography (normal result), hemoglobin measurement (10.3 gm/dL), cervical screening for gonorrhea and chlamydia, and normal cervical cytology. Her only sibling had been healthy until she recently received a diagnosis of pulmonary embolus at age 35 years. The most appropriate first-line therapy to treat heavy menstrual bleeding in this patient is

      (A) combination oral contraceptives
*   (B) levonorgestrel intrauterine device (IUD)
      (C) copper IUD
      (D) endometrial ablation
      (E) tranexamic acid

The International Federation of Gynecology and Obstetrics recently recommended abandoning terms, such as "menorrhagia" and "metrorrhagia," to describe abnormal uterine bleeding. The preferred terminology to describe disturbances in menstrual flow include "heavy menstrual bleeding," "heavy and prolonged menstrual bleeding," and "light menstrual bleeding." *Heavy menstrual bleeding* is the most common symptom, defined as "excessive menstrual blood loss that interferes with the woman's physical, emotional, social, and material quality of life." Heavy and prolonged menstrual bleeding is a less common symptom. Its distinction from heavy menstrual bleeding is important because these two symptomatic components may have different etiologies and may respond differently to the same therapies. Light menstrual bleeding is rarely related to pathology, but often is a cultural symptom in communities where a heavy, "red" menses are valued as a perceived sign of health.

The levonorgestrel IUD is a first-line drug treatment for heavy menstrual bleeding, providing the patient plans to delay childbearing for at least 12 months. Contraindications to the levonorgestrel IUD are uterine malformations, infections, existing carcinoma, and contraindications to progestin. The levonorgestrel IUD is safe and cost-effective, and can be prescribed by primary care clinicians. In 2009, the U.S. Food and Drug Administration approved the levonorgestrel IUD for heavy menstrual bleeding for patients who desire an IUD for contraception. In a phase III clinical trial, 85% of patients treated with the levonorgestrel IUD for heavy menstrual bleeding had the menstrual blood loss normalized or reduced by at least 50%. The levonorgestrel IUD is highly effective in preventing pregnancy and normalizing heavy menstrual bleeding, which makes it the best choice for this patient.

Tranexamic acid is approved by the U.S. Food and Drug Administration for the treatment of heavy menstrual bleeding. The endometria of women with heavy menstrual bleeding have increased levels of plasminogen activators, the enzymes that cause fibrinolysis or dissolution of clots. Tranexamic acid reduces levels of tissue plasminogen activator and plasmin activity in peripheral blood, in menstrual fluid, and in the endometrium. Clinical trials show that two 650-mg tablets of tranexamic acid taken three times daily during the first 5 days of the menses reduce menstrual flow by 39%. However, tranexamic acid will not provide contraception. It is not the best choice for this patient who does not desire pregnancy. Product labeling for tranexamic acid in the United States contains a warning against prescribing it in combination with combined hormonal contraceptive methods because of concerns regarding increasing risk of venous thromboembolism. Also, it is contraindicated in patients with identified thrombophilias.

This patient's previously healthy sister recently received a diagnosis a pulmonary embolus at age 35 years. This would raise concern for the sister and the patient for an increased risk of thrombophilias, most commonly heterozygote factor V Leiden mutation. Given this family history, the patient requires screening for thrombophilias before initiating combination hormonal contraceptive methods. Therefore, combination oral contraceptives would not be the best choice for her.

The copper IUD will provide effective contraception, but will not address the patient's symptoms of heavy menstrual bleeding and resulting anemia. Although definitive evidence of the increased effectiveness of the levonorgestrel IUD over surgical procedures, such as endometrial ablation, is lacking, many experts suggest drug therapy over surgical interventions as first-line therapy for heavy menstrual bleeding. Additionally, endometrial ablation alone does not provide contraception.

Fraser IS, Critchley HO, Broder M, Munro MG. The FIGO recommendations on terminologies and definitions for normal and abnormal uterine bleeding. Semin Reprod Med 2011;29:383–90.

Kaunitz AM, Meredith S, Inki P, Kubba A, Sanchez-Ramos L. Levonorgestrel-releasing intrauterine system and endometrial ablation in heavy menstrual bleeding: a systematic review and meta-analysis. Obstet Gynecol 2009;113:1104–16.

Middleton LJ, Champaneria R, Daniels JP, Bhattacharya S, Cooper KG, Hilken NH, et al. Hysterectomy, endometrial destruction, and levo-norgestrel releasing intrauterine system (Mirena) for heavy menstrual bleeding: systematic review and meta-analysis of data from individual patients. International Heavy Menstrual Bleeding Individual Patient Data Meta-analysis Collaborative Group. BMJ 2010;341:c3929.

Nelson AL. Levonorgestrel intrauterine system: a first-line medical treatment for heavy menstrual bleeding. Womens Health (Lond Engl) 2010;6:347–56.

Shaaban MM, Zakherah MS, El-Nashar SA, Sayed GH. Levonorgestrel-releasing intrauterine system compared to low dose combined oral contraceptive pills for idiopathic menorrhagia: a randomized clinical trial [published erratum appears in Contraception 2011;84:112]. Contraception 2011;83:48–54.

84

Outpatient management of pelvic inflammatory disease

A 16-year-old patient comes to the emergency department with lower abdominal pain for 48 hours. She has no nausea, vomiting, diarrhea, or dysuria. She reports a normal appetite. Over the past year, she has had three sexual partners. She is currently not using any birth control. Her last menstrual period was 5 weeks ago. Physical examination shows a well-nourished young woman in no acute distress. She has a mildly tender lower abdomen, left more than right, purulent discharge per cervical os, and left adnexal tenderness. Oral temperature is 38.1°C (100.5°F). Laboratory tests reveal a total leukocyte count of 10,540 per microliter and a positive pregnancy test result. Ultrasonography of the abdomen and pelvis yields a negative result for appendicitis or fluid in the cul-de-sac. The contraindication to outpatient therapy in this patient is

* (A) pregnancy
  (B) leukocyte count
  (C) body temperature
  (D) her age
  (E) left adnexal tenderness

Pelvic inflammatory disease (PID) includes inflammatory disorders of the upper female genital tract, comprising any combination of endometritis, salpingitis, tubo-ovarian abscess, and pelvic peritonitis. Sexually transmitted organisms, such as *Neisseria gonorrhoeae* and *Chlamydia trachomatis* have been implicated in many cases of PID. However, microorganisms that are part of the vaginal flora (such as anaerobes, *Gardnerella vaginalis, Haemophilus influenzae*, enteric Gram-negative rods, and *Streptococcus agalactiae*) also have been associated with PID. The Centers for Disease Control and Prevention recommends that all women with acute PID be tested for *N gonorrhoeae, C trachomatis*, and human immunodeficiency virus (HIV).

This patient has PID based on her lower abdominal pain and the examination findings of abdominal tenderness and cervical motion tenderness. The clinical diagnosis of PID has been shown to be highly sensitive. Box 84-1 shows the criteria for the diagnosis of PID. Outpatient management is appropriate if the patient has a mild to moderate clinical severity of illness and does not have any indications for inpatient management (Box 84-2).

The abdominal pain in this patient cannot be explained by appendicitis given a normal ultrasonographic result, a pain that is mostly left sided, and the absence of nausea and vomiting. The diagnosis of PID can be established based on the presence of abdominal pain, adnexal tenderness, and purulent cervical discharge in a sexually active female at risk for sexually transmitted infections. It is appropriate to treat her empirically for PID. The only contraindication to outpatient treatment would be pregnancy.

The Centers for Disease Control and Prevention has recommended the initiation of empiric treatment for PID in women who are sexually active and at risk for sexually transmitted diseases with abdominal pain, if no other cause can be found to explain the pain. The preferred outpatient antibiotic regimen includes single-dose intramuscular ceftriaxone and 14 days of oral doxycycline with

BOX 84-1

Criteria for the Diagnosis of Pelvic Inflammatory Disease

Pelvic or lower abdominal pain or one or more of the following minimal criteria on pelvic examination:
- Cervical motion tenderness
- Uterine tenderness
- Adnexal tenderness

Confirmatory criteria for pelvic inflammatory disease:
- Endometrial biopsy that shows evidence of endometritis
- Imaging study that reveals hydrosalpinges, with or without free pelvic fluid, or tubo–ovarian abscess, or Doppler ultrasonographic studies that suggest pelvic infection
- Laparoscopic evidence of pelvic inflammatory disease

The presence of the following factors will enhance the specificity of diagnosing the disease:
- Oral temperature greater than 38.3°C (101°F)
- Abnormal cervical or vaginal mucopurulent discharge
- Presence of abundant white blood cells on saline microscopy of vaginal fluid
- Elevated erythrocyte sedimentation rate
- Elevated C-reactive protein levels
- Laboratory documentation of cervical infection with *Neisseria gonorrhoeae* or *Chlamydia trachomatis*

Modified from Workowski KA, Berman S. Sexually transmitted diseases treatment guidelines, 2010. Centers for Disease Control and Prevention [published erratum appears in MMWR Morb Mortal Wkly Rep 2011;60:18]. MMWR Recomm Rep 2010;59:1–110.

BOX 84-2

Indications for Inpatient Management of Pelvic Inflammatory Disease

- A surgical emergency, such as appendicitis, cannot be ruled out.
- The patient is pregnant.
- The patient does not respond clinically to oral antimicrobial therapy.
- The patient is unable to adhere to or tolerate an outpatient oral regimen.
- Severe illness, nausea and vomiting, or high fever is present.
- A tubo–ovarian abscess is present.

appears normal and no leukocytes are observed on the wet prep of vaginal fluid, the diagnosis of PID is unlikely. An elevated serum leukocyte count, as in this case, is not a contraindication to outpatient therapy of PID.

A high-grade fever is an indication for inpatient management. However, as long as the patient has mild to moderate clinical illness and does not appear severely ill, PID in a patient with low-grade fever can be managed on an outpatient basis.

The fact that this patient is an adolescent is not an indication for inpatient management. The data are lacking to show that inpatient treatment is superior to outpatient treatment, and adolescents should be treated in the same manner as adults.

Adnexal tenderness also is a sign of PID. However, it is not an indication for inpatient treatment. By contrast, tubo–ovarian abscess is an indication for inpatient treatment. However, it cannot be inferred from adnexal tenderness that a tubo–ovarian abscess is present.

Gaitán H, Angel E, Diaz R, Parada A, Sanchez L, Vargas C. Accuracy of five different diagnostic techniques in mild-to-moderate pelvic inflammatory disease. Infect Dis Obstet Gynecol 2002;10:171–80.

Workowski KA, Berman S. Sexually transmitted diseases treatment guidelines, 2010. Centers for Disease Control and Prevention [published erratum appears in MMWR Morb Mortal Wkly Rep 2011;60:18]. MMWR Recomm Rep 2010;59:1–110.

or without oral metronidazole. The preferred inpatient antibiotic regimen is intravenous cefotetan or cefoxitin with doxycycline (Appendix J).

The finding of mucopurulent discharge from the cervical os with predominance of leukocytes visualized on microscopy is a sign of PID. If the cervical discharge

85

Postmenopausal bleeding with hormone therapy

A 54-year-old woman, gravida 3, para 2, comes to your office for evaluation of postmenopausal bleeding. Approximately 6 months ago, she started continuous combined estrogen and progestin therapy for postmenopausal symptoms. She states that her hot flushes and vaginal dryness have improved since she began the hormone therapy (HT). She reports 1 week of light spotting and no other symptoms. You schedule her for pelvic ultrasonography, which reveals an endometrial thickness of 3 mm. The most appropriate management with respect to her medication is to

     (A) stop the medication
     (B) switch to cyclic progestin
*   (C) continue the same dose of HT
     (D) add another form of estrogen
     (E) increase the dose of HT

Postmenopausal bleeding is a frequent adverse effect of HT. Up to 51% of patients report intermittent bleeding with the initiation of HT compared with 5% of patients who take placebo. Bleeding most commonly occurs in the first 6–12 months after initiation of HT. Studies also have shown that the bleeding profiles vary based on the type of hormone regimen. In the Postmenopausal Estrogen/ Progestin Interventions Trial, women who took conjugated equine estrogen plus cyclical micronized progestin had fewer excess bleeding episodes in the first 6 months than women who took continuous conjugated equine estrogen plus medroxyprogesterone acetate. However, after 1 year, women who took continuous regimens reported less bleeding.

Although studies have shown that patients are more likely to self-discontinue their medication secondary to bleeding, health care providers should advise patients that bleeding during the first few months of initiation of HT is common and is likely to be benign. The risk of endometrial cancer in women who took combined estrogen and progestin therapy was similar to that in women who took placebo. In the described patient, the medication has been effective in treating her symptoms, and the current dose should be continued. Switching to cyclic progestin would not be effective because studies have shown that cyclic progestin is associated with irregular bleeding. In

a large Swedish study, the use of continuous progestin rather than sequential progestin was shown to reduce the risk of endometrial cancer.

Increasing the dose of the medication is unnecessary because the patient already has adequate relief of vasomotor symptoms. Experts agree that patients should receive the lowest possible dose of estrogen to manage their symptoms in order to limit the potential risks. If pelvic ultrasonography demonstrates an endometrial thickness of 4 mm or less, the patient can be reassured that the risk of endometrial neoplasia is low and continued on the same dose. If the endometrial thickness is greater than 4 mm, endometrial sampling should be considered.

Anderson GL, Judd HL, Kaunitz AM, Barad DH, Beresford SA, Pettinger M, et al. Effects of estrogen plus progestin on gynecologic cancers and associated diagnostic procedures: the Women's Health Initiative randomized trial. Women's Health Initiative Investigators. JAMA 2003;290:1739–48.

Beral V, Bull D, Reeves G. Endometrial cancer and hormone-replacement therapy in the Million Women Study. Million Women Study Collaborators. Lancet 2005;365:1543–51.

Jaakkola S, Lyytinen H, Pukkala E, Ylikorkala O. Endometrial cancer in postmenopausal women using estradiol-progestin therapy. Obstet Gynecol 2009;114:1197–204.

Lindenfeld EA, Langer RD. Bleeding patterns of the hormone replacement therapies in the postmenopausal estrogen and progestin interventions trial. Obstet Gynecol 2002;100:853–63.

86

Recalcitrant condyloma

A 32-year-old immunocompetent woman is referred to you for further treatment of a genital condyloma. She has been treated for genital condylomas (warts) by her family health care practitioner initially using imiquimod followed by trichloroacetic acid for incomplete lesion resolution over the past 6 months. Currently, the patient notes a continued "lump" on the mons pubis. Her vulva appears as shown in Fig. 86-1 (see color plate). The next step in management is

* (A) excisional biopsy
  (B) laser ablation
  (C) office cryotherapy
  (D) re-treatment with imiquimod
  (E) treatment with podophyllin resin

Human papillomavirus (HPV) is the most common sexually transmitted infection in the United States. Infection with HPV is so common that at least 50% of men and women will contract the disease at some time in their lives. For most affected individuals, the virus remains subclinical and clears spontaneously. However, HPV infection may result in a broad spectrum of vulvar disease, including warts, dysplasia, and invasive cancer. Approximately 1% of women will develop a condyloma, and a few women will develop dysplasia.

More than 180 HPV types are known, of which approximately 40 affect the lower genital tract and 15 are oncogenic (high-risk HPV types); HPV genotype 6 and HPV genotype 11 are low-risk types and are associated with 90% of genital warts. Transmission of HPV is enhanced by irritation, abrasion, and microtrauma. In addition to limited epidermal host immune response, the virus induces a local immune deficiency, which allows prolonged viral manifestations in some individuals.

Although commonly they are asymptomatic, genital warts can cause itching, burning, pain, or bleeding. Their morphologic appearance can range from flat-topped papules to flesh colored, dome-shaped papules, keratotic warts, or classic wart-like lesions. Typically, they occur on the moist surfaces of the vulva, introitus, and perianal areas.

Spontaneous regression occurs in up to 30% of patients with genital warts. However, regression does not necessarily herald viral clearance. Viral genomes can be detected in normal epithelium for months to years after resolution of visible disease.

Generally, the goal of treating genital warts has been physical destruction or removal of visible disease, rather than eradication of HPV infection, as evidenced by the currently recommended treatment regimens. Treatments include patient-applied podofilox solution or gel, imiqui-

mod, sinecatechins ointment, and physician-administered cryotherapy with podophyllin resin, trichloroacetic, or bichloracetic acid, surgical removal, and laser therapy (Box 86-1). Although the therapies are equivalent in terms of clearance rates, recurrence is common. The fact that many therapies are available for the treatment of HPV-associated lesions underscores the reality that no single treatment is ideal for all patients or for all warts.

The best option for the described patient is excisional biopsy. Distinguishing warts from vulvar dysplasia based

---

BOX 86-1

Recommended Regimens for External Genital Warts

- Patient-applied
  Podofilox 0.5% solution or gel, or
  Imiquimod 5% cream, or
  Sinecatechins 15% ointment

- Physician-administered
  Cryotherapy with liquid nitrogen or cryoprobe; repeat applications every 1–2 weeks, or
  Podophyllin resin 10–25% in a compound tincture of benzoin, or
  Trichloroacetic acid or bichloracetic acid 80%–90%, or
  Surgical removal by either tangential scissor excision, tangential shave excision, curettage, or electrosurgery

Workowski KA, Berman S. Sexually transmitted diseases treatment guidelines, 2010. Centers for Disease Control and Prevention [published erratum appears in MMWR Morb Mortal Wkly Rep 2011;60:18]. MMWR Recomm Rep 2010;59:1–110.

on appearance alone is not always possible. Thus, hyperpigmented, indurated, fixed, or ulcerative lesions should be biopsied. In addition, lesions that do not respond to treatment or worsen during treatment, require biopsy for diagnosis. Evaluation for immune competency may be indicated for patients with recalcitrant disease. Each of the other treatment modalities may be considered once dysplasia or malignancy has been excluded.

Edwards L, Lynch PJ. Genital dermatology atlas. First edition. Philadelphia (PA): Lippincott Williams & Wilkins; 2004.

Kennedy CM, Boardman LA. New approaches to external genital warts and vulvar intraepithelial neoplasia. Clin Obstet Gynecol 2008; 51:518–26.

Stanley MA. Genital human papillomavirus infections: current and prospective therapies. J Gen Virol 2012;93:681–91.

Workowski KA, Berman S. Sexually transmitted diseases treatment guidelines, 2010. Centers for Disease Control and Prevention [published erratum appears in MMWR Morb Mortal Wkly Rep 2011;60:18]. MMWR Recomm Rep 2010;59:1–110.

87

Breast abscess

A 27-year-old woman, gravida 1, para 1, comes to your office at 8 weeks postpartum. Two weeks previously, you diagnosed puerperal mastitis in this patient. At that time you prescribed dicloxacillin and advised her to continue breastfeeding. Currently, she has a fever of 39°C (102°F) and you observe a painful firm erythematous lump 2 cm in diameter in the lateral aspect of the right breast. The most appropriate next step in management is

*   (A) ultrasonography-guided needle aspiration
       (B) breast milk culture
       (C) warm compress therapy
       (D) change to different antibiotic therapy
       (E) incision and drainage

The incidence of puerperal or lactational mastitis has been reported to range from 2% to 10%, which makes health care provider familiarity with this condition important in general practice. Lactational or puerperal mastitis is the most common inflammatory breast disorder. It is characterized by a localized cellulitis caused by introduction of bacteria through an inflamed or fissured nipple. Frequently, it is preceded by milk stasis. Risk factors include prior lactational mastitis, prolonged unilateral engorgement, poor milk drainage, and cracking or excoriation of the nipple. Onset usually occurs after the second postpartum week and may be precipitated by milk stasis. Although it may manifest in both breasts, unilateral infection is more common and is characterized by the following signs and symptoms:

- Breast tenderness or warmth to the touch (dolor and calor)
- General malaise
- Swelling of the breast
- Pain or a burning sensation while breastfeeding
- Skin erythema, often in a wedge-shaped pattern
- Pyrexia with fever of 38.3°C (101°F) or greater
- A "lumpy" consistency to the affected breast

The most common etiologic organism that causes puerperal mastitis is *Staphylococcus aureus*, although other organisms, including *Streptococcus pyogenes*, *Escherichia coli*, and *Bacteroides* species, also may be encountered. Because a significant percentage of these organisms are penicillin- or ampicillin-resistant, dicloxacillin typically is the first-line agent chosen for treatment.

Despite early and aggressive treatment of mastitis, sequelae, such as an abscess, occur in a small number of patients. Breast abscess typically occurs as a result of keratin plugging of affected milk ducts. Conservative management of breast abscess with antibiotics and continued breastfeeding usually are unsuccessful and surgical management is required.

The best management for the described clinical scenario is ultrasonography-guided needle aspiration with culture of aspirated fluid. Ultrasonography helps identify loculations and assures complete drainage of the abscess. The described patient has clinical examination findings that clearly demonstrate a localized area of concern for abscess. She has failed initial antibiotic therapy management of mastitis; therefore, more aggressive treatment is warranted. Needle drainage as treatment for this small breast abscess will likely correct the problem and allow continued lactation, which is critical to treatment success. Additionally, it may spare patients the potential discomfort and scarring that may be associated with incision and drainage.

Breast milk culture is unlikely to yield positive results because this patient has completed a course of antibiotics before re-presentation, and her milk will likely be sterile despite the presence of an infected collection in the breast. Warm compresses alone in the presence of an abscess may offer some symptomatic relief but will not resolve the infection. Changing antibiotics empirically without draining the abscess by some means will not likely improve her clinically. Although surgical incision and drainage will treat the abscess, such a procedure has high rates of discontinuation of lactation because of associated pain. This procedure is best reserved for larger abscesses or those that are refractory to prior treatment.

Eryilmaz R, Sahin M, Hakan Tekelioglu M, Daldal E. Management of lactational breast abscesses. Breast 2005;14:375–9.

Schwarz RJ, Shrestha R. Needle aspiration of breast abscesses. Am J Surg 2001;182:117–9.

World Health Organization Department of Child and Adolescent Health and Development. Mastitis: causes and management. Geneva: WHO; 2000. Available at: http://whqlibdoc.who.int/hq/2000/WHO_FCH_CAH_00.13.pdf. Retrieved June 6, 2013.

88
Endometriosis

A 34-year-old woman, gravida 3, para 3, comes to your office for a second opinion. She has had three laparoscopic procedures for endometriosis-associated pelvic pain over the past 4 years. The procedures have not helped to decrease her symptoms of dysmenorrhea, dyspareunia, and noncyclic pelvic pain although all of the endometriotic tissue was removed each time. Her gynecologist has recommended a hysterectomy and bilateral salpingo-oophorectomy (BSO). She does not desire preservation of fertility. In the past year, she has been treated for six episodes of urinary tract infections with symptoms of urgency, frequency, and pain. Culture was performed during her last episode and showed negative results. She has no gastrointestinal symptoms. Bimanual examination reveals severe, diffuse tenderness. The best next step in management is

      (A) hysterectomy and BSO
      (B) depot leuprolide treatment
      (C) colonoscopy
      (D) laparoscopy
  * (E) cystoscopy

Strong evidence supports the association of endometriosis and dysmenorrhea, dyspareunia, and noncyclic pelvic pain (chronic pelvic pain). Observational data suggest that hysterectomy and BSO with removal of all endometriotic lesions has significant efficacy for the relief of pain symptoms associated with endometriosis.

For the described patient, to proceed with hysterectomy and BSO without further evaluation would be inappropriate. The patient has undergone multiple laparoscopic treatments for endometriosis without achieving any degree of pain relief. Randomized placebo-controlled trials of laparoscopic surgical treatment suggest that 85–90% of women obtained significant pain relief that usually lasted 1 year or longer. It is important to remember that endometriosis may be asymptomatic, even when severe, and that finding it in a patient with chronic pelvic pain does not automatically imply an etiologic relationship. In the described scenario, the lack of any improvement of pain symptoms with a history of three operative laparoscopic procedures strongly suggests the lack of etiologic relationship.

Evidence suggests that gonadotropin-releasing hormone agonists are effective in the treatment of endometriosis-associated pelvic pain. Treatment with a gonadotropin-releasing hormone agonist in this clinical scenario is not necessarily inappropriate, but it is not the best option because endometriosis does not seem to be the source of pain in this patient. Her history suggests that she has interstitial cystitis.

A number of studies have shown the high prevalence of irritable bowel syndrome (IBS) in women with chronic pelvic pain, including women with endometriosis. In this case, no symptoms suggest IBS. Patients with IBS present with pain or discomfort associated with changes in bowel frequency or quality or pain or discomfort relieved by defecation. If a patient has these symptoms, referral to a gastroenterologist for evaluation of chronic abdominal pelvic pain would be appropriate. Referral simply for colonoscopy or barium enema is not indicated. No symptoms suggestive of inflammatory bowel disease, diverticular disease, or any other organic gastrointestinal pathology that would require a colonoscopy are present in this case.

Given the described patient's history of three prior operative laparoscopic procedures and no relief of pain symptoms, another laparoscopy is not likely to be helpful either with diagnosis or treatment.

In patients with endometriosis-associated pelvic pain, a number of studies have shown a high prevalence of other pelvic pain-related diagnoses, especially interstitial cystitis (IC) and IBS. The simultaneous presence of IC–painful bladder syndrome and endometriosis ranges from 30–90%.

Interstitial cystitis is defined as chronic bladder pain in the absence of an identifiable etiology and usually is associated with urinary urge and frequency, in addition to bladder pain. The symptoms often lead to repeated treatment of suspected urinary tract infections without confirmation of infection by positive urine cultures. The described patient's history suggests IC. A pelvic pain urgency frequency questionnaire is used to assess clinical symptoms associated with IC (Fig. 88-1). Current thinking is that clinical diagnosis often is sufficient and cystoscopic hydrodistention is not always needed for diagnosis; the criterion standard for diagnosis remains the finding of glomerulations at the time of cystoscopic hydrodistention.

In addition to the history of pelvic pain, urinary urgency and frequency, and possibly recurrent urinary tract infections, physical examination often will reveal

Patient's name:_____   Today's date:_____

Pelvic Pain and Urgency/Frequency Patient Symptom Scale

Please circle the answer that best describes how you feel for each question.

	0	1	2	3	4	Symptom Score	Bother Score
1. How many times do you go to the bathroom during the day?	3–6	7–10	11–14	15–19	20+		
2. a. How many times do you go to the bathroom at night?	0	1	2	3	4+		
b. If you get up at night to go to the bathroom, does it bother you?	Never	Occasionally	Usually	Always			
3. a. Do you now or have you ever had pain or symptoms during or after sexual intercourse?	Never	Occasionally	Usually	Always			
b. Has pain or urgency ever made you avoid sexual intercourse?	Never	Occasionally	Usually	Always			
4. Do you have pain associated with your bladder or in your pelvis (vagina, labia, lower abdomen, urethra, perineum, testes, or scrotum)?	Never	Occasionally	Usually	Always			
5. a If you have pain, is it usually		Mild	Moderate	Severe			
b. Does your pain bother you?	Never	Occasionally	Usually	Always			
6. Do you still have urgency after going to the bathroom?	Never	Occasionally	Usually	Always			
7. a. If you have urgency, is it usually		Mild	Moderate	Severe			
b. Does your urgency bother you?	Never	Occasionally	Usually	Always			
8. Are you sexually active? Yes____ No____							

Symptom Score = (1, 2a, 3a, 4, 5a, 6, 7a)		
Bother Score = (2b, 3b, 5b, 7b)		
Total Score (Symptom Score + Bother Score) =		

FIG. 88-1. Pelvic pain urgency and frequency patient symptom scale questionnaire. (Reprinted from Urology, Volume 60, Parsons CL, Dell J, Stanford EJ Bullen M, Kahn BS, Waxell T, Koziol JA. Increased prevalence of interstitial cystitis: previously unrecognized urologic and gynecologic cases identified using a new symptom questionnaire and intravesical potassium sensitivity, pages 573–8, Copyright 2002, with permission from Elsevier and © 2000 C. Lowell Parsons, MD. Used with permission.)

significant tenderness of the bladder base, urethra, and pelvic floor musculature. Urinalysis and urine cultures usually will yield negative results. Postvoid residual urine volume should be normal. Cystoscopy may need to be performed to exclude any other conditions, especially bladder cancer. Some clinicians use the potassium sensitivity test for diagnostic evaluation, which involves filling the bladder with a potassium solution, but most experts do not recommend this as a routine test.

Oral pentosan polysulfate sodium and intravesical dimethylsulfoxide have been approved by the U.S. Food and Drug Administration as medical treatments for IC. Treatments not approved by the U.S. Food and Drug Admminstration include oral tricyclic antidepressants, oral antihistamines, intravesical local anesthetic agents, intravesical heparin, and dietary changes, such as avoidance of alcohol, caffeine, citrus fruit, and spicy food.

Abbott J, Hawe J, Hunter D, Holmes M, Finn P, Garry R. Laparoscopic excision of endometriosis: a randomized, placebo-controlled trial. Fertil Steril 2004;82:878–84.

Chung MK, Chung RR, Gordon D, Jennings C. The evil twins of chronic pelvic pain syndrome: endometriosis and interstitial cystitis. JSLS 2002;6:311–4.

Droz J, Howard FM. Use of the Short-Form McGill Pain Questionnaire as a diagnostic tool in women with chronic pelvic pain. J Minim Invasive Gynecol 2011;18:211–7.

Ling FW. Randomized controlled trial of depot leuprolide in patients with chronic pelvic pain and clinically suspected endometriosis. Pelvic Pain Study Group. Obstet Gynecol 1999;93:51–8.

Shakiba K, Bena JF, McGill KM, Minger J, Falcone T. Surgical treatment of endometriosis: a 7-year follow-up on the requirement for further surgery [published erratum appears in Obstet Gynecol 2008;112:710]. Obstet Gynecol 2008;111:1285–92.

Sutton CJ, Ewen SP, Whitelaw N, Haines P. Prospective, randomized, double-blind, controlled trial of laser laparoscopy in the treatment of pelvic pain associated with minimal, mild, and moderate endometriosis. Fertil Steril 1994;62:696–700.

89

Perioperative care of a patient with diabetes mellitus

An obese woman with type 2 diabetes mellitus is scheduled for a total abdominal hysterectomy for large, symptomatic uterine myomas. She takes 40 units of long-acting insulin every evening and 1,000 mg of metformin daily. The preoperative hemoglobin A_{1c} level is 6.8%. Hysterectomy takes 4 hours to perform and is complicated by an estimated blood loss of 750mL. On postoperative day 1, her vital signs are stable, and the urine output is 10 mL/hr. She is nauseated and is not eager to resume oral intake. In addition to glucose-containing intravenous (IV) fluids, the best management plan for postoperative glucose control in this patient is

(A) insulin regimen and metformin
(B) metformin alone
(C) long-acting insulin alone
* (D) long-acting insulin plus sliding scale
(E) metformin with an insulin sliding scale

Women with diabetes mellitus have an increased risk of perioperative infection and postoperative cardiovascular morbidity and mortality. Preoperatively, a patient with diabetes mellitus should undergo an assessment of cardiac risk and glycemic control and evaluation of possible sequelae of diabetes mellitus, such as chronic kidney disease, cerebrovascular disease, and neuropathy. Preoperative testing should include baseline cardiac function assessment based on symptoms and electrocardiography. Additional cardiac noninvasive testing should be reserved for patients with abnormal electrocardiography results, uncontrolled hypertension, or a creatinine level greater than 2 mg/dL. Glycemic control is assessed with hemoglobin A_{1c} monitoring, range of blood glucose level monitoring, and medication regimen and timing.

Surgery and general anesthesia cause a stress response that leads to insulin resistance, decreased peripheral glucose use, impaired insulin secretion, lipolysis, and protein catabolism that contributes to hyperglycemia. Postoperative nausea, vomiting, and anorexia can lead to poor caloric intake and hypoglycemia. The postoperative goal is to maintain fluid and electrolyte balance and avoid hyperglycemia and hypoglycemia. The American Diabetes Association recommends achieving fasting glucose level of less than 140 mg/dL and random glucose levels of less than 180 mg/dL for hospitalized patients.

Women with type 2 diabetes mellitus who take only oral hypoglycemic agents should stop taking oral medications on the morning of surgery. The regimen should be restarted when patients resume eating. Glucose levels should be monitored and a sliding scale for short-acting insulin administration should be instituted to maintain glycemic control. Metformin is contraindicated with renal hypoperfusion, which can lead to lactate accumulation and tissue hypoxia.

Women who use injectable insulin should continue with the long-acting insulin therapy and receive glucose-containing IV fluids until they can resume a normal diet. An additional administration of short-acting insulin on a sliding scale can optimize blood sugar levels, with correction used for blood glucose levels greater than 150 mg/dL.

The described patient is receiving oral and injectable hypoglycemics. She had significant blood loss, and her low urine output suggests renal hypoperfusion. Metformin is contraindicated under these conditions. However, she should be given the long-acting insulin along with glucose-containing IV fluids. Once she has a normal urine output, is fully resuscitated, and has resumed her

usual diet, metformin can be restarted. In the meantime, for optimal glucose management, she should receive an insulin regimen that includes glucose-containing IV fluid, her home dose of long-acting insulin, and additional insulin administered on a sliding scale, with the goal to maintain blood sugar levels below 180 mg/dL.

King JT Jr, Goulet JL, Perkal MF, Rosenthal RA. Glycemic control and infections in patients with diabetes undergoing noncardiac surgery. Ann Surg 2011;253:158–65.

Moghissi ES, Korytkowski MT, DiNardo M, Einhorn D, Hellman R, Hirsch IB, et al. American Association of Clinical Endocrinologists and American Diabetes Association consensus statement on inpatient glycemic control. American Association of Clinical Endocrinologists and American Diabetes Association. Diabetes Care 2009;32:1119–31.

Salpeter SR, Greyber E, Pasternak GA, Salpeter EE. Risk of fatal and nonfatal lactic acidosis with metformin use in type 2 diabetes mellitus. Cochrane Database of Systematic Reviews 2010, Issue 4. Art. No.: CD002967. DOI: 10.1002/14651858.CD002967.pub4.

90

Endometrial ablation

A 44-year-old woman, gravida 3, para 3, has heavy, irregular menses and mild right lower quadrant discomfort. The patient has declined hormonal management in the past because her mother has a history of breast cancer. She is interested in endometrial ablation. She has a history of cesarean delivery. On bimanual examination, she has mild right adnexal tenderness. Transvaginal ultrasonography shows a retroverted uterus with a sagittal length of 9.5 cm, endometrial echo of 6 mm, a 2-cm submucosal and fundal myoma, normal ovaries, and no free fluid. Endometrial biopsy reveals disordered, proliferative phase endometrium and acute endometritis with the presence of plasma cells. The absolute contraindication to endometrial ablation in this patient is

(A) history of cesarean delivery
(B) retroverted uterus
(C) submucosal myoma
* (D) pelvic inflammatory disease
(E) uterine length greater than 8 cm

Endometrial ablation is targeted destruction of the endometrium. The endometrial cavity can be ablated either with a resectoscopic or nonresectoscopic device. Nonresectoscopic devices appear to require less training and experience than resectoscopic devices. Currently, five different nonresectoscopic endometrial ablative techniques are approved by the U.S. Food and Drug Administration. The different destructive techniques are 1) tissue freezing, 2) radiofrequency electricity, 3) microwaves, and heated fluid, 4) either freely circulating within the endometrial cavity or 5) within a balloon. None of these techniques has been shown to be more efficacious than the others.

The most common indication for endometrial ablation is heavy menstrual bleeding in premenopausal women who have no desire for future childbearing. The endometrium must be sampled and the histopathologic results reviewed before the procedure.

The gynecologist may prescribe preoperative preparatory drugs, such as a gonadotropin-releasing hormone analog or a hormonal contraceptive that produces a thinned (atrophic) lining, which results in a more favorable environment for performing an endometrial ablation than intact endometrium (a thinned endometrium is easier to destroy and devascularize). Alternatively, the procedure may be scheduled in the early proliferative phase of the patient's menstrual cycle or the patient may undergo dilation and curettage immediately before endometrial ablation.

Contraindications to endometrial ablation are endometrial cancer, endometrial hyperplasia, viable intrauterine pregnancy or future desire for pregnancy, acute pelvic inflammatory disease, and postmenopausal bleeding. An unfavorable positioning of the long axis of the uterus, a thin myometrial wall, and submucosal myomas are not absolute contraindications to nonresectoscopic endometrial ablation. Extreme uterine retroversion, anteversion, or flexion may obviate correct placement of the device within the endometrial cavity. A relatively thin myometrial wall, ie, from prior cesarean delivery, myomectomy, or endometrial ablation, may increase the risk of transmural thermal injury to the adjacent bladder or bowel.

Submucosal myomas can be hysteroscopically resected before endometrial ablation. Alternatively, some global endometrial ablation devices have shown success in treating submucosal myomas based on the size and location of the myoma. Appendix E shows a classification system of submucosal myomas based on their depth of penetration into the myometrium. Type 0 submucosal myomas are best treated by hysteroscopic resection.

Global endometrial ablation initially showed similar efficacy with lower cost and complication rates compared with hysterectomy. However, these outcomes appear to diminish over time, and some studies have reported that up to 30% of patients have required hysterectomy within 4 years after ablation. Failure leading to hysterectomy is predominant in patients younger than 40 years. Other factors that decrease the success of endometrial ablation include dysmenorrhea, adenomyosis, hyperplasia, and uterine length greater than 10 cm. Nonresectoscopic endometrial ablation is not recommended in women with a uterine cavity length that exceeds device limitations. The maximum uterine length is 10–14 cm based on the device.

Pelvic inflammatory disease (PID) represents a spectrum of inflammatory disorders of the upper genital tract, including any combination of endometritis, salpingitis, tubo–ovarian abscess, and pelvic peritonitis. The features that suggest acute PID in this patient are right lower quadrant pain and pathologic diagnosis of acute endometritis. Acute PID may be difficult to diagnose because many women with PID have subtle or mild symptoms. Delay in diagnosis and treatment of PID contributes to rates of chronic pelvic pain and infertility. Appropriate treatment includes broad-spectrum oral or parenteral antibiotics. If, after this treatment, abnormal bleeding persists, endometrial ablation is a reasonable option and is no longer contraindicated.

AAGL practice report: practice guidelines for the diagnosis and management of submucous myomas. American Association of Gynecologic Laparoscopists (AAGL): Advancing Minimally Invasive Gynecology Worldwide. J Minim Invasive Gynecol 2012;19:152–71.

Baggish MS, Valle RF, Guedj H, editors. Hysteroscopy: visual perspectives of uterine anatomy, physiology and pathology. 3rd ed. Philadelphia (PA): Wolters Kluwer/Lippincott Williams & Wilkins; 2007.

Dickersin K, Munro MG, Clark M, Langenberg P, Scherer R, Frick K, et al. Hysterectomy compared with endometrial ablation for dysfunctional uterine bleeding: a randomized controlled trial. Surgical Treatments Outcomes Project for Dysfunctional Uterine Bleeding (STOP-DUB) Research Group. Obstet Gynecol 2007;110:1279–89.

Endometrial ablation. ACOG Practice Bulletin No. 81. American College of Obstetricians and Gynecologists. Obstet Gynecol 2007;109:1233–48.

Workowski KA, Berman S. Sexually transmitted diseases treatment guidelines, 2010. Centers for Disease Control and Prevention [published erratum appears in MMWR Morb Mortal Wkly Rep 2011;60:18]. MMWR Recomm Rep 2010;59:1–110.

91

Vascular supply of the pelvis

A 47-year-old woman, gravida 3, para 3, comes to your office with symptoms of stress urinary incontinence. The patient undergoes placement of a tension-free vaginal tape with cystoscopy. During the procedure, the patient is noted to have brisk bleeding from the trocar sites and becomes hypotensive. The vessel that has been shown to have the closest mean distance to the lateral aspect of the tension-free vaginal tape trocar is the

   (A) superficial epigastric
* (B) obturator
   (C) inferior epigastric
   (D) external iliac
   (E) femoral

Stress urinary incontinence can be effectively managed on an outpatient basis with methods, such as the tension-free vaginal tape (TVT) procedure, which has shown cure rates of 74–85% at 4–6 years of follow-up. The TVT procedure involves the placement of a tape under the midurethra by passing stainless steel trocars from the vagina through the retropubic space upward to the anterior abdominal wall. The tape is not sutured in place and, therefore, is labeled tension-free. This helps decrease anatomic distortion and urinary dysfunction. In some instances, the procedure may be performed under local anesthesia.

Complications of the TVT procedure include bladder injury, intraoperative hemorrhage, infection, bowel perforation, nerve injury, and postoperative hematoma. Trocar insertion into the bladder is one of the most common complications (2.7%). Routine cystoscopy at the time of the procedure aids in identification of bladder perforations.

Vascular injuries that involve the obturator, femoral, external iliac, and inferior epigastric vessels have been reported. Injury to the obturator vessels during the TVT procedure constitutes the most common injury. Arterial bleeding will present intraoperatively or in the immediate postoperative period with acute hemodynamic instability. Intraoperative bleeding typically is managed with pressure, electrocautery, and packing. Pelvic imaging during the postoperative period will demonstrate a retropubic hematoma. In one study of 336 consecutive TVT procedures, excessive intraoperative blood loss was noted in 2.1% of patients.

Venous bleeding usually is self-limited and typically will present postoperatively with the presence of a hema-

toma on examination. Patients may be asymptomatic or may have pain, ecchymosis, and possibly an inability to void. Small hematomas (blood loss of less than 100 mL) tend to have minimal symptoms and do not require intervention. Large hematomas (blood loss of 200 mL or greater) can cause moderate to severe pain and significant urinary symptoms and often necessitate drainage. Generally, development of a hematoma does not appear to affect the overall success rate of the incontinence procedure. Postoperative retropubic hematoma was reported in 4.1% of patients.

A thorough understanding of the pelvic anatomy is needed for safe placement of the TVT trocars. In one study, the mean distance from the TVT trocar to the obturator vessels was closest at 3.2 cm, followed by superficial epigastric (3.9 cm), inferior epigastric (3.9 cm), and the external iliac vessels (4.9 cm) (Fig. 91-1). Aiming the TVT trocar in a plane from the mid-labia majora toward the ipsilateral shoulder, while maintaining the trocar directly posterior to the pubic bone, aids in decreasing vascular injuries. Lateral deviation of the trocar can occur in an attempt to avoid the bladder.

Flock F, Reich A, Muche R, Kreienberg R, Reister F. Hemorrhagic complications associated with tension-free vaginal tape procedure. Obstet Gynecol 2004;104:989–94.

Karram MM, Segal JL, Vassallo BJ, Kleeman SD. Complications and untoward effects of the tension-free vaginal tape procedure. Obstet Gynecol 2003;101:929–32.

Muir TW, Tulikangas PK, Fidela Paraiso M, Walters MD. The relationship of tension-free vaginal tape insertion and the vascular anatomy. Obstet Gynecol 2003;101:933–6.

Walters MD, Tulikangas PK, LaSala C, Muir TW. Vascular injury during tension-free vaginal tape procedure for stress urinary incontinence. Obstet Gynecol 2001;98:957–9.

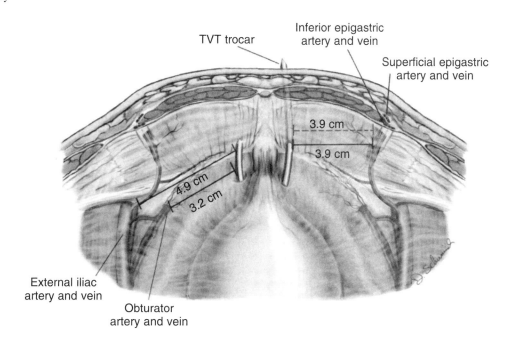

FIG. 91-1. The relationship of the tension-free vaginal tape (TVT) trocar to the vascular anatomy of the anterior abdominal wall and retropubic space. Numbers represent the mean distance from the lateral aspect of the TVT trocar to the medial edge of the vessels. (Muir TW, Tulikangas PK, Fidela Paraiso M, Walters MD. The relationship of tension-free vaginal tape insertion and the vascular anatomy. Obstet Gynecol 2003;101:933–6.)

92

Lichen sclerosus

A 58-year-old woman has been treated for several months for chronic candidiasis despite negative vaginal culture results. Your partner performed a vulvar biopsy 2 weeks ago that showed lichen sclerosus. The patient has intense vulvar pruritus and moderate dyspareunia (numeric rating scale pain score, 4 out of 10). On examination, you find the presence of significant adhesions at the clitoris that were not previously documented. Your next step in the treatment of this patient should be

* (A) topical clobetasol propionate
   (B) lysis of the clitoral adhesions
   (C) triamcinolone hexacetonide injection
   (D) repeat biopsy
   (E) pimecrolimus cream

Lichen sclerosus is a benign, chronic skin condition that causes symptoms of pruritus and pain. Most cases of lichen sclerosus occur in the anogenital region. Although it can occur at any age, vulvar lichen sclerosus most often occurs in prepubertal girls and perimenopausal or postmenopausal women. Its etiology is not known. Vulvar disease may be asymptomatic but usually causes intense pruritus that may even affect sleep. Pain and dyspareunia may be present, especially later in the course of the disease. Anal lichen sclerosus causes intense pruritus but also can cause rectal bleeding, anal fissures, and painful defecation.

Physical examination usually reveals white, atrophic papules or plaques of the labia minora or majora. Hemorrhagic, purpuric, or ulcerated lesions or fissures may be present. Scratching may lead to lichenification and edema. Later in the disease, a loss of normal anatomic architecture may occur with fusing of the labia majora and minora or burying of the clitoris under a fused clitoral hood. Introital and perineal shrinkage may occur, which leads to significant dyspareunia. Lichen sclerosus does not involve the vagina.

The diagnosis is based on histologic findings. Most experts recommend vulvar biopsy before initiating therapy to establish the diagnosis and exclude other diagnoses, such as lichen simplex, vulvar intraepithelial neoplasia, and malignancy. One well-chosen 3–4-mm punch biopsy is sufficient for diagnosis and exclusion of malignancy. Histology usually shows thinned epidermis with acanthosis and elongation of rete pegs, areas of hyperkeratosis, and hyalinization of the upper dermis with lymphocytes below. Clinical judgment should be used if the biopsy yields negative or nondiagnostic results. Evaluation for coexisting infections, especially *Candida,* should be performed in all cases. Repeat biopsies are performed only for new, worrisome lesions or those that

are resistant to treatment. Therefore, repeat biopsy is not warranted for this patient.

Consensus is lacking on the treatment of lichen sclerosus, but most experts recommend patient education, good vulvar hygiene, and superpotent corticosteroid therapy to control symptoms and preserve anatomy. In the case of associated vulvovaginal atrophy in postmenopausal women, vaginal estrogen treatment may be helpful, especially for dyspareunia. Patient education is important because lichen sclerosus is a chronic, progressive disease that requires long-term treatment. Risk of malignancy must be emphasized to ensure adequate regular follow-up. Superpotent topical ointments, particularly clobetasol propionate and halobetasol propionate 0.05%, have been shown in small clinical trials to be effective, and to be more effective than progesterone or testosterone. Progesterone and testosterone are no longer recommended for treatment. Ointments are preferred over creams because creams contain alcohol, which may act as an irritant on application. Therefore, topical clobetasol ointment is the best recommendation for the described patient. Clobetasol or halobetasol used nightly for 6–12 weeks provides symptomatic relief in approximately 95% of women and generally reverses hyperkeratosis, fissures, and ecchymoses. Long-term maintenance treatment 2–3 times per week often is needed once remission is achieved.

Surgical treatment is not recommended as first-line therapy because lesions often resolve with medical therapy. Although not first-line therapy, intralesional injections of corticosteroids, such as triamcinolone hexacetonide, are sometimes needed to treat hypertrophic plaques that have not responded to topical steroid ointment treatment. Other medications, such as retinoids and calcineurin inhibitors (tacrolimus and pimecrolimus), appear to be efficacious. However, they are not as well studied as clobetasol and halobetasol and tend to have more significant adverse effects and risks. Such medications are used as second-line therapy.

Ayhan A, Guven S, Guvendag Guven ES, Sakinci M, Gultekin M, Kucukali T. Topical testosterone versus clobetasol for vulvar lichen sclerosus. Int J Gynaecol Obstet 2007;96:117–21.

Bornstein J, Heifetz S, Kellner Y, Stolar Z, Abramovici H. Clobetasol dipropionate 0.05% versus testosterone propionate 2% topical appli-

cation for severe vulvar lichen sclerosus. Am J Obstet Gynecol 1998;178:80–4.

Funaro D. Lichen sclerosus: a review and practical approach. Dermatol Ther 2004;17:28–37.

McPherson T, Cooper S. Vulval lichen sclerosus and lichen planus. Dermatol Ther 2010;23:523–32.

Rouzier R, Haddad B, Deyrolle C, Pelisse M, Moyal-Barracco M, Paniel BJ. Perineoplasty for the treatment of introital stenosis related to vulvar lichen sclerosus. Am J Obstet Gynecol 2002;186:49–52.

93

Ectopic pregnancy

A 23-year-old woman, gravida 2, para 0, comes to the emergency department with spotting. The time of her last menstrual period is unknown. Her history is significant for an ectopic pregnancy 2 years ago treated by laparoscopic salpingectomy. Examination reveals height 1.57 m (5 ft 2 in), weight 61.2 kg (135 lb), blood pressure 112 mm Hg systolic and 65 mm Hg diastolic, pulse 72 beats per minute, and respiratory rate 16 breaths per minute. Her abdomen is soft and nontender. The uterus is slightly enlarged, nontender with a palpable right adnexal mass. Laboratory results reveal a quantitative human chorionic gonadotropin (hCG) level of 2,392 mIU/mL and hematocrit of 36%; the blood type is O positive. Ultrasonography reveals an endometrial thickness of 17.8 mm with no intrauterine gestational sac. Both ovaries are visualized, and a 3-cm complex mass in the right ovary is identified. No other adnexal masses are noted. No fluid is present in the cul-de-sac. The best next step in management is

      (A) methotrexate sodium
      (B) dilation and curettage
      (C) diagnostic laparoscopy
      (D) serum progesterone level
*   (E) hCG level measurement in 48 hours

This patient is at an increased risk of an ectopic pregnancy. However, the failure to identify an intrauterine pregnancy on ultrasonography, even when the hCG level exceeds the discriminatory zone, is not diagnostic of an ectopic pregnancy. The *discriminatory zone* generally is defined as an hCG level of 1,500–2,000 mIU/mL, which is associated with the appearance on transvaginal ultrasonography of a normal singleton pregnancy. Approximately 4.5% of pregnant women with an initial hCG level greater than 2,000 mIU/mL with no visualized intrauterine fluid collection subsequently are found to have a viable intrauterine pregnancy. This is particularly true with multiple gestations. The presence of a complex mass in the ovary in the described patient is more consistent with a corpus luteum than an ectopic pregnancy. The definitive diagnosis of an ectopic pregnancy requires identification of either a yolk sac or a fetus, with or without cardiac activity, outside of the normal intrauterine location. Additionally, the finding of a thickened endometrium is more suggestive of an intrauterine pregnancy

than an ectopic pregnancy. A single hCG level determination with nondiagnostic ultrasonography is not sufficient for the diagnosis of an ectopic pregnancy. Thus, a patient who is clinically stable, as in this case, does not require immediate treatment with methotrexate, dilation and curettage, or laparoscopy.

The described patient has a diagnosis of a pregnancy of unknown location and, therefore, methotrexate sodium should be withheld until the diagnosis of an ectopic pregnancy is likely. Methotrexate is an antimetabolite that binds to the catalytic site of dihydrofolate reductase and interrupts the synthesis of purine nucleotides and the amino acids serine and methionine, thus inhibiting DNA synthesis and cell replication. It affects actively proliferating tissues, such as bone marrow, buccal and intestinal mucosa, respiratory epithelium, malignant cells, and trophoblastic tissue.

Systemic methotrexate is used in the management of ectopic pregnancy with an overall success rate that ranges on average from 71.2% to 94.2%. The success rate is affected by the treatment protocol, gestational age, and hCG level. Single-dose regimens have been shown to have a failure rate of 14.3% or higher when pretreatment hCG levels are greater than 5,000 mIU/mL compared with 3.7% for pretreatment hCG levels less than 5,000 mIU/mL. Candidates for medical management with methotrexate are patients with confirmed or high clinical suspicion of ectopic pregnancy who are hemodynamically stable with no evidence of rupture, a mass 3.5 cm or less in size, and, preferably, no fetal cardiac activity. In addition, they must be able to comply with follow-up surveillance. Treatment protocols with systemic methotrexate are listed in Box 93-1.

Contraindications to the use of methotrexate are shown in Box 93-2. Before administering methotrexate, a woman should undergo screening for contraindications. Adherence with the protocol should be ensured. Normal serum creatinine and liver transaminase levels should be confirmed. No bone marrow dysfunction indicated by significant anemia, leukopenia, or thrombocytopenia should be present.

Serum progesterone level measurement has been suggested for evaluation of patents with ectopic pregnancy. Levels higher than 25 ng/mL usually are associated with normal intrauterine pregnancy. A serum progesterone level less than 5 ng/mL was found in 11% of women with nor-

---

BOX 93-1

Methotrexate Treatment Protocols

Single-dose regimen*:

Single dose MTX 50 mg/m^2 IM day 1

Measure hCG level on posttreatment days 4 and 7.

Check for 15% hCG decrease between days 4 and 7.

Then measure hCG level weekly until reaching the nonpregnant level.

If results are less than the expected 15% decrease, readminister MTX 50 mg/m^2 and repeat hCG measurement on days 4 and 7 after second dose. This can be repeated as necessary.

If, during follow-up, hCG levels plateau or increase, consider repeating MTX.

Two-dose regimen[†]:

Administer 50 mg/m^2 IM on day 0.

Repeat 50 mg/m^2 IM on day 4.

Measure hCG levels on days 4 and 7, and expect a 15% decrease between days 4 and 7.

If the decrease is greater than 15%, measure hCG levels weekly until reaching nonpregnant level.

If less than a 15% decrease in hCG levels, readminister MTX 50 mg/m^2 on days 7 and 11, measuring hCG levels.

If hCG levels decrease 15% between days 7 and 11, continue to monitor weekly until nonpregnant hCG levels are reached.

If the decrease is less than 15% between days 7 and 11, consider surgical treatment.

Fixed multidose regimen[‡]:

Administer MTX 1 mg/kg IM (on days 1, 3, 5, 7), alternate daily with folinic acid 0.1 mg/kg IM (on days 2, 4, 6, 8).

Measure hCG levels on MTX dose days and continue until hCG has decreased by 15% from its previous measurement.

The hCG level may increase initially above pretreatment value, but after 15% decrease, monitor hCG levels weekly until reaching the nonpregnant level.

If the hCG level plateaus or increases, consider repeating MTX using the regimen described.

Abbreviations: hCG indicates human chorionic gonadotropin; IM, intramuscular; MTX, methotrexate.

*Stovall TG, Ling FW. Single-dose methotrexate: an expanded clinical trial. Am J Obstet Gynecol 1993;168:1759–62; discussion 1762–5.

[†]Barnhart K, Hummel AC, Sammel MD, Menon S, Jain J, Chakhtoura N. Use of "2-dose" regimen of methotrexate to treat ectopic pregnancy. Fertil Steril 2007;87:250–6.

[‡]Rodi IA, Sauer MV, Gorrill MJ, Bustillo M, Gunning JE, Marshall JR, et al. The medical treatment of unruptured ectopic pregnancy with methotrexate and citrovorum rescue: preliminary experience. Fertil Steril 1986;46:811–3.

Medical management of ectopic pregnancy. ACOG Practice Bulletin No. 94. American College of Obstetricians and Gynecologists. Obstet Gynecol 2008;111:1479–85.

mal pregnancies. Levels between 5 ng/mL and 25 ng/mL are nondiscriminatory. Thus, serum progesterone level measurement is of limited value.

BOX 93-2

Contraindications to Methotrexate

Absolute contraindications
- Breastfeeding
- Overt or laboratory evidence of immuno-deficiency
- Alcoholism, alcoholic liver disease, or other chronic liver disease
- Preexisting blood dyscrasias, such as bone marrow hypoplasia, leukopenia, thrombocytopenia, or significant anemia
- Known sensitivity to methotrexate
- Active pulmonary disease
- Peptic ulcer disease
- Hepatic, renal, or hematologic dysfunction

Relative contraindications
- Gestational sac larger than 3.5 cm
- Embryonic cardiac motion

Medical management of ectopic pregnancy. ACOG Practice Bulletin No. 94. American College of Obstetricians and Gynecologists. Obstet Gynecol 2008;111:1479–85.

In early pregnancy, an increase in serum hCG level of less than 53% in 48 hours confirms an abnormal pregnancy with 99% sensitivity. In the absence of an ultrasonographic diagnosis of ectopic pregnancy in the described patient, evaluation of hCG level in 48 hours would be the best next step. If serum hCG doubles, it would be suggestive of an intrauterine pregnancy. Repeat ultrasonography correlated with serial hCG levels would be indicated to determine if this were an intrauterine or ectopic pregnancy.

Barnhart K, van Mello NM, Bourne T, Kirk E, Van Calster B, Bottomley C, et al. Pregnancy of unknown location: a consensus statement of nomenclature, definitions, and outcome. Fertil Steril 2011;95:857–66.

Barnhart KT, Sammel MD, Rinaudo PF, Zhou L, Hummel AC, Guo W. Symptomatic patients with an early viable intrauterine pregnancy: HCG curves redefined. Obstet Gynecol 2004;104:50–5.

Brown DL, Doubilet PM. Transvaginal sonography for diagnosing ectopic pregnancy: positivity criteria and performance characteristics. J Ultrasound Med 1994;13:259–66.

Doubilet PM, Benson CB. Further evidence against the reliability of the human chorionic gonadotropin discriminatory level. J Ultrasound Med 2011;30:1637–42.

Medical management of ectopic pregnancy. ACOG Practice Bulletin No. 94. American College of Obstetricians and Gynecologists. Obstet Gynecol 2008;111:1479–85.

Spandorfer SD, Barnhart KT. Endometrial stripe thickness as a predictor of ectopic pregnancy. Fertil Steril 1996;66:474–7.

Stovall TG, Ling FW. Single-dose methotrexate: an expanded clinical trial. Am J Obstet Gynecol 1993;168:1759–62; discussion 1762–5.

94

Vaginal intraepithelial neoplasia

A 51-year-old woman comes to your office for her annual gynecologic examination. Her history is significant for hysterectomy for cervical intraepithelial neoplasia (CIN) 3 at age 45 years. Her Pap test results have been normal since her hysterectomy, and her last normal Pap test was performed 1 year ago. In regard to the possible need for further screening, you advise her that she needs

      (A) no further cytologic screening

      (B) biennial thin-layer cytology with reflex human papillomavirus (HPV) testing

*   (C) thin-layer cytology and HPV cotesting every 5 years

      (D) annual HPV testing

      (E) annual thin-layer cytology

Infection with HPV is associated with neoplasia of the cervix, vagina, vulva, anus, and nasopharynx. Vaginal intraepithelial neoplasia (VAIN) is less common than CIN, with an incidence of approximately 2–3 per million women. Approximately 50–90% of women with VAIN have or have had CIN or cancer of the cervix or vulva. The most common HPV serotypes seen with VAIN are HPV 16 and HPV 18. The natural history of VAIN is not well characterized, but progression of VAIN 3 to invasive cancer has been reported. As with CIN 3, treatment of VAIN 3 is recommended to prevent progression to invasive disease.

Although hysterectomy is considered definitive therapy for CIN, women who have had a hysterectomy for CIN 2 or CIN 3 remain at risk to develop VAIN. The incidence of VAIN has been reported to be 1–7% in women who have undergone a hysterectomy for CIN. Detection of VAIN often occurs months to years after hysterectomy. The described patient remains at risk of development of VAIN. It would be inappropriate for her to have no further cytologic testing. However, the ideal screening strategy for patients with a history of CIN is not entirely clear.

In 2012, the American Society for Colposcopy and Cervical Pathology (ASCCP) published guidelines for the prevention and early detection of cervical cancer (Appendix H), and these guidelines were updated in 2013 (Appendix I). The ASCCP recommended age-appropriate screening guidelines to detect cervical precancerous lesions. The guidelines specifically do not address special populations, such as immunocompromised women and women who have had hysterectomy for CIN. However,

given the paucity of data for this population and the relative rarity of the disease, women who have undergone hysterectomy for CIN should continue screening for VAIN and vaginal cancer.

The ASCCP guidelines for women older than 30 years recommend thin-layer cytology and HPV co-testing every 5 years. Such testing will detect the patient who remains HPV positive and, thus, who remains at risk of HPV-related VAIN. Testing more frequently, either with cytology alone, HPV alone, or with reflex HPV testing, has not been shown to decrease the incidence of invasive vaginal cancer.

Dodge JA, Eltabbakh GH, Mount SL, Walker RP, Morgan A. Clinical features and risk of recurrence among patients with vaginal intraepithelial neoplasia. Gynecol Oncol 2001;83:363–9.

Massad LS, Einstein MH, Huh WK, Katki HA, Kinney WK, Schiffman M, et al. 2012 updated consensus guidelines for the management of abnormal cervical cancer screening tests and cancer precursors. 2012 ASCCP Consensus Guidelines Conference. J Obstet Gynecol 2013;121:829–46.

Saslow D, Solomon D, Lawson HW, Killackey M, Kulasingam SL, Cain J, et al. American Cancer Society, American Society for Colposcopy and Cervical Pathology, and American Society for Clinical Pathology screening guidelines for the prevention and early detection of cervical cancer. American Cancer Society, American Society for Colposcopy and Cervical Pathology and American Society for Clinical Pathology. Am J Clin Pathol 2012;137:516–42.

Schockaert S, Poppe W, Arbyn M, Verguts T, Verguts J. Incidence of vaginal intraepithelial neoplasia after hysterectomy for cervical intraepithelial neoplasia: a retrospective study. Am J Obstet Gynecol 2008;199:113.e1–5.

Yalcin OT, Rutherford TJ, Chambers SK, Chambers JT, Schwartz PE. Vaginal intraepithelial neoplasia: treatment by carbon dioxide laser and risk factors for failure. Eur J Obstet Gynecol Reprod Biol 2003; 106:64–8.

95

Adnexal mass in a postmenopausal woman

A 60-year-old woman comes to your office for a preventive health visit. She reports no significant interval medical history. Her family history includes her paternal grandmother with ovarian cancer and a maternal cousin with postmenopausal breast cancer. The patient underwent a screening mammography and colonoscopy within the last year, both with normal results. Breast, abdominal, and rectal examinations yield normal results. A right adnexal mass is palpated on bimanual examination. Transvaginal ultrasonography shows the finding as shown in Figure 95-1. A CA 125 level is 11 units/mL and hemoglobin level is 12.7 g/dL. The best next step in the management is

     (A) laparoscopy
     (B) laparotomy
*   (C) repeat ultrasonography in 3–6 months
     (D) gynecologic oncologist evaluation
     (E) *BRCA1* and *BRCA2* testing

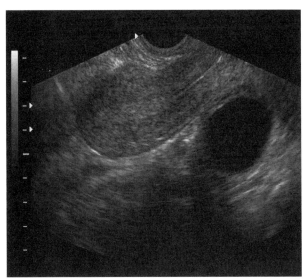

FIG. 95-1

Evaluation of a postmenopausal woman with an adnexal mass includes transvaginal ultrasonography and serum CA 125 level measurement. Simple ovarian cysts have the following benign characteristics: oval or round, anechoic, smooth, thin walls, no solid component or septation, posterior acoustic enhancement, and no internal flow. Cyst characteristics concerning for malignancy include thick (greater than 3 mm), irregular septations and nodules with blood flow.

An elevated CA 125 level in a postmenopausal woman with an adnexal mass raises suspicion for ovarian cancer. In a prospective study of 158 patients who underwent laparotomy for a pelvic mass, the positive predictive value of an elevated CA 125 level was 98% in postmenopausal women (cancer prevalence 63%) compared with 49% in premenopausal women.

Simple cysts up to 10 cm in diameter as measured by ultrasonography are almost universally benign and may safely be monitored without intervention, even in postmenopausal patients. No studies have been conducted to determine the ideal interval length between ultrasonographic evaluations. Most experts advocate an interval of 3–6 months between evaluations. Serum CA 125 level measurements do not need to be repeated in postmenopausal patients with simple adnexal cysts.

This patient does not require a referral to a gynecologic oncologist. Box 95-1 lists the American College of Obstetricians and Gynecologists and the Society of Gynecologic Oncologists' referral guidelines for a newly diagnosed pelvic mass in a postmenopausal woman (older than age 50 years). Malignancy in the case of a simple

---

BOX 95-1

American College of Obstetricians and Gynecologists and Society of Gynecologic Oncologists' Referral Guidelines for a Newly Diagnosed Pelvic Mass in a Postmenopausal Woman (Older Than 50 Years)

- Elevated CA 125 levels
- Ascites
- Nodular or fixed pelvic mass
- Evidence of abdominal or distant metastasis (by results of examination or imaging study)
- Family history or breast or ovarian cancer (in a first-degree relative)

Hereditary breast and ovarian cancer syndrome. ACOG Practice Bulletin No. 103. American College of Obstetricians and Gynecologists and Society of Gynecologic Oncologists. Obstet Gynecol 2009;113:957–66.

cyst is highly unlikely. Thus, surgical management by laparoscopy or laparotomy is not needed. Surgery should be considered for the patient if she develops pain, in the case of interval growth, or if changes are noted in the characteristics of the cyst.

This patient does not meet the criteria for genetic testing for hereditary breast and ovarian cancer syndrome. Genetic testing could be offered to a patient in the following circumstances:

- If multiple family members have breast cancer, ovarian cancer, or both

- Breast and ovarian cancer are present in a single individual

- If the breast cancer was characterized by early age of onset

Box 95-2 lists criteria for genetic risk assessment for breast cancer.

Bailey CL, Ueland FR, Land GL, DePriest PD, Gallion HH, Kryscio RJ, et al. The malignant potential of small cystic ovarian tumors in women over 50 years of age. Gynecol Oncol 1998;69:3–7.

Hereditary breast and ovarian cancer syndrome. ACOG Practice Bulletin No. 103. American College of Obstetricians and Gynecologists and Society of Gynecologic Oncologists. Obstet Gynecol 2009;113:957–66.

Levine D, Brown DL, Andreotti RF, Benacerraf B, Benson CB, Brewster WR, et al. Management of asymptomatic ovarian and other adnexal cysts imaged at US Society of Radiologists in Ultrasound consensus conference statement. Society of Radiologists in Ultrasound. Ultrasound Q 2010;26:121–31.

Management of adnexal masses. ACOG Practice Bulletin No. 83. American College of Obstetricians and Gynecologists. Obstet Gynecol 2007;110:201–14.

Nezhat C, Cho J, King LP, Hajhosseini B, Nezhat F. Laparoscopic management of adnexal masses. Obstet Gynecol Clin North Am 2011;38:663–76.

BOX 95-2

Criteria for Genetic Risk Assessment for Breast Cancer

Patients with greater than an approximate 20–25% chance of having an inherited predisposition to breast cancer and ovarian cancer and for whom genetic risk assessment is recommended:

- Women with a personal history of both breast-cancer and ovarian cancer*

- Women with ovarian cancer* and a close relative[†] with ovarian cancer or premenopausal breast cancer or both

- Women with ovarian cancer* who are of Ashkenazi Jewish ancestry

- Women with breast cancer at age 50 years or younger and a close relative[†] with ovarian cancer* or male breast cancer at any age

- Women of Ashkenazi Jewish ancestry in whom breast cancer was diagnosed at age 40 years or younger

- Women with a close relative[†] with a known BRCA 1 or BRCA 2 mutation

Patients with greater than an approximate 5–10% chance of having an inherited predisposition to breast cancer and ovarian cancer and for whom genetic risk assessment may be helpful:

- Women with breast cancer at age 40 years or younger

- Women with ovarian cancer, primary peritoneal cancer, or fallopian tube cancer of high grade, serous histology at any age

- Women with bilateral breast cancer (particularly if the first case of breast cancer was diagnosed at age 50 years or younger)

- Women with breast cancer at age 50 years or younger and a close relative[†] with breast cancer at age 50 years or younger

- Women of Ashkenazi Jewish ancestry with breast cancer at age 50 years or younger

- Women with breast cancer at any age and two or more close relatives[†] with breast cancer at any age (particularly if at least one case of breast cancer was diagnosed at age 50 years or younger)

- Unaffected women with a close relative[†] that meets one of the previous criteria

*Cancer of the peritoneum and fallopian tubes should be considered a part of the spectrum of the hereditary breast and ovarian cancer syndrome.

[†]Close relative is defined as a first-degree relative (mother, sister, daughter) or second-degree relative (grandmother, granddaughter, aunt, niece).

Hereditary breast and ovarian cancer syndrome. ACOG Practice Bulletin No. 103. American College of Obstetricians and Gynecologists and Society of Gynecologic Oncologists. Obstet Gynecol 2009;113:957–66.

96

Intraoperative hypotension

A 21-year-old woman is undergoing a laparotomy for a cystectomy of a 20-cm teratoma on her right ovary. Her medical history is otherwise unremarkable and her only medication is an oral contraceptive. During the surgery, after lifting the right ovary off the right pelvic sidewall, the anesthesiologist reports significant hypotension, tachycardia, hypoxemia, and decreased end-tidal carbon dioxide. The most likely diagnosis is

        (A) acute blood loss anemia
*   (B) pulmonary embolus
        (C) acute myocardial infarction
        (D) septic shock

The diagnosis of acute pulmonary embolus should be considered in a patient with a clinical description, such as that described. Acute pulmonary embolus would be the most likely diagnosis. The most common anesthesia findings include hypotension, tachycardia, hypoxemia, and decreased end-tidal carbon dioxide. These findings are consistent with a fixed cardiopulmonary defect that can lead to shock and cardiac collapse. Early identification, supportive care, and anticoagulation can lead to improved outcomes. Risk factors for this patient include surgery, age, immobility, and oral contraceptive use. Appendix F provides a list of risk factors for venous thromboembolism.

In the operating room, the most important concern is the safety of the patient. In a situation of hemodynamic instability without a clear etiology, continuation of the surgery may add another variable and potential complications to her recovery. Aggressive anticoagulation for a presumed pulmonary embolus may be limited by surgical site bleeding.

Acute anemia often is found in those patients with extensive blood loss in the perioperative period. An open cystectomy in an otherwise healthy patient is unlikely to lead to acute blood loss anemia.

Myocardial infarction and septic shock should be considered for patients with a history of an acute cardiopulmonary event in the operating room. Atypical cardiac findings in a young patient without other cardiac risk factors would favor a pulmonary embolus compared with a new onset myocardial infarction. Levels of cardiac enzymes may be abnormal in a patient with a significant pulmonary embolus that causes cardiopulmonary instability, but they are secondary to the pulmonary strain. Sepsis also can lead to cardiopulmonary collapse; however, in this patient, little supporting history is present to suggest an infectious etiology.

Desciak MC, Martin DE. Perioperative pulmonary embolism: diagnosis and anesthetic management. J Clin Anesth 2011;23:153–65.

Martino MA, Borges E, Williamson E, Siegfried S, Cantor AB, Lancaster J, et al. Pulmonary embolism after major abdominal surgery in gynecologic oncology. Obstet Gynecol 2006;107:666–71.

Prevention of deep vein thrombosis and pulmonary embolism. ACOG Practice Bulletin No. 84. American College of Obstetricians and Gynecologists. Obstet Gynecol 2007;110:429–40.

Raghav KP, Makkuni P, Figueredo VM. A review of electrocardiography in pulmonary embolism: recognizing pulmonary embolus masquerading as ST-elevation myocardial infarction. Rev Cardiovasc Med 2011;12:157–63.

97

Recommendations to prevent osteoporosis

A 66-year-old postmenopausal woman presents for follow-up after bone density screening. Her T-score was –0.9. She takes daily vitamin D and calcium. Her past medical history is significant for deep vein thrombosis after delivery of her second child 30 years ago. She currently reports treatment for gastroesophageal reflux disease and osteoarthritis. She takes a daily antacid and acetaminophen as needed. She recently was treated with an oral steroid taper for 10 days because of an urticarial skin reaction. The best recommendation to maintain her bone mineral density is

    (A) oral estrogen and progestin
    (B) selective estrogen receptor modulators
    (C) bisphosphonates
*   (D) calcium-rich foods and strength-building exercise

Osteoporosis is characterized by excessive loss of protein and mineral content of bones, leading to fragility and risk of fracture. It is more common in women, particularly after menopause (because of accelerated loss of bone mass), than in men. Approximately 13–18% of U.S. women aged 50 years and older have osteoporosis and another 37–50% of U.S. women have low bone mass (osteopenia). Common fractures with the most morbidity are hip and thoracic fractures. Furthermore, it is important to recognize that the risk of osteoporosis varies by race (Table 97-1).

Bone mineral density (BMD) is measured to diagnose osteoporosis and osteopenia on the basis of resultant Z-score (compared with a reference population stratified by age, sex, and race) or T-score (Table 97-2). Several tests are used to screen for BMD and, therefore, the parameters for each test should be considered individually.

TABLE 97-1. Association Between Screening for Osteoporosis and Hip Fractures Overall and by Subgroup

Variable	Sample Size (n) Screened Group	Sample Size (n) Usual Care Group	Hip Fractures (n) Screened Group	Hip Fractures (n) Usual Care Group	Incidence of Hip Fractures per 1,000 Person-years Screened Group	Incidence of Hip Fractures per 1,000 Person-years Usual Care Group	Hazard of Hip Fractures (95% Confidence Interval) Screened Group Versus Usual Care Group Unadjusted	Hazard of Hip Fractures (95% Confidence Interval) Screened Group Versus Usual Care Group Adjusted*
Overall	1,422	1,685	33	69	4.8	8.2	0.59 (0.39–0.89)	0.64 (0.41–0.99)
Sex								
Women	768	959	20	47	5.3	9.7	0.55 (0.32–0.92)	0.61 (0.35–1.06)
Men	654	726	13	22	4.2	6.3	0.68 (0.34–1.36)	0.68 (0.32–1.42)
Age (Years)								
65–74	598	758	7	16	2.3	4.1	0.57 (0.24–1.42)	0.61 (0.29–1.87)
75–84	724	812	23	35	6.6	8.8	0.76 (0.45–1.28)	0.82 (0.47–1.44)
Greater than 85	100	115	3	18	8.1	38.6	0.22 (0.06–0.73)	0.22 (0.06–0.79)
Race								
White	1,133	1,442	31	67	5.6	9.3	0.61 (0.40–0.94)	0.62 (0.39–0.97)
Black	289	243	2	2	1.4	1.7	0.82 (0.12–5.84)	Not given[†]

*Adjusted for sex and the propensity to be screened; results stratified by sex were adjusted only for the propensity to be screened.

[†]There were too few events (less than 20) to allow for adjustment.

Kern LM, Powe NR, Levine MA, Fitzpatrick AL, Harris TB, Robbins J, et al. Association between screening for osteoporosis and the incidence of hip fracture. Ann Intern Med 2005;142:173–81.

TABLE 97-2. Diagnosing Osteoporosis Using Bone Densitometry Criteria Developed by the World Health Organization

Category	T-Score*
Normal	Greater than or equal to –1.0
Low Bone Mass (osteopenia)	Less than –1 to greater than –2.5
Osteoporosis	Less than or equal to –2.5

*T-score is the number of standard deviations above or below the mean average bone density value for young adult women.

Osteoporosis. Practice Bulletin No. 129. American College of Obstetricians and Gynecologists. Obstet Gynecol 2012;120: 718–34.

Dual-energy X-ray absorptiometry is preferred because it measures BMD at the at-risk sites for fracture, and has high precision, accuracy, and minimal radiation exposure. Other modalities that may be useful screening options are ultrasonography and computed tomography. Bone mineral density testing is recommended for the following postmenopausal groups: women greater than age 65 years, women younger than 65 years with one or more risk factor for osteoporosis, and women who have had a bone fracture. Such testing should be considered in premenopausal women with medical conditions or treatments associated with osteoporosis. Screening interval should be no more often than every 2 years, although recent data may support longer intervals.

Risk factors for osteoporosis include estrogen deficiency, risk factors for falls, smoking and alcohol abuse, nutritional deficiencies, certain chronic medical conditions, and drug therapy (Table 97-3). Corticosteroids are associated with increased risk of osteoporosis, but this patient only took a short limited course of therapy.

Although estrogen therapy improves BMD, it carries potential risks of venous thromboembolic cardiovascular events and breast cancer. Therefore, a decision to use estrogen therapy should be based on individual factors and the need for management of vasomotor symptoms. Nutritional supplementation with calcium and vitamin D along with lifestyle changes, such as weight-bearing exercises, cessation of tobacco use, and moderation in alcohol intake, should be discussed. This patient would benefit most from a calcium-rich diet and weight-bearing exercise. However, a review of recent studies showed that calcium supplementation is not helpful for BMD and may carry some risks of coronary disease.

Bisphosphonate therapy and selective estrogen receptor modulators (SERMs) can be used for the prevention and treatment of osteoporosis. Human recombinant parathyroid hormone also may be used for treatment of osteoporosis. Secondary causes of bone mineral deficiency should be ruled out. The World Health Organization's online Fracture Risk Assessment Tool accounts for geographical, racial, and lifestyle factors along with BMD (Appendix B). Treatment should be considered with a 3% risk of hip fracture or a 20% risk of a major osteoporotic fracture (forearm, hip, shoulder, or clinical spine) or both in the next 10 years.

The described patient has neither osteopenia nor osteoporosis and does not meet criteria for treatment. She should continue with her calcium and vitamin D supplementation as a strategy to prevent osteoporosis. If she did have osteoporosis, because of her history of venous thromboembolism, she may not choose estrogen or SERM therapy; however, SERM therapy also may cause vasomotor symptoms. Bisphosphonates are poorly absorbed and may cause upper gastrointestinal tract adverse effects. They are contraindicated in women with gastroesophageal reflux disease and other esophageal abnormalities.

Gourlay ML, Fine JP, Preisser JS, May RC, Li C, Lui LY, et al. Bone-density testing interval and transition to osteoporosis in older women. Study of Osteoporotic Fractures Research Group. N Engl J Med 2012;366:225–33.

Osteoporosis. Practice Bulletin No. 129. American College of Obstetricians and Gynecologists. Obstet Gynecol 2012;120:718–34.

World Health Organization Collaborating Centre for Metabolic Bone Diseases. WHO Fracture Risk Assessment Tool (FRAX). Sheffield, United Kingdom: University of Sheffield; 2013. Available at: http://www.shef.ac.uk/FRAX/. Retrieved June 21, 2013.

TABLE 97-3. Conditions, Diseases, and Medications That Cause or Contribute to Osteoporosis and Fractures

Lifestyle Factors		
Alcohol abuse	High salt intake	Falling
Low calcium intake	Inadequate physical activity	Excessive thinness
Vitamin D insufficiency	Immobilization	
Excessive vitamin A level	Smoking (active or passive)	

Genetic Factors		
Cystic fibrosis	Homocystinuria	Osteogenesis imperfecta
Ehlers–Danlos syndrome	Hypophosphatasia	Parental history of hip fracture
Gaucher disease	Idiopathic hypercalciuria	Porphyria
Glycogen storage diseases	Marfan syndrome	Riley–Day syndrome
Hemochromatosis	Menkes steely hair syndrome	

Hypogonadal States		
Androgen insensitivity	Hyperprolactinemia	Premature ovarian failure
Anorexia nervosa and bulimia	Premature menopause	Athletic amenorrhea
Turner syndrome and Klinefelter syndrome	Panhypopituitarism	

Endocrine Disorders		
Adrenal insufficiency	Cushing syndrome	Central adiposity
Diabetes mellitus type 1 and diabetes mellitus type 2	Hyperparathyroidism	Thyrotoxicosis

Gastrointestinal Disorders		
Celiac disease	Inflammatory bowel disease	Primary biliary cirrhosis
Gastric bypass	Malabsorption	
Gastrointestinal surgery	Pancreatic disease	

Hematologic Disorders		
Multiple myeloma	Monoclonal gammopathies	Sickle cell disease
Hemophilia	Leukemia and lymphomas	Systemic mastocytosis
Thalassemia		

Rheumatologic and Autoimmune Diseases		
Ankylosing spondylitis	Lupus	Rheumatoid arthritis
Other rheumatic and autoimmune diseases		

Central Nervous System Disorders		
Epilepsy	Parkinson disease	Stroke
Multiple sclerosis	Spinal cord injury	

Miscellaneous Conditions and Diseases		
Acquired immunodeficiency syndrome and human immunodeficiency virus	Congestive heart failure	Muscular dystrophy
Alcoholism	Depression	Posttransplantation bone disease
Amyloidosis	End-stage renal disease	Sarcoidosis
Chronic metabolic acidosis	Hypercalciuria	Weight loss
Chronic obstructive pulmonary disease	Idiopathic scoliosis	

(continued)

TABLE 97-3. Conditions, Diseases, and Medications That Cause or Contribute to Osteoporosis and Fractures *(continued)*

Medications		
Aluminum (in antacids)	Cyclosporine A and tacrolimus	Proton pump inhibitors
Anticoagulants (heparin)	Depot medroxyprogesterone acetate for premenopausal contraception	Selective serotonin reuptake inhibitors
Anticonvulsants	Glucocorticoids (5 mg/day or more of prednisone or equivalent for 3 months or more)	Tamoxifen citrate for premenopausal use
Aromatase inhibitors	Gonadotropin-releasing hormone antagonists and agonists	Thiazolidinediones
Barbiturates	Lithium	Thyroid hormones (in excess)
Chemotherapy	Methotrexate sodium	Parenteral nutrition

National Osteoporosis Foundation. Clinician's guide to prevention and treatment of osteoporosis. Washington, DC: NOF; 2013. Available at: http://www.nof.org/files/nof/public/content/resource/913/files/580.pdf. Retrieved August 29, 2013.

Reprinted with permission from Clinician's Guide to Prevention and Treatment of Osteoporosis, pages 14–15, 2013 National Osteoporosis Foundation, Washington, DC 20037. All rights reserved. From U.S. Department of Health and Human Services. Bone Health and Osteoporosis: A Report of the Surgeon General. Rockville, MD: 2004. U.S. Department of Health and Human Services, Office of the Surgeon General; 2004 with modifications.

98

Indications for risk-reducing surgery

A 29-year-old woman is referred to you for reproductive health counseling. She was treated with a total colectomy at age 19 years for right-sided colon cancer. The cancer was associated with an *MLH1* mismatch repair mutation by immunohistochemistry studies. She is adamant that she does not want to get pregnant. The most appropriate risk-reducing strategy is

   (A) progestin-containing intrauterine device
   (B) permanent tubal occlusion
   (C) vaginal hysterectomy
 * (D) hysterectomy with bilateral salpingo-oophorectomy (BSO)
   (E) BSO

Although it accounts for only 2–3% of all colorectal cancer cases, colon cancer associated with Lynch II syndrome or a hereditary nonpolyposis colorectal cancer (HNPCC) occurs frequently in individuals of young age, tends to be right-sided, and can be metachronous. Approximately 90% of cancer patients have mutations in one of the mismatch repair genes (*MLH1, MSH2, MSH6,* and *PMS2*), which can be measured by immunohistochemical analysis or a measurement of deficient DNA repair known as microsatellite instability. Women with a congenital mismatch repair mutation are at high risk of colon, endometrial, ovarian, urinary tract, stomach, pancreas, biliary tract, or small bowel cancer. Two variants of HNPCC also exist, Turcot syndrome and Muir–Torre syndrome. Turcot syndrome also includes brain cancer, and Muir–Torre syndrome includes sebaceous gland

adenomas and keratoacanthomas. Familial adenomatous polyposis is another inherited colon cancer syndrome; it is caused by a germline mutation in the *adenomatous polyposis coli* gene and accounts for only 1% of colorectal cancer cases. In contrast with patients with HNPCC, individuals affected by this mutation have greater than 100 colon polyps and a nearly 100% lifetime risk of colon cancer but do not have an increased risk of gynecologic cancer.

The revised Amsterdam criteria can be useful for identifying candidate families with HNPCC, ie, of three relatives with the associated cancer that occur in two generations, one relative with cancer that occured before age 50 years will identify 60% of HNPCC families (Appendix K-1). The revised Bethesda criteria (Appendix K-2) have higher specificity than the Amsterdam criteria for identification of families with mismatch repair gene mutations. Instead of relying on clinical criteria, many institutions use immunohistochemical evaluation of candidate cases when they occur in young men or women.

The Society of Gynecologic Oncologists recommends referral to a familial cancer program for women with:

- Endometrial or ovarian cancer with a synchronous or metachronous colorectal or other HNPCC-associated cancer with the first case of cancer diagnosed in an individual at any age
- Endometrial or colorectal cancer diagnosed in an individual younger than 50 years
- Endometrial or colorectal cancer and those that fulfill the modified Amsterdam criteria
- First- or second-degree relative who meets the above criteria

Individuals who have an inherited predisposition to HNPCC should be monitored closely and be considered for risk-reducing surgery. Box 98-1 shows the National Comprehensive Cancer Network's screening strategies for HNPCC-associated cancer. The lifetime risk of endometrial cancer approaches 60%, and this cancer occurs frequently in premenopausal women. In addition to transvaginal ultrasonography, which is insensitive in detecting endometrial cancer in premenopausal women, annual endometrial sampling is recommended for women who have not yet completed childbearing. The risk of endometrial cancer is not decreased by use of progestins or ovulatory menses. Whereas the lifetime risk of ovarian cancer is only 12%, this represents a nearly 10-fold increase over the risk of the general population.

According to a comprehensive analysis conducted by the French Cancer Genetics Network, the lifetime risk of ovarian cancer varies according to the inherited mutation, ie, lifetime risks are 20%, 24%, and 1% for the *MLH1*, *MSH2*, and *MSH6* mutations, respectively. The analysis also showed that ovarian cancer was unlikely after age 30 years. Ovarian cancer screening by ultrasonography with or without CA 125 measurement remains a recommended but unproved test for women at high risk of ovarian cancer.

Definitive risk-reducing surgery, with hysterectomy and BSO when childbearing is complete remains the best plan for an affected woman. Timing of this surgery often occurs before age 40 years because the risk of endometrial cancer is increased at the time. Hysterectomy alone does not address this patient's increased risk of ovarian cancer.

Tubal ligation and BSO are associated with a decreased risk of ovarian cancer, but do not decrease the risk of endometrial cancer in either the general population or in women at increased risk because of a genetic mutation. Because the described patient is at average risk of breast cancer and has no contraindication to hormone

---

BOX 98-1

National Comprehensive Cancer Network's Screening Strategies for Hereditary Nonpolyposis Colorectal Cancer-Associated Cancer

Colon cancer

- Colonoscopy at age 20–25 years or 2–5 years before the earliest case of colon cancer in family if it is diagnosed in a relative before age 25 years; repeat every 1–2 years

Extracolonic cancer

Endometrial and ovarian cancer

- Prophylactic hysterectomy and bilateral salpingo-oophorectomy is a risk-reducing option that should be considered by women who have completed childbearing.
- Patients must be aware that dysfunctional uterine bleeding warrants evaluation.
- No evidence clearly supports screening for endometrial cancer as a way to screen for hereditary nonpolyposis colorectal cancer (HNPCC)-associated cancer. However, annual office endometrial sampling is an option.
- Although clinicians may find screening helpful in certain circumstances, data do not support routine ovarian screening for HNPCC-associated cancer. Transvaginal ultrasonography for ovarian and endometrial cancer has not been shown to be sufficiently sensitive or specific to support a positive recommendation but may be considered at the clinician's discretion. Serum CA 125 level measurement is an additional ovarian screening test with caveats similar to transvaginal ultrasonography.

Gastric and small bowel cancer

- No evidence clearly supports screening for gastric and small bowel cancer as way to screen for HNPCC-associated cancer; however, the clinician may consider esophagogastroduodenoscopy with extended duodenoscopy (to distal duodenum and into the jejunum) at 2- to 3-year intervals beginning at age 30–35 years.

Urothelial cancer

- Annual urinalysis should be considered starting at age 25–30 years.

Central nervous system cancer

- Annual physical examination starting at age 25–30 years; no additional screening recommendations have been made.

Pancreatic cancer

- Because of limited data, no recommendation is possible at this time.

National Comprehensive Cancer Network. NCCN guidelines. Fort Washington (PA): NCCN; 2013. Available at: http://www.nccn.org/professionals/physician_gls/f_guidelines.asp. Retrieved June 7, 2013.

therapy, she should be offered estrogen-only therapy postoperatively to avoid the consequences of premature menopause.

Bonadona V, Bonaïti B, Olschwang S, Grandjouan S, Huiart L, Longy M, et al. Cancer risks associated with germline mutations in MLH1, MSH2, and MSH6 genes in Lynch syndrome. JAMA 2011;305:2304–10.

Guillem JG, Wood WC, Moley JF, Berchuck A, Karlan BY, Mutch DG, et al. ASCO/SSO review of current role of risk-reducing surgery in common hereditary cancer syndromes. ASCO and SSO. J Clin Oncol 2006;24:4642–60.

Lancaster JM, Powell CB, Kauff ND, Cass I, Chen LM, Lu KH, et al. Society of Gynecologic Oncologists Education Committee statement on risk assessment for inherited gynecologic cancer predispositions. Society of Gynecologic Oncologists Education Committee. Gynecol Oncol 2007;107:159–62.

Lindor NM, Petersen GM, Hadley DW, Kinney AY, Miesfeldt S, Lu KH, et al. Recommendations for the care of individuals with an inherited predisposition to Lynch syndrome: a systematic review. JAMA 2006;296:1507–17.

99

Ovarian preservation or removal at the time of hysterectomy

A 44-year-old woman with symptomatic myomas comes to your office for a preoperative evaluation. She is not at an increased genetic risk of ovarian cancer. As part of the hysterectomy informed consent, you discuss the risks and benefits of ovary retention at the time of surgery. You explain that, compared with the general population, if she has a hysterectomy with ovarian retention, the time at which she is likely to experience menopause is

      (A) at a similar age
      (B) at an older age
      (C) immediately postoperatively
*   (D) at a younger age

Approximately 460,000–600,000 hysterectomies are performed in the United States annually, making hysterectomy the most common major nonobstetric surgical procedure performed on women. More than one half of these procedures occur in women younger than 44 years. Since 2000, the rates of oophorectomy at the time of hysterectomy for benign disease have been decreasing. Age, route of hysterectomy, and indication for surgery affect rates of bilateral salpingo-oophorectomy. Women are more likely to retain their ovaries if they are younger than 40 years; undergo vaginal hysterectomy; or have surgery for myomas, abnormal uterine bleeding, or prolapse. Factors that favor oophorectomy and ovary retention are listed in Box 99-1.

Inherited susceptibility to ovarian cancer is the greatest risk factor for development of ovarian cancer. Women with a genetically identified increased risk of ovarian cancer should undergo risk-reducing bilateral salpingo-oophorectomy at the time of hysterectomy. This should include inspection of the peritoneal cavity, pelvic washings, and ligation of the ovarian vessels at the pelvic brim.

A study that used decision analysis found that bilateral oophorectomy at the time of hysterectomy for benign disease was associated with a decreased risk of breast and

---

BOX 99-1

Oophorectomy Versus Ovarian Preservation at the Time of Hysterectomy

Factors favoring oophorectomy

- Genetic susceptibility for ovarian carcinoma based on family history or genetic testing
- Bilateral ovarian neoplasms
- Severe endometriosis
- Pelvic inflammatory disease or bilateral tubo-ovarian abscesses
- Postmenopausal status

Factors favoring ovarian preservation

- Premenopausal status
- Desire for fertility
- Impact on sexual function, libido, and quality of life in young women
- Osteopenia, osteoporosis, or risk factors for osteoporosis (if premenopausal)

Elective and risk-reducing salpingo-oophorectomy. ACOG Practice Bulletin No. 89. American College of Obstetricians and Gynecologists. Obstet Gynecol 2008;111:231–41.

ovarian cancer. This study also showed an increased risk of all-cause mortality, fatal and nonfatal coronary heart disease, and lung cancer.

In the short term, most women do not lose ovarian function after hysterectomy with ovary retention. Two prospective studies noted a proportional excess risk over the study periods and not abruptly after hysterectomy. After 4 years of follow-up, women with hysterectomy experienced ovarian failure 1.9–3.7 years earlier than control participants.

The causal pathway of earlier menopause in women who undergo premenopausal hysterectomy with ovary retention is unknown. One hypothesis is that hysterectomy causes compromise of blood flow to the ovaries and may lead to a reduced production of hormones. Additionally, the uterus may have an inhibitory influence on pituitary follicle-stimulating hormone secretions, and its removal may allow levels to increase, which accelerates follicular depletion. Another hypothesis is that the

underlying conditions that led to surgery, ie, abnormal uterine bleeding, myomas, and endometriosis may increase the risk of ovarian failure. When discussing hysterectomy for benign disease with a patient, physicians should incorporate the potential for earlier menopause into their discussions.

Elective and risk-reducing salpingo-oophorectomy. ACOG Practice Bulletin No. 89. American College of Obstetricians and Gynecologists. Obstet Gynecol 2008;111:231–41.

Jacoby VL, Vittinghoff E, Nakagawa S, Jackson R, Richter HE, Chan J, et al. Factors associated with undergoing bilateral salpingo-oophorectomy at the time of hysterectomy for benign conditions. Obstet Gynecol 2009;113:1259–67.

Moorman PG, Myers ER, Schildkraut JM, Iversen ES, Wang F, Warren N. Effect of hysterectomy with ovarian preservation on ovarian function. Obstet Gynecol 2011;118:1271–9.

Parker WH, Broder MS, Chang E, Feskanich D, Farquhar C, Liu Z, et al. Ovarian conservation at the time of hysterectomy and long-term health outcomes in the nurses' health study. Obstet Gynecol 2009;113:1027–37.

100

Recurrent urinary incontinence

A 55-year-old multiparous woman is evaluated for urinary incontinence. She underwent a transobturator tape procedure 3 years ago for the clinical diagnosis of stress urinary incontinence. The patient reports some incontinence with activity and Valsalva maneuvers but no urgency. Urodynamic testing is significant for a maximal urethral closing pressure of less than 40 cm H_2O. The most likely diagnosis for urinary incontinence in this patient is

      (A) overactive bladder
      (B) vesicovaginal fistula
*   (C) intrinsic sphincter deficiency
      (D) overflow incontinence
      (E) recurrent stress incontinence

Persistent or recurrent urinary incontinence can occur in up to 20% of women who have had surgery to correct stress urinary incontinence. It is important that women with recurrent or persistent symptoms undergo a thorough evaluation, including urodynamic testing. Women who have a body mass index greater than 30 (calculated as weight in kilograms divided by height in meters squared), diabetes mellitus, or concomitant pelvic organ prolapse are more likely to have an unsuccessful outcome of primary surgery. Additionally, urodynamic testing can identify women who are likely to have mixed urinary incontinence, overactive bladder, or intrinsic sphincter deficiency.

The initial evaluation of a woman with persistent or recurrent urinary incontinence includes obtaining history

and a physical examination. In evaluating the patient, the health care provider should consider the following questions:

- Does the patient have the same symptoms as she did preoperatively?
- Are the current symptoms urge related?
- Is infection present?
- Is overflow incontinence present from overcorrection of urethral hypermobility?
- Is a fistula present?
- How severe are her symptoms?

Urodynamic testing is important to evaluate the patient for intrinsic sphincter deficiency and detrusor instability if pelvic examination, urinalysis, and postvoid residual are normal. Minimally invasive suburethral sling procedures are the most common procedures for stress urinary incontinence; they supplant the pubovaginal sling and colposuspension. Tension-free vaginal tape (TVT) and transobturator tape procedures have similar efficacy for women with stress urinary incontinence without intrinsic sphincter deficiency. The transobturator tape method is preferred by some experts to the TVT method because of its lower incidence of injury to the bladder, pelvic vessels, and bowel. Recent reports have suggested that the TVT procedure has better long-term cure rates than the transobturator tape procedure for women with stress urinary incontinence and intrinsic sphincter deficiency. Women with recurrent stress urinary incontinence with intrinsic sphincter deficiency whose symptoms are bothersome enough to consider an additional surgical procedure would be candidates for the TVT procedure.

The described patient has a low maximal urethral closing pressure, which indicates intrinsic sphincter deficiency. Although she still has stress urinary incontinence based on medical history, the urodynamic profile demonstrates intrinsic sphincter deficiency. Her history and urodynamic findings do not suggest fistula, detrusor overactivity, or overflow incontinence.

Houwert RM, Venema PL, Aquarius AE, Bruinse HW, Roovers JP, Vervest HA. Risk factors for failure of retropubic and transobturator midurethral slings. Am J Obstet Gynecol 2009;201:202.e1–8.

Schierlitz L, Dwyer PL, Rosamilia A, Murray C, Thomas E, De Souza A, et al. Three-year follow-up of tension-free vaginal tape compared with transobturator tape in women with stress urinary incontinence and intrinsic sphincter deficiency. Obstet Gynecol 2012;119:321–7.

Schierlitz L, Dwyer PL, Rosamilia A, Murray C, Thomas E, De Souza A, et al. Effectiveness of tension-free vaginal tape compared with transobturator tape in women with stress urinary incontinence and intrinsic sphincter deficiency: a randomized controlled trial. Obstet Gynecol 2008;112:1253–61.

101

Prophylactic antibiotics for abdominal surgery

A 45-year-old woman with a body mass index of 24 (calculated as weight in kilograms divided by height in meters squared) undergoes a total abdominal hysterectomy for asymptomatic uterine fibroids. She receives intravenous cefazolin 1 hour before skin incision. The procedure is complicated by extensive adhesiolysis, repair of a small bowel injury, and cystotomy. Estimated blood loss is 700 mL, and the procedure is completed in 4.5 hours. The patient is extubated without difficulty and transferred to the recovery area. During quality improvement review, the patient is noted to have received inadequate prophylactic antibiotics during the procedure. The most likely source of the inadequacy was

* (A) lack of antibiotic administration at the time of cystotomy repair
* (B) timing of preoperative antibiotics
* * (C) length of surgical procedure
* (D) amount of estimated blood loss

Acquisition of a surgical site infection increases morbidity, cost, and mortality in patients who undergo surgical procedures. In 2006, the Surgical Care Improvement Project published guidelines to provide standard quality measures and track standards of care regarding prevention of surgical infection, including during the perioperative period (Box 101-1). Table 101-1 lists recommendations for antibiotic prophylaxis in gynecologic procedures, and Appendix G lists factors to be considered by the health care practitioner when choosing a prophylactic antimicrobial agent.

Prophylactic antibiotics are not required for every surgical procedure. Decisions regarding the need for antibiotics in gynecologic surgery are based on surgical wound classification, ie, clean, clean–contaminated, contaminated, dirty–infected (Box 101-2). Although modern aseptic technique has been associated with a dramatic decrease in surgical site infections, bacterial contamination of the surgical site is inevitable. Systemic antibiotic prophylaxis is based on the concept that antibiotics in the host tissues can augment natural immune-defense mechanisms and help kill any bacteria that are inoculated into the wound. Only a narrow window of antimicrobial efficacy is available, which requires the administration of antibiotics either shortly before or at the time of bacterial inoculation (eg, when the incision is made, the vagina is entered, or the pedicles are clamped). Most studies have shown that no particular regimen is superior to others.

Individual hospital policies should be considered when deciding the best possible regimen. An increased dose of preoperative antibiotics may be required in obese patients.

Additional intraoperative doses of prophylactic antibiotics are indicated in several instances. In lengthy procedures, additional intraoperative doses, given at intervals of one to two times the half-life of the drug will maintain adequate levels of medication throughout the operation. For cefazolin, a second dose should be administered if the surgical time exceeds 3 hours. A second dose also is appropriate in surgical cases when the estimated blood loss exceeds 1,500 mL. Additional prophylactic antibiotics should be given if a surgical case becomes contaminated with large bowel flora.

This patient had preoperative antibiotics at the appropriate time and her estimated blood loss did not meet criteria for additional prophylactic antibiotics. Her visceral injuries were to the bladder and small bowel, which do not require such additional antibiotics. This patient should have received an additional dose of prophylactic antibiotics because the procedure time exceeded 3 hours.

Antibiotic prophylaxis for gynecologic procedures. ACOG Practice Bulletin No. 104. American College of Obstetricians and Gynecologists. Obstet Gynecol 2009;113:1180–9.

Rosenberger LH, Politano AD, Sawyer RG. The surgical care improvement project and prevention of post-operative infection, including surgical site infection. Surg Infect (Larchmt) 2011;12:163–8.

BOX 101-1

Guidelines for Use of Prophylactic Antibiotics in the Perioperative Period*

- Prophylactic antibiotics should be
  - received 1 hour prior to surgical incision
  - selected for activity against the most probable antimicrobial contaminants
  - always given for hysterectomy
  - discontinued within 24 hours after surgery end
- Euglycemia should be maintained with well-controlled morning glucose levels on the first 2 postoperative days.
- Hair at the surgical site should be removed with clippers or by depilatory methods, not with a blade.
- Urinary catheters should be removed within the first 2 postoperative days.
- Normothermia should be maintained perioperatively.

*Each hospital should consider community prevalence and resistance of pathogens in making individual choices of antibiotics. Prophylactic antibiotics are indicated in women who have induced abortion or hysterosalpingography that shows dilated fallopian tubes. Prophylactic antibiotics can be given after completion of the procedure.

Rosenberger LH, Politano AD, Sawyer RG. The surgical care improvement project and prevention of postoperative infection, including surgical site infection. Surg Infect (Larchmt) 2011;12:163–8. The publisher for this copyrighted material is Mary Ann Liebert, Inc. publishers.

BOX 101-2

Surgical Wound Classification System

Class I/Clean: An uninfected operative wound in which no inflammation is encountered and the alimentary, genital, and uninfected urinary tract is not entered. In addition, clean wounds are primarily closed and, if necessary, drained with closed drainage.

Class II/Clean-contaminated: An operative wound in which the alimentary, genital, or urinary tracts are entered under controlled conditions and without unusual contamination. Specifically, operations involving the appendix and vagina are included in this category, provided there is no evidence of infection or major break in technique is encountered.

Class III/Contaminated: Operations with major breaks in sterile technique or gross spillage from the gastrointestinal tract, and incisions in which acute, nonpurulent inflammation is encountered.

Class IV/Dirty-infected: Operative sites involving existing clinical infection or perforated viscera. This definition suggests that the organisms causing the postoperative infection were present in the operative field before the operation.

Antibiotic prophylaxis for gynecologic procedures. ACOG Practice Bulletin No. 104. American College of Obstetricians and Gynecologists. Obstet Gynecol 2009;113: 1180–9.

TABLE 101-1. Antimicrobial Prophylactic Antibiotic Regimens by Procedure*

Procedure	Antibiotic	Dose (single dose)
Hysterectomy	Cefazolin[†]	1 g or 2g[‡] IV
Urogynecology procedures, including those involving mesh	Clindamycin[§] plus gentamicin or quinolone[‖] or aztreonam	600 mg IV 1.5 mg/kg IV 400 mg IV 1 g IV
	Metronidazole[§] plus gentamicin or quinolone[‖]	500 mg IV 1.5 mg/kg IV 400 mg IV
Laparoscopy Diagnostic Operative Tubal sterilization	None	
Laparotomy	None	
Hysteroscopy Diagnostic Operative Endometrial ablation Essure	None	
Hysterosalpingography or Chromotubation	Doxycycline[¶]	100 mg orally, twice daily for 5 days
IUD insertion	None	
Endometrial biopsy	None	
Induced abortion/dilation and evacuation	Doxycycline Metronidazole	100 mg orally 1 hour before procedure and 200 mg orally after procedure 500 mg orally twice daily for 5 days
Urodynamics	None	

Abbreviations: IUD indicates intrauterine device; IV, intravenously.

*A convenient time to administer antibiotic prophylaxis is just before induction of anesthesia.

[†]Acceptable alternatives include cefotetan, cefoxitin, cefuroxime, or ampicillin–sulbactam.

[‡]A 2-g dose is recommended in women with a body mass index greater than 35 or weight greater than 100 kg or 220 lb.

[§]Antimicrobial agents of choice in women with a history of immediate hypersensitivity to penicillin

[‖]Ciprofloxacin or levofloxacin or moxifloxacin

[¶]If patient has a history of pelvic inflammatory disease or procedure demonstrates dilated fallopian tubes; no prophylaxis is indicated for a study without dilated tubes.

Antibiotic prophylaxis for gynecologic procedures. ACOG Practice Bulletin No. 104. American College of Obstetricians and Gynecologists. Obstet Gynecol 2009;113:1180–9.

102

Premalignant and in situ breast disease

A 46-year-old woman has been treated with breast-conserving surgery and radiotherapy for ductal carcinoma in situ of the breast. Her medical oncologist recommends that she take adjuvant tamoxifen citrate therapy. The benefit of tamoxifen therapy for this patient is that it will decrease her risk of

      (A) endometrial cancer
      (B) death from breast cancer
      (C) ipsilateral recurrent ductal carcinoma in situ (DCIS)
*   (D) invasive breast cancer
      (E) ovarian cancer

Ductal carcinoma in situ of the breast occurs in approximately 35 per 100,000 women in the United States. In approximately 90% of women who have DCIS, the tumor is detected only on imaging studies. Although the detection rate of DCIS has increased substantially over the past several decades through the widespread use of screening mammography, invasive cancer is four times as common as DCIS.

The risk of developing DCIS increases with age and is reported to be 1.3 per 1,000 screened women older than 70 years. The risk factors for DCIS are similar to the risk factors for invasive breast cancer, ie, family history of breast cancer, *BRCA1* and *BRCA2* mutations, increased breast density, obesity, nulliparity, and late age at first birth. Women with DCIS have an excellent prognosis, but one half of all local–regional recurrences are invasive. The goal of DCIS treatment is to prevent future invasive breast cancer.

The treatment of DCIS can be mastectomy or breast-conserving surgery with or without breast radiotherapy. The risk of recurrence over 10 years is 1% for mastectomy, 20% for breast-conserving surgery, and 10% for breast-conserving surgery followed by radiotherapy. Long-term survival is similar for all of these therapies. Sentinel lymph node sampling is not routinely performed for women with DCIS but can be considered in women with extensive DCIS that requires mastectomy.

The role of antiestrogen therapy for DCIS is not clear. Tamoxifen citrate has been most studied. In women with invasive breast cancer, tamoxifen has been shown to be associated with a reduction in breast cancer recurrence, reduction in contralateral breast cancer, and improvement in survival. For women with DCIS, a meta-analysis of two large clinical trials showed that tamoxifen reduced the risk of ipsilateral invasive cancer and contralateral DCIS but did not decrease breast cancer-specific mortality or overall mortality. Adjuvant tamoxifen therapy is best used for women with estrogen receptor-positive DCIS who have had breast-conserving surgery and postoperative radiotherapy. The decision to use tamoxifen must be weighed against the risks of tamoxifen.

Tamoxifen is a competitive inhibitor of estrogen receptors. In the uterus, it functions as an unopposed estrogen. In menopausal women, the risks for endometrial hyperplasia, endometrial cancer, and uterine sarcoma are increased. Other effects include hot flushes, stimulation of uterine myomas, growth of endometrial polyps, and increased risk of venous thromboembolism.

For the described patient, who has been treated with breast-conserving surgery and radiotherapy for DCIS of the breast, tamoxifen therapy is reasonable to consider and will decrease her risk of invasive breast cancer. Use of tamoxifen in the perimenopausal woman will increase her risk of endometrial cancer. It will not improve her overall survival or her breast cancer-specific survival, and it will not decrease her risk of ipsilateral DCIS. Tamoxifen will have no effect on her risk of ovarian cancer.

Fisher B, Dignam J, Wolmark N, Wickerham DL, Fisher ER, Mamounas E, et al. Tamoxifen in treatment of intraductal breast cancer: National Surgical Adjuvant Breast and Bowel Project B-24 randomised controlled trial. Lancet 1999;353:1993–2000.

Petrelli F, Barni S. Tamoxifen added to radiotherapy and surgery for the treatment of ductal carcinoma in situ of the breast: a meta-analysis of 2 randomized trials. Radiother Oncol 2011;100:195–9.

Wapnir IL, Dignam JJ, Fisher B, Mamounas EP, Anderson SJ, Julian TB, et al. Long-term outcomes of invasive ipsilateral breast tumor recurrences after lumpectomy in NSABP B-17 and B-24 randomized clinical trials for DCIS. J Natl Cancer Inst 2011;103:478–88.

103
Obesity

A 48-year-old woman comes to your office for a preventive health care visit. She expresses frustration about her weight and her difficulty in losing weight. Her body mass index (BMI) is 40 (calculated as weight in kilograms divided by height in meters squared). The serum thyroid-stimulating hormone level is normal. You recommend that in addition to exercise, the most effective dietary plan to lose weight is to maintain a diet that is

    (A) low in fat
    (B) low in carbohydrates
    (C) high in proteins
*   (D) calorie-reduced

Obesity is defined as a BMI of 30 or greater and represents an excessive accumulation of fat in the body. Overweight is defined as a BMI of 25–29.9. These definitions may vary by geographic location and over time. Worldwide, an estimated 1.5 billion adults are overweight and 400 million are obese. Obesity is associated with increased rates of mortality in patients with ischemic heart disease, stroke, diabetes mellitus, cancer (liver, kidney, breast, endometrial, prostate, and colon), and respiratory disease.

Body weight change occurs with an imbalance between the energy content of consumed food and energy expended by the body. *Exercise*, defined as intentional physical activity for improving health and fitness, increases energy expenditure. Exercise and physical activity decrease blood pressure; improve lipoprotein profile, C-reactive protein, and other coronary heart disease biomarkers; and enhance insulin sensitivity. Weight-bearing exercise and physical activity preserve bone mass and reduce the risk of falls in older adults. In addition, exercise prevents and improves mild to moderate depressive disorders and anxiety, and it enhances well-being, quality of life, and cognitive function. However, exercise interventions in overweight and obese patients result in great individual variation in body weight response even when adherence to the exercise intervention is maintained. This may be caused by compensation by increasing caloric intake.

Energy intake consists of the macronutrient groups—protein, fat, and carbohydrate—and, to a lesser extent, alcohol. Early studies reached conflicting findings regarding which calorie-restricted macronutrient ratio was most effective in treating overweight and obese patients, including vegetarian and Mediterranean-style diets. These studies were limited by small samples, underrepresentation of men, limited generalizability, a lack of blinded ascertainment of the outcome, a lack of data regarding adherence to assigned diets, duration of 12 months or less, and a large loss to follow-up. One study placed patients on different ratios of macronutrients and followed them for 2 years; the authors concluded that participants lost on average 10% of their initial body weight, regardless of the macronutrient ratio. The most effective dietary plan is to lose weight with a calorie-reduced diet that contains a range of macronutrients. Hence, a diet with a specific macronutrient composition is not advantageous.

The glycemic index is a number assigned to individual food items based on their overall effect on blood sugar levels. Items with low glycemic index provide a slower and more sustained release of glucose to the bloodstream, stimulating less insulin release compared with items with high glycemic index. Items with low glycemic index modulate circulating levels of insulin by increasing insulin sensitivity. Studies have shown mixed results concerning weight loss in overweight or obese individuals consuming low glycemic index–reduced calorie diets compared with high glycemic index–reduced calorie diets.

After weight loss achieved with a calorie-reduced diet, most obese individuals relapse and regain the weight. A strong physiologic basis exists for the weight gain. Caloric restriction results in a reduction in energy expenditure and an increase in appetite. The homeostatic regulation of body weight is complex and involves the hypothalamus and circulating peripheral hormones released from the gastrointestinal tract, pancreas, and adipose tissue. Circulating levels of leptin are markedly reduced, as are peptide YY31 and cholecystokinin. One study showed changes in levels of leptin, ghrelin, peptide YY, gastric inhibitory polypeptide, pancreatic polypeptide, amylin, and cholecystokinin and changes in appetite that encourage weight regain and persist for 12 months after initial weight reduction. Future strategies for prevention of obesity relapse may be designed to counteract these physiologic adaptations.

Casazza K, Fontaine KR, Astrup A, Brown AW, Bohan Brown MM, Durant N, et al. Myths, presumptions, and facts about obesity. N Engl J Med 2013;368:446–54.

Garber CE, Blissmer B, Deschenes MR, Franklin BA, Lamonte MJ, Lee IM, et al. American College of Sports Medicine position stand. Quantity and quality of exercise for developing and maintaining cardiorespiratory, musculoskeletal, and neuromotor fitness in apparently healthy adults: guidance for prescribing exercise. American College of Sports Medicine. Med Sci Sports Exerc 2011;43:1334–59.

Gardner CD, Kiazand A, Alhassan S, Kim S, Stafford RS, Balise RR, et al. Comparison of the Atkins, Zone, Ornish, and LEARN diets for change in weight and related risk factors among overweight premenopausal women: the A TO Z Weight Loss Study: a randomized trial. JAMA 2007;297:969–77.

Hall KD, Heymsfield SB, Kemnitz JW, Klein S, Schoeller DA, Speakman JR. Energy balance and its components: implications for body weight regulation. Am J Clin Nutr 2012;95:989–94.

Sacks FM, Bray GA, Carey VJ, Smith SR, Ryan DH, Anton SD, et al. Comparison of weight-loss diets with different compositions of fat, protein, and carbohydrates. N Engl J Med 2009;360:859–73.

Sumithran P, Prendergast LA, Delbridge E, Purcell K, Shulkes A, Kriketos A, et al. Long-term persistence of hormonal adaptations to weight loss. N Engl J Med 2011;365:1597–604.

Thomas D, Elliott EJ, Baur L. Low glycaemic index or low glycaemic load diets for overweight and obesity. Cochrane Database of Systematic Reviews 2007, Issue 3. Art. No.: CD005105. DOI: 10.1002/14651858. CD005105.pub2.

104

Complex endometrial hyperplasia

A 55-year-old woman, gravida 3, para 3, with type 2 diabetes mellitus and a body mass index of 35 (calculated as weight in kilograms divided by height in meters squared), comes to your office for her annual well-woman examination. At that time, a Pap test is completed and the result is remarkable for atypical glandular cells. She also reports intermittent vaginal bleeding. An office endometrial biopsy demonstrates complex atypical hyperplasia. The most appropriate next step is

    (A) pelvic ultrasonography
    (B) progestin therapy
    (C) levonorgestrel intrauterine device
    (D) dilation and curettage
*   (E) hysterectomy

Endometrial hyperplasia is a histologic diagnosis, which encompasses a broad spectrum of entities. It is characterized by proliferating glands, which result in an increased gland–stromal ratio compared with normal endometrium. The spectrum of changes varies from slightly crowded and dilated glands (simple hyperplasia) to nearly back-to-back glands (complex hyperplasia) and abnormal nuclei. The more progressive lesions often are indistinguishable from a well-differentiated endometrioid adenocarcinoma. The transition from simple to complex proliferation to an invasive histology is hypothesized to be a continuum. The management of endometrial hyperplasia is dependent on multiple factors, including patient age, medical history, desired fertility, and most importantly severity of hyperplasia. As a result, an accurate classification for endometrial hyperplasia is essential to optimize clinical management and to avoid either undertreatment or overtreatment.

The World Health Organization classification is most widely used to interpret endometrial hyperplasia and is based on two criteria: 1) glandular crowding and 2) nuclear appearance. The classification recognizes four histologic subtypes, including simple and complex hyperplasia with or without atypia. However, this classification requires a pathologist to subjectively assess the diagnostic criteria. Multiple studies have demonstrated a low reproducibility of the World Health Organization classification, which may have significant clinical impact. Recent investigations have not only demonstrated the diagnostic dilemmas and discrepancies associated with endometrial hyperplasia, but also the high rate of concurrent endometrial cancer in patients with complex atypical hyperplasia.

A Gynecologic Oncology Group study estimated the prevalence of concurrent endometrial cancer in women with a community diagnosis of atypical complex hyperplasia. A panel of three experienced gynecologic pathologists reviewed the biopsy specimen and hysterectomy, which was completed within 12 weeks of the endometrial sampling without any intervention. This study demonstrated a low rate of concurrence with the referring biopsy specimen of 39%, and a prevalence of carcinoma of 43% (most patients had stage I, grade 1 disease). This prospective cohort provides additional evidence that a modification in the widely accepted classification of endometrial hyperplasia may be warranted and that conservative management for complex atypical hyperplasia, such as hormonal therapy, may need to be reconsidered.

Risk factors for endometrial hyperplasia are the same as for endometrial cancer (ie, unopposed estrogen, late menopause, nulliparity, obesity, chronic anovulation, diabetes mellitus, and tamoxifen citrate use). The most common sources of unopposed estrogen are chronic anovulation, which is a feature of both polycystic ovary syndrome and perimenopause, and obesity from peripheral conversion of androgens. Typically, endometrial hyperplasia presents as abnormal uterine bleeding especially in perimenopausal or postmenopausal woman, although 80% of the time this bleeding is due to a benign process.

The treatment of simple or complex hyperplasia without atypia is essential to control abnormal bleeding and to prevent progression to cancer. Progestins have been demonstrated to be effective in the treatment of endometrial hyperplasia. Response rates are highest in patients without atypia and for treatment duration of at least 12 days per month. In a premenopausal woman, medroxyprogesterone acetate, 10 mg daily for 12–14 days per month for 3–6 months is effective. Response rates have been demonstrated to be as high as 80% if no atypia is present. Ovulation induction or a levonorgestrel IUD can be considered as alternatives. In patients who do not desire future fertility or who are not willing to follow-up for surveillance endometrial sampling, a hysterectomy should be considered.

In postmenopausal women with endometrial hyperplasia without atypia, progestin therapy can be considered for 3 months followed by a repeat sampling. If atypia is present, in light of the high rates of concurrent endometrial cancer, hysterectomy is the recommended treatment. However, a gynecologic oncologist should be available at the time of hysterectomy to assess whether surgical staging is warranted if an endometrial cancer is identified. Because this patient is postmenopausal and has complex atypical hyperplasia, neither pelvic ultrasonography nor dilation and curettage would be the most appropriate option. In this patient, hormonal treatment with a levonorgestrel IUD might be appropriate if she was not suited for the surgical approach.

Lacey JV Jr, Chia VM. Endometrial hyperplasia and the risk of progression to carcinoma. Maturitas 2009;63:39–44.

Lacey JV Jr, Ioffe OB, Ronnett BM, Rush BB, Richesson DA, Chatterjee N, et al. Endometrial carcinoma risk among women diagnosed with endometrial hyperplasia: the 34-year experience in a large health plan. Br J Cancer 2008;98:45–53.

Reed SD, Voigt LF, Newton KM, Garcia RH, Allison HK, Epplein M, et al. Progestin therapy of complex endometrial hyperplasia with and without atypia. Obstet Gynecol 2009;113:655–62.

Trimble CL, Kauderer J, Zaino R, Silverberg S, Lim PC, Burke JJ 2nd, et al. Concurrent endometrial carcinoma in women with a biopsy diagnosis of atypical endometrial hyperplasia: a Gynecologic Oncology Group study. Cancer 2006;106:812–9.

Ushijima K, Yahata H, Yoshikawa H, Konishi I, Yasugi T, Saito T, et al. Multicenter phase II study of fertility-sparing treatment with medroxyprogesterone acetate for endometrial carcinoma and atypical hyperplasia in young women. J Clin Oncol 2007;25:2798–803.

105

Fibrocystic breast disease

A 38-year-old woman reports bilateral breast tenderness and heaviness. Her discomfort is primarily in the lateral aspects of both breasts. She has no family history of breast cancer, is otherwise healthy, and takes no medications. She has not detected a breast mass nor has she noted any nipple discharge or skin changes. The breast and axillary examinations yield normal results with some generalized fullness and lumpiness in the upper outer quadrants of both breasts. The most appropriate next step is

* (A) reassurance
  (B) breast magnetic resonance imaging
  (C) bilateral mammography
  (D) low-dose combined oral contraceptives
  (E) tamoxifen citrate

Clinicians must be able to distinguish between benign and malignant conditions, attempt to alleviate symptoms associated with benign breast disorders, identify patients at high risk of breast cancer, and implement risk-reducing strategies when appropriate.

Breast pain, also known as mastalgia, is a common symptom and accounts for almost one-half of all breast-related visits to physicians. Mastalgia may be cyclical or noncyclical and affects reproductive-aged and postmenopausal patients, including women who are not taking hormone therapy. The first step in the evaluation of a patient with breast pain is obtaining a medical history and performing a physical examination. The history should focus on the timing, frequency, severity, and location of the pain with attention to recent activities or trauma that may have caused or exacerbated the pain. A physical examination should evaluate discrete or concerning abnormalities of the breast and abnormalities of the chest wall separate from the breast. If a palpable breast mass is identified, imaging should be performed. In this patient with mastalgia without concerning findings on physical examination, providing reassurance and observation is the most appropriate next step. Breast cancer is rarely identified in patients who have mastalgia with no other findings.

Once reassured, most patients do not seek additional treatment. Options for management include well-fitted and supportive bras; dietary changes, such as restriction of methylxanthines and caffeine, fat, and salt intake; and intermittent use of diuretics. However, none of these interventions has been conclusively proved to improve mastalgia.

Although users of combined oral contraceptives generally are less likely to report mastalgia than nonusers, initiation of oral contraceptives is not a proven treatment for mastalgia. Postmenopausal women who develop mastalgia after initiation of hormone therapy may benefit from discontinuation of the therapy or decreasing the estrogen dose.

Bilateral mammography and breast magnetic resonance imaging are not appropriate options. No radiologic findings are associated with mastalgia alone. In the absence of obvious clinical findings, such as erythema or a mass, breast imaging is not useful. Tamoxifen citrate is not approved by the U.S. Food and Drug Administration for the treatment of benign mastalgia, although some evidence exists that tamoxifen can be helpful to treat the condition. In one trial, most patients reported decreased mastalgia when they took tamoxifen, 10 mg, daily, for 3 months. However, tamoxifen would not be the most appropriate next step because few patients with mastalgia need treatment for their symptoms. Most are seeking reassurance that they do not have breast cancer. Other medical interventions that may be helpful if a patient seeks treatment include mild analgesic agents, such as acetaminophen, nonsteroidal antiinflammatory drugs, or aspirin. For refractory cases, danazol and gonadotropin-releasing hormone agonists may be used.

Miltenburg DM, Speights VO Jr. Benign breast disease. Obstet Gynecol Clin North Am 2008;35:285–300, ix.

Neal L, Tortorelli CL, Nassar A. Clinician's guide to imaging and pathologic findings in benign breast disease. Mayo Clin Proc 2010; 85:274–9.

Pearlman MD, Griffin JL. Benign breast disease. Obstet Gynecol 2010;116:747–58.

Santen RJ, Mansel R. Benign breast disorders. N Engl J Med 2005; 353:275–85.

106

Thrombophilias and contraception

At her first gynecologic visit, a 20-year-old healthy woman requests combination oral contraceptives. She has irregular cycle intervals of 21–34 days. Her menstrual periods last up to 5 days and are characterized by heavy blood flow. She recently became sexually active. Her family history is unremarkable except for her mother who had a confirmed diagnosis of deep vein thrombosis. You advise her that before starting oral contraceptives she should undergo

    (A) an endometrial biopsy
    (B) cervical cytology screening
 *   (C) a factor V Leiden test
    (D) pelvic ultrasonography
    (E) serum testing for thyroid-stimulating hormone

This patient should be screened for thrombophilias before initiation of a combination oral contraceptive. Users of combined oral contraceptives are at an increased risk of venous thromboembolism (VTE) compared with nonusers. The risk of VTE with the use of combination oral contraceptives is approximately 0.9–14 events per 10,000 woman-years. By contrast, the risk of VTE associated with pregnancy is 10 events per 10,000 woman-years, and the risk of VTE associated with the puerperium is 50 events per 10,000 woman-years. This is a more appropriate comparison for patients who are assessing their thrombotic risk and who wish to avoid pregnancy. It is important to evaluate a patient's risk of VTE with the use of combination oral contraceptives. Screening for thrombophilias is based on the prevalence of each inherited thrombophilia and the association of each with the risk of thrombosis. Universal screening for all patients before initiating combination oral contraceptives is not recommended. Careful evaluation for a personal or family history of thrombosis should be performed, and directed screening should be considered on an individualized basis.

Factor V Leiden mutation is the most common genetic risk factor for VTE. The highest prevalence of factor V Leiden mutation is among European populations, ranging from 2% to 7%. In the United States, the mutation is carried in heterozygous form by approximately 5% of the white population and is less frequent among Hispanic Americans (2.2%), African Americans (1.2%), and Asian Americans (0.45%). Users of combination oral contraceptives who have the factor V Leiden mutation have an increased risk of VTE and cerebral vein and cerebral sinus thrombosis compared with nonusers with the mutation. This patient's family history of a first-degree relative with VTE is an indication for screening for thrombophilias.

Because a specific thrombophilia has not been identified in the patient's mother, screening for factor V Leiden mutation is indicated based on its prevalence. Screening for specific abnormalities, such as protein C, protein S, *prothrombin* gene mutations, and *MTHFR* abnormalities, is reserved for instances when the specific gene abnormality is identified in the family member.

Other thrombotic risk factors include obesity, immobility, prolonged land and air travel, and cigarette smoking. If a patient receives a diagnosis of an inherited thrombophilia, she should not be given combination oral contraceptives because of her increased thrombotic risk. Nonestrogen-containing contraceptive methods would be safer options. Cervical cytology screening should be initiated at age 21 years; therefore, such screening is not indicated in the described patient before starting contraception. This patient reports that her cycle interval is 21–34 days with menses that last up to 5 days and are characterized by heavy bleeding. The acceptable range for cycle interval is 21–35 days; her cycle interval is normal and does not require additional evaluation. Menses that last up to 7 days are normal, even if on some days the bleeding is described as heavy. Her menstrual cycle pattern does not warrant further investigation with either a serum thyroid-stimulating hormone screening for thyroid disease or pelvic ultrasonography. An endometrial biopsy is indicated in women older than 35 years who report irregular or heavy menstrual bleeding or in patients with prolonged periods of unopposed estrogen. This patient's age precludes the need for an endometrial biopsy to investigate endometrial pathology.

Blickstein D, Blickstein I. Oral contraception and thrombophilia. Curr Opin Obstet Gynecol 2007;19:370–6.

Dietrich JE, Yee DL. Thrombophilic conditions in the adolescent: the gynecologic impact. Obstet Gynecol Clin North Am 2009;36:163–75.

Mohllajee AP, Curtis KM, Martins SL, Peterson HB. Does use of hormonal contraceptives among women with thrombogenic mutations increase their risk of venous thromboembolism? A systematic review. Contraception 2006;73:166–78.

Raymond EG, Burke AE, Espey E. Combined hormonal contraceptives and venous thromboembolism: putting the risks into perspective. Obstet Gynecol 2012;119:1039–44.

Trenor CC 3rd, Chung RJ, Michelson AD, Neufeld EJ, Gordon CM, Laufer MR, et al. Hormonal contraception and thrombotic risk: a multidisciplinary approach. Pediatrics 2011;127:347–57.

107

Patient with sexual partner who has genital herpes

A newly-married 26-year-old woman tells you that her husband informed her he previously received a diagnosis of genital herpes but has been asymptomatic for several years. She has never had any lesions. Her pelvic examination is normal. The most appropriate recommendation in the management of this patient is that she

      (A) start suppressive therapy
      (B) recommend her partner start suppressive therapy
*   (C) undergo type-specific serologic testing
      (D) consider suppressive therapy in pregnancy
      (E) undergo serologic testing only if she becomes pregnant

It is estimated that more than 50 million Americans are infected with genital herpes. Patients often are asymptomatic; serologic testing shows that approximately 25% of reported primary infections are actually recurrent episodes. Most commonly, genital infections are the result of herpes simplex virus type 2 (HSV-2); however, the incidence of herpes simplex virus type 1 (HSV-1) is increasing, particularly in third-world countries. Skin-to-skin contact is the predominant mode of transmission for HSV. Although transmission is more likely in patients with active lesions, asymptomatic shedding can occur at any time. Patients should be counseled that consistent condom use and avoiding intercourse during outbreaks can decrease transmission.

Suppressive therapy should be considered in women with recurrent and frequent outbreaks. Studies have shown that daily suppressive therapy may decrease occurrences by 70–80%. In addition, pregnant women with genital HSV are recommended to use suppressive therapy at the end of pregnancy to decrease viral shedding and decrease the chance of an outbreak in order to increase their ability to have a vaginal delivery. Research also has shown that use of suppressive therapy by the infected individual with either acyclovir or valacyclovir can decrease transmission to HSV-naïve partners.

The described patient should undergo serologic testing for HSV-1 and HSV-2. Because her partner is known to have genital herpes, it is possible that he has already transmitted the infection to the patient and she is an asymptomatic carrier. In this case, suppressive therapy for the husband would be unnecessary. If the patient was found to be HSV negative, her husband should consider starting suppressive therapy to decrease the chance of transmission to his wife.

The American College of Obstetricians and Gynecologists recommends suppressive therapy for pregnant women with active recurrent genital herpes. Without a diagnosis, empiric suppression could lead to unnecessary exposure to medication, potential adverse effects, and increased medical costs. In addition, delaying serologic testing until the time of pregnancy could decrease the potential for inhibiting transmission.

Garber CE, Blissmer B, Deschenes MR, Franklin BA, Lamonte MJ, Lee IM, et al. American College of Sports Medicine position stand. Quantity and quality of exercise for developing and maintaining cardiorespiratory, musculoskeletal, and neuromotor fitness in apparently healthy adults: guidance for prescribing exercise. American College of Sports Medicine. Med Sci Sports Exerc 2011;43:1334–59.

Gardner CD, Kiazand A, Alhassan S, Kim S, Stafford RS, Balise RR, et al. Comparison of the Atkins, Zone, Ornish, and LEARN diets for change in weight and related risk factors among overweight premenopausal women: the A TO Z Weight Loss Study: a randomized trial. JAMA 2007;297:969–77.

Hall KD, Heymsfield SB, Kemnitz JW, Klein S, Schoeller DA, Speakman JR. Energy balance and its components: implications for body weight regulation. Am J Clin Nutr 2012;95:989–94.

Sacks FM, Bray GA, Carey VJ, Smith SR, Ryan DH, Anton SD, et al. Comparison of weight-loss diets with different compositions of fat, protein, and carbohydrates. N Engl J Med 2009;360:859–73.

Sumithran P, Prendergast LA, Delbridge E, Purcell K, Shulkes A, Kriketos A, et al. Long-term persistence of hormonal adaptations to weight loss. N Engl J Med 2011;365:1597–604.

Thomas D, Elliott EJ, Baur L. Low glycaemic index or low glycaemic load diets for overweight and obesity. Cochrane Database of Systematic Reviews 2007, Issue 3. Art. No.: CD005105. DOI: 10.1002/14651858. CD005105.pub2.

108

Frequent urination

Two weeks after an uncomplicated total abdominal hysterectomy for uterine myomas, a 48-year-old woman comes to your office and reports frequent urination. She reports that she has "leaking day and night," and that it is worse in the morning. The problem started 2 days ago. Pelvic examination reveals clear fluid at the vaginal introitus. Urinalysis result is significant for microscopic hematuria. The most likely diagnosis is

* (A) postoperative urinary tract infection
* (B) vesicovaginal fistula
* (C) stress urinary incontinence
* (D) overactive bladder syndrome

Vesicovaginal fistula should be suspected in postoperative patients with painless urinary incontinence after surgery. Injuries to the urinary tract include bladder and ureteral injuries. Such injuries have been reported in up to 4% of women with a history of uncomplicated hysterectomy for benign indications.

An office-based evaluation is appropriate for workup in the postoperative patient. Indigo carmine dye is a blue dye that can be mixed with sterile water or saline to help as a contrast agent for patients with suspected vesicovaginal fistula. Insertion of a temporary Foley catheter with 200 mL of blue dye and a tampon placed vaginally is a relatively inexpensive diagnostic technique. Limitations of this method of evaluation include the inability to identify higher urinary tract injury involving the ureter. Use of oral phenazopyridine may assist with identifying ureteral injuries. Intravenous pyelography and delayed contrast computed tomography also may assist with identification of the kidneys, ureters, and bladder for confirmation. Vesicovaginal fistulas may not be as easily diagnosed in patients who undergo computed tomography or intravenous pyelography because of the potential for radiographic scatter found in the pelvis due to the pelvic bones. Diagnostic cystoscopy or cystography also may be considered for diagnosis of vesicovaginal fistula.

Postoperative urinary tract infection is one of the most common infections in the postoperative period and often presents with dysuria within the first week of surgery.

Stress urinary incontinence may be reported to be worsened with an increase in pelvic pressure with coughing and lifting; however, it is rare in the immediate postoperative period. Overactive bladder syndrome is another potential diagnosis that could lead to increased urination. Overactive bladder with the symptoms of urgency and frequency often is diagnosed in the preoperative period and is unlikely to manifest only in the postoperative period. Therefore, a vesicovaginal fistula is the most likely cause of the described patient's symptoms.

Fletcher SG, Lemack GE. Clarifying the role of urodynamics in the preoperative evaluation of stress urinary incontinence. Scientific World Journal 2008;8:1259–68.

Gilmour DT, Das S, Flowerdew G. Rates of urinary tract injury from gynecologic surgery and the role of intraoperative cystoscopy. Obstet Gynecol 2006;107:1366–72.

Hoffman CP, Kennedy J, Borschel L, Burchette R, Kidd A. Laparoscopic hysterectomy: the Kaiser Permanente San Diego experience. J Minim Invasive Gynecol 2005;12:16–24.

Irwin DE, Milsom I, Hunskaar S, Reilly K, Kopp Z, Herschorn S, et al. Population-based survey of urinary incontinence, overactive bladder, and other lower urinary tract symptoms in five countries: results of the EPIC study. Eur Urol 2006;50:1306–14; discussion 1314–5.

Jelovsek JE, Chiung C, Chen G, Roberts SL, Paraiso MF, Falcone T. Incidence of lower urinary tract injury at the time of total laparoscopic hysterectomy. J Soc Laparoendosc Surg 2007;11:422–7.

109

Postoperative delirium in an elderly patient

A 75-year-old woman, gravida 2, para 2, with an unremarkable medical history underwent an uncomplicated total abdominal hysterectomy and bilateral salpingo-oophorectomy. On postoperative day 2, you are contacted by a nurse regarding this patient's new onset confusion. On evaluation, the patient is in moderate distress and her vital signs are significant for elevated blood pressure of 140 mm Hg systolic and 90 mm Hg diastolic and a heart rate of 80 beats per minute. She is alert and oriented to herself but not to place or time. Examination yields unremarkable results with clear breath sounds, normal heart rate, and positive bowel sounds with appropriate incision tenderness. Electrocardiography performed at the bedside produces unchanged results from those of her preoperative electrocardiography performed 2 weeks before surgery. Complete blood count and metabolic electrolytes levels are in the normal range. The best next step in her care is to

　　　(A) order complete cardiac workup
*　　(B) review her current medications to limit sedating drugs
　　　(C) order a computed tomography of the head
　　　(D) order neurology consultation

Delirium is defined as a disturbance of consciousness with inattention that is accompanied by changes in cognition or perceptual disturbance. It has an acute onset and a fluctuating course. Postoperative delirium is a common neurologic complication that affects up to 18% of geriatric patients who have undergone elective surgery. It should be considered as a possible diagnosis in elderly patients who have no other clear etiology for confusion. Risk factors for postoperative delirium include patient's age and preoperative cognitive impairment. The risk of development of subsequent postoperative delirium increases to approximately 37% in high-risk groups.

Medications are the most common cause of postoperative delirium in the older patients with exposure to anesthesia, narcotics, and potentially sedating antiemetics listed as potential culprits. Thus, the most reasonable next step in this patient's care would be to review her current medications to limit sedating drugs.

Older women do not always present with the classical symptoms of myocardial infarction. In the postoperative period, myocardial infarction should be considered as a diagnosis for any patient who displays clinical deterioration (eg, reduced oxygenation and poor vital signs). However, given the described patient's stable clinical presentation, a complete cardiac workup is not indicated at this time.

Strokes are relatively uncommon in the postoperative period and generally would show other examination findings consistent with acute neurologic deficits. Strokes have been reported in approximately 0.5–1% of patients who undergo elective noncardiac surgery and would not be the first consideration in this patient who has an unremarkable history, examination, and laboratory data. Therefore, consultation with a neurologist is not indicated at this time.

Devereaux PJ, Yang H, Yusuf S, Guyatt G, Leslie K, Villar JC, et al. Effects of extended-release metoprolol succinate in patients undergoing non-cardiac surgery (POISE trial): a randomised controlled trial. POISE Study Group. Lancet 2008;371:1839–47.

Kalisvaart KJ, Vreeswijk R, de Jonghe JF, van der Ploeg T, van Gool WA, Eikelenboom P. Risk factors and prediction of postoperative delirium in elderly hip-surgery patients: implementation and validation of a medical risk factor model. J Am Geriatr Soc 2006;54:817–22.

Nishikawa K, Nakayama M, Omote K, Namiki A. Recovery characteristics and post-operative delirium after long-duration laparoscope-assisted surgery in elderly patients: propofol-based vs. sevoflurane-based anesthesia. Acta Anaesthesiol Scand 2004;48:162–8.

Patti R, Saitta M, Cusumano G, Termine G, Di Vita G. Risk factors for postoperative delirium after colorectal surgery for carcinoma. Eur J Oncol Nurs 2011;15:519–23.

Vaurio LE, Sands LP, Wang Y, Mullen EA, Leung JM. Postoperative delirium: the importance of pain and pain management. Anesth Analg 2006;102:1267–73.

110

Levonorgestrel intrauterine device with missing strings

A 19-year-old nulligravid patient presents for a follow-up appointment after levonorgestrel intra-uterine device (IUD) placement 6 weeks ago. During the speculum examination, the strings from the system are not visible and cannot be teased from the cervix with a cytobrush. Ultrasonography is performed and does not demonstrate the levonorgestrel IUD in the endometrial cavity. The most appropriate next step is to perform

(A) pelvic magnetic resonance imaging
(B) abdominal–pelvic computed tomography
(C) diagnostic laparoscopy
(D) dilation and curettage and hysteroscopy
* (E) radiography of the abdomen

Patients should be seen after an insertion of a levonorgestrel IUD to check for the presence of strings at the cervix. If the strings are not easily identified, a cytobrush can be used to try to "tease" the strings from the endocervical canal. In any patient with missing strings, it becomes imperative to identify the location of the device. The levonorgestrel IUD may have perforated the uterine wall or have been expelled. Back up contraception should be initiated until evaluation is complete.

Although it is an uncommon complication, levonorgestrel IUD perforation through the uterine wall into the pelvic or peritoneal cavity occurs in up to 1 per 1,000 insertions. The incidence of uterine perforation is directly related to the skill of the performing clinician and the size, shape, and position of the uterus. Previously unde-tected uterine anomalies increase the likelihood of uterine perforation. Uterine perforation is associated with method failure and pelvic adhesive disease. Perforation occurs most commonly at the time of insertion but also can occur later or during the puerperium. Patients with uterine per-foration may be asymptomatic or report abdominal pain or vaginal bleeding. If a pregnancy occurs in a patient who uses a levonorgestrel IUD, uterine perforation must be ruled out. A levonorgestrel IUD may only partially penetrate the uterine wall. Partial perforation also must be addressed because it may lead to method failure, abnor-mal bleeding, and abdominal or pelvic pain.

Another explanation for missing strings may be expul-sion. The risk of levonorgestrel IUD expulsion during the first year of use ranges between 2% and 10%. Expulsion is associated with method failure. Risk factors for expul-sion include nulliparity, heavy menstrual bleeding, and severe dysmenorrhea.

Vaginal ultrasonography is the first step in identifying the location of a misplaced levonorgestrel IUD. Pelvic ultrasonography provides precise imaging of the uterus and its cavity, including the location of the device and its relation to the uterus. If the device is not localized to the uterine cavity, perforation or expulsion should be considered. The most appropriate next step is to order radiography of the upper and lower abdomen. The levo-norgestrel IUD is radiopaque; thus, if the device is within the peritoneal cavity, it will be easily identified. If the levonorgestrel IUD is not seen on the radiograph, expul-sion is confirmed.

Pelvic magnetic resonance imaging and abdominal–pelvic computed tomography are not appropriate next steps. Radiography of the abdomen will suffice; it can be more rapidly obtained and interpreted and is more cost-effective. After pelvic ultrasonography does not con-firm intrauterine location of the levonorgestrel IUD, the intraperitoneal location of the misplaced levonorgestrel IUD should be confirmed. Moving directly to diagnostic laparoscopy without checking the intraperitoneal loca-tion would not be the best option because the device may have been expelled. Dilation and curettage and hysteros-copy would offer no clinical benefit because the pelvic ultrasonography confirmed that the device was not in the endometrial cavity.

American College of Obstetricians and Gynecologists. ACOG Practice Bulletin No. 121. Long-acting reversible contraception: implants and intrauterine devices. Obstet Gynecol 2011;118:184–96.

Gill RS, Mok D, Hudson M, Shi X, Birch DW, Karmali S. Laparoscopic removal of an intra-abdominal intrauterine device: case and systematic review. Contraception 2012;85:15–8.

Markovitch O, Klein Z, Gidoni Y, Holzinger M, Beyth Y. Extrauterine mislocated IUD: is surgical removal mandatory? Contraception 2002; 66:105–8.

111
Wound dehiscence

You are completing the abdominal closure after a cesarean delivery in a multigravid woman with an antenatal course complicated by smoking and gestational diabetes mellitus. Her body mass index is 40 (calculated as weight in kilograms divided by height in meters squared). The thickness of the subcutaneous adipose tissue is 6 cm. The step most likely to prevent separation of the skin and superficial tissues in the setting of cesarean delivery is

* (A) closure of the subcutaneous tissue
  (B) placement of a closed subcutaneous drain
  (C) placement of pressure dressing
  (D) placement of surgical staples

Wound separation is one of the most common complications after cesarean delivery. It is more common in patients who have risk factors for inadequate healing, such as obesity, diabetes mellitus, and smoking. Obstetricians who provide care to patients with a high-risk antenatal history must identify surgical techniques to reduce the likelihood of postoperative complications in this patient population.

A meta-analysis of studies in women after they underwent cesarean delivery demonstrates that closure of the subcutaneous fat with thickness greater than 2 cm results in a 34% decrease in subsequent wound disruption. Therefore, in the described patient, closure of the subcutaneous tissue is the technique that would most likely prevent separation of the skin and superficial tissues. Placement of a subcutaneous drain has been shown to increase and decrease rates in different studies. Although pressure dressings are commonly used, they have not been shown to significantly reduce rates of wound separation.

Studies that have compared subcuticular sutures and metal staples for closure of Pfannenstiel incisions have demonstrated that staples have been associated with a higher risk of wound separation. However, the studies often are limited by the timing of staple removal, which often occurs approximately on day 3 or day 4 after cesarean delivery. Therefore, these findings do not support the use of staples instead of subcuticular sutures to help reduce the risk of wound separation. A recent randomized clinical trial of women who underwent cesarean delivery found a wound disruption rate for wound closure with staples of 13.4% compared with 3.5% for closure with a subcuticular suture.

Chelmow D, Rodriguez EJ, Sabatini MM. Suture closure of subcutaneous fat and wound disruption after cesarean delivery: a meta-analysis. Obstet Gynecol 2004;103:974–80.

Figueroa D, Jauk VC, Szychowski JM, Garner R, Biggio JR, Andrews WW, et al. Surgical staples compared with subcuticular suture for skin closure after cesarean delivery: a randomized controlled trial. Obstet Gynecol 2013;121:33–8.

Mackeen AD, Berghella V, Larsen M. Techniques and materials for skin closure in caesarean section. Cochrane Database of Systematic Reviews 2012, Issue 11. Art. No.: CD003577. DOI: 10.1002/14651858. CD003577.pub3.

112

Emergency contraception

An 18-year-old patient asks you for a prescription for levonorgestrel-containing emergency contraception. Her last menstrual period was 5 weeks ago and she has a history of irregular menses. Recently, she received a diagnosis of chlamydial infection and has not completed her prescribed antibiotics. She has missed several of her progestin-only contraceptive pills during the current cycle. The urine pregnancy test yields a positive result. Her body mass index is 32 (calculated as weight in kilograms divided by height in meters squared), and she is known to have a heterozygous factor V Leiden mutation. You advise her that a contraindication to prescribing emergency contraception for her is

        (A) current antibiotic use
        (B) poor compliance
*   (C) positive urine pregnancy test result
        (D) heterozygosity for factor V Leiden mutation
        (E) obesity

Emergency contraception should be offered or made available to women who have unprotected or inadequately protected sexual intercourse and who do not desire pregnancy. The World Health Organization's document *Medical Eligibility Criteria for Contraception Use*, Fourth edition, states that the benefits of emergency contraception outweigh the risks. Reproductive-aged women who are victims of sexual assault should always be offered emergency contraception.

This patient is already pregnant; thus, emergency contraception is contraindicated because it would not be effective. Although emergency contraception is not considered harmful to a pregnant woman or a developing fetus, the effect of emergency contraception on a pregnant woman and a developing fetus has not been studied prospectively. To date, no evidence has been produced to show that increased dose formulations of combination oral contraceptives pose increased risk to a pregnant woman or a developing fetus. In addition, no evidence exists that the use of emergency contraception increases the risk of a subsequent ectopic pregnancy. As with all forms of contraception, emergency contraception decreases ectopic pregnancy rates by decreasing overall pregnancy rates. A urine pregnancy test is not required before the use of levonorgestrel-containing emergency contraception.

Single-dose emergency contraception contains 1.5 mg of levonorgestrel. Alternative regimens include 0.75 mg of levonorgestrel, two doses taken 12–24 hours apart. Emergency contraception reduces the risk of an unexpected pregnancy by at least 74%. It can be offered up to 120 hours after exposure, but is most effective when used within 72 hours. The progestin-only regimens are preferred over the combination methods because they are more effective and cause less nausea and vomiting. Emergency contraception is considered safe; no deaths or serious adverse events have been causally linked to emergency contraception. The most common adverse effects are nausea and vomiting and irregular vaginal bleeding.

Obesity is not a contraindication to emergency contraception; no special dosing is required and no evidence exists of decreased efficacy in overweight or obese patients. Sexually transmitted diseases, including chlamydial infection, also are not a contraindication to hormonal contraceptive use. Because the single-dose regimen is progestin-only, thrombophilias, such as factor V Leiden mutation are not a contraindication. The patient's poor adherence would not preclude prescribing emergency contraception. Current antibiotic use is not a contraindication to emergency contraception and does not decrease efficacy. Although not appropriate in this patient because of her current chlamydial infection and pregnancy, the copper intrauterine device is another effective form of emergency contraception and can be inserted up to 5 days after unprotected intercourse. Another medical option is ulipristal acetate, an emergency contraceptive recently approved by the U.S. Food and Drug Administration. It is a single-dose agent that is available by prescription only. Ulipristal acetate is a progestin-receptor modulator that should be taken as soon as possible, within 5 days of unprotected intercourse. Because the effects of the drug on the developing fetus and a breastfeeding infant are unknown, the use of ulipristal acetate should be avoided in pregnant and breastfeeding women.

Curtis KM, Jamieson DJ, Peterson HB, Marchbanks PA. Adaptation of the World Health Organization's medical eligibility criteria for contraceptive use for use in the United States. Contraception 2010;82:3–9.

Duffy K, Gold MA. Adolescents and emergency contraception: update 2011. Curr Opin Obstet Gynecol 2011;23:328–33.

Emergency contraception. Practice Bulletin No. 112. American College of Obstetricians and Gynecologists. Obstet Gynecol 2010;115:1100–9.

Langston A. Emergency contraception: update and review. Semin Reprod Med 2010;28:95–102.

113

Heavy menstrual bleeding

A 42-year-old woman, gravida 1, para 1, reports fatigue and menstrual cycles with heavy menstrual bleeding. Her menstrual interval is every 30 days with 4 days of heavy bleeding; she frequently soils her clothes due to the heavy flow. She takes a nonsteroidal antiinflammatory drug during the menses for painful cramping. She has been prescribed a daily diuretic for management of hypertension but has difficulty remembering to take it. On physical examination, her height is 1.6 m (64 in); weight, 105.2 kg (140 lb); blood pressure, 150 mm Hg systolic and 95 mm Hg diastolic; and pulse, 72 beats per minute. The pelvic examination is notable for a small anteverted uterus and no pelvic masses. The hemoglobin level is 9.5 g/dL and thyroid-stimulating hormone level is 2.5 mIU/L. Endometrial biopsy and pelvic ultrasonography yield normal results, and she has no personal or family history of excessive bruising or epistaxis. The patient declines the use of the levonorgestrel intrauterine device for the management of heavy bleeding because she is fearful of a foreign body inside her. The best medical option for this patient is

        (A) transdermal contraceptive patch
        (B) oral contraceptives
*   (C) tranexamic acid
        (D) progestin-only minipill

Heavy menstrual bleeding adversely affects reproductive-aged women through diminished quality of life and adverse effects of anemia. Tranexamic acid is an antifibrinolytic medication that works by reversibly blocking lysine-binding sites on plasminogen, thus preventing fibrin degradation. It has been used for decades outside of the United States and was recently approved by the U.S. Food and Drug Administration for management of heavy menstrual bleeding. Previous formulations of tranexamic acid have been found to cause adverse gastrointestinal events. The current formulation approved by the U.S. Food and Drug Administration is a modified release formulation that has been found to be safe and effective with less gastrointestinal effects. Women with significant uterine or reproductive tract pathology or history of thrombosis, cerebrovascular accident, or myocardial infarction were excluded from this research. This medication is contraindicated in women with personal histories or an intrinsic risk of thrombosis. The risk of thrombosis may increase further if tranexamic acid is administered in conjunction with hormonal contraceptives, particularly in women who are obese or smoke cigarettes.

Tranexamic acid is used for a maximum of 5 days per month during menstrual bleeding so it does not require a daily commitment on the part of the patient. The treatment regimen can be titrated to a maximum dosage based on an individual woman's needs. The dosage should be adjusted in women with renal impairment. Tranexamic acid does not affect fertility. Unlike oral contraceptives or the transdermal contraceptive patch, it may be used in women who have medical conditions, such as uncontrolled hypertension, as in the described patient. The levonorgestrel IUD may be an option for a woman such as this patient who has concurrent medical conditions and cannot remember to take daily medications. However, the described patient declined this option. The patient has no medical contraindications to the progestin-only minipill, but it requires daily administration. A randomized controlled trial of women with heavy menstrual bleeding showed a decrease in menstrual blood loss of 40.4% among women who received tranexamic acid versus an 8.2% decrease in menstrual blood loss among women who received placebo. Therefore, although tranexamic acid may not lead to significant decrease in bleeding or amenorrhea compared with hormonal options, it is the best medical option for initial treatment of heavy menstrual bleeding in this patient.

Freeman EW, Lukes A, VanDrie D, Mabey RG, Gersten J, Adomako TL. A dose-response study of a novel, oral tranexamic formulation for heavy menstrual bleeding. Am J Obstet Gynecol 2011;205:319.e1–7.

Lukes AS, Freeman EW, Van Drie D, Baker J, Adomako TL. Safety of tranexamic acid in women with heavy menstrual bleeding: an open-label extension study. Womens Health (Lond Engl) 2011;7:591–8.

Lukes AS, Moore KA, Muse KN, Gersten JK, Hecht BR, Edlund M, et al. Tranexamic acid treatment for heavy menstrual bleeding: a randomized controlled trial. Obstet Gynecol 2010;116:865–75.

Wellington K, Wagstaff AJ. Tranexamic acid: a review of its use in the management of menorrhagia. Drugs 2003;63:1417–33.

114

First-trimester pregnancy loss

A 36-year-old woman comes to your office for an initial prenatal visit. She states that her last menstrual period occurred 10 weeks ago. She does not report any bleeding or problems with nausea and vomiting. On bimanual examination, you note a small uterus. Ultrasonography confirms an empty gestational sac consistent with an embryonic pregnancy loss. You counsel her regarding the risks and benefits of medical versus surgical treatment of pregnancy loss as they pertain to blood loss, infection, treatment follow-up, and patient accessibility. You inform her that use of misoprostol is advantageous to surgical evacuation because it

*   (A) provides easier patient access
       (B) leads to decreased blood loss
       (C) has a decreased risk of infection
       (D) requires no follow-up

First-trimester pregnancy loss is a common obstetric complication that occurs in approximately 20% of pregnancies. Management options should be tailored to the individual. Traditionally, women have been offered surgical intervention with dilation and curettage.

Medical management has been shown to be a safe alternative to surgical intervention. In a randomized study of 652 women who received a diagnosis of first-trimester pregnancy loss, high-dose vaginal misoprostol was shown to be an effective alternative to surgical evacuation. Of the 491 women randomized to receive 800 micrograms of vaginal misoprostol, success rates of 71% at day 3 and 84% by day 8 were observed. Secondary analysis noted that women who reported vaginal bleeding and abdominal cramping before the use of misoprostol had completion rates of 92%. Follow-up should occur 1–2 weeks after administration of misoprostol to determine the outcome of treatment.

Misoprostol can be administered orally, vaginally, or bucally. Medical management with misoprostol has numerous advantages to surgical intervention. Misoprostol is inexpensive, does not require refrigeration, physician administration, or initial surgical intervention. Women

are able to take the medication at a time that they deem most convenient and in the privacy of their home. The medication has been shown to be effective for incomplete abortions and missed abortions.

The disadvantage of medical management with misoprostol is that it takes more time for pregnancy resolution than surgical intervention. Medical management may take days to weeks as opposed to surgical management, which can be completed in less than 1 hour. Studies have shown that vaginal bleeding is characteristically heavier and lasts longer with medical management than with surgical management. Women who use misoprostol typically can expect heavy bleeding for 3–4 days and lighter bleeding that often lasts a total of 1–2 weeks. In some studies, hemoglobin levels have been shown to be decreased in patients after medical management, although clinical significance was small. Women who undergo surgical intervention have less blood loss than those taking misoprostol. Infection rates appear to be similar in both treatment groups.

Women who undergo medical and surgical intervention should undergo follow-up within 1–2 weeks of treatment. Bleeding, signs of infection, retained products of conception, and other potential complications should be assessed at the follow-up visit. In addition, this is a crucial time to review individual birth control plans.

Medical management with misoprostol allows for increased access for care. The World Health Organization has estimated that approximately 67,000 women die annually secondary to the lack of adequate health care for spontaneous and induced abortions. Alternative options are crucial in third-world countries where women may have to travel great distances and supplies and health care providers are limited.

Creinin MD, Huang X, Westhoff C, Barnhart K, Gilles JM, Zhang J. Factors related to successful misoprostol treatment for early pregnancy failure. National Institute of Child Health and Human Development Management of Early Pregnancy Failure Trial. Obstet Gynecol 2006; 107:901–7.

Davis AR, Hendlish SK, Westhoff C, Frederick MM, Zhang J, Gilles JM, et al. Bleeding patterns after misoprostol vs surgical treatment of early pregnancy failure: results from a randomized trial. National Institute of Child Health and Human Development Management of Early Pregnancy Failure Trial. Am J Obstet Gynecol 2007;196:31.e1–7.

Misoprostol for postabortion care. ACOG Committee Opinion No. 427. American College of Obstetricians and Gynecologists. Obstet Gynecol 2009;113:465–8.

Zhang J, Gilles JM, Barnhart K, Creinin MD, Westhoff C, Frederick MM. A comparison of medical management with misoprostol and surgical management for early pregnancy failure. National Institute of Child Health Human Development (NICHD) Management of Early Pregnancy Failure Trial. N Engl J Med 2005;353:761–9.

115

Recurrent urinary tract infection

A 29-year old woman presents to your office following treatment for a fourth urinary tract infection (UTI) after sexual intercourse in the past year. She has a test-of-cure result that indicates that her last course of therapy was successful and she is asymptomatic today. You discuss with her a number of approaches to reduce the risk of such infections, including prophylactic antibiotics, daily ingestion of cranberry juice, voiding immediately after intercourse, postcoital douching, and daily ingestion of D-mannose. She would prefer to avoid antibiotics because antibiotic therapy for her UTIs has led to monilial vaginitis on two occasions. You inform her that the method with the best evidence to support reduction in risk of recurrent urinary tract infections is

* (A) prophylactic antibiotics
  (B) daily cranberry juice
  (C) postcoital voiding
  (D) postcoital douching
  (E) daily D-mannose

Urinary tract infections are among the most common infections in women; more than 50% of women will experience an acute UTI during their lifetime. Furthermore, among healthy young women, the risk of recurrence is high. In one study of college women, 27% experienced another episode within 6 months of the initial infection. *Recurrent UTI* is defined as either greater than or equal to two uncomplicated UTIs within 6 months or three or more positive urine cultures within 1 year. *Escherichia coli* is responsible for approximately 80% of recurrent UTIs. Other organisms, such as *Staphylococcus saprophyticus, Klebsiella pneumoniae, Enterococcus faecalis*, and *Streptococcus agalactiae* (group B streptococci), may also be found on culture.

Frequency of sexual intercourse is a significant risk factor for recurrent UTIs in young women. In a case–control study, women aged 18–30 years with a sexual intercourse frequency of four to eight episodes per month had a significantly greater risk of recurrent UTIs than women who had no prior history of recurrent UTIs. Thus, because of this high risk of recurrent infection, effective preventive strategies are important.

A number of nonantibiotic approaches have been suggested to reduce the risk of postcoital UTIs. The daily ingestion of cranberry juice theoretically could work because laboratory studies show the juice inhibits adherence of uropathogens to uroepithelial cells. However, despite several clinical studies that examined whether cranberry juice provides a benefit in this situation, none of them have convincingly demonstrated the efficacy of cranberry juice in the prevention of recurrent UTIs. Similarly, voiding immediately after sexual intercourse would seem to be beneficial because intercourse could push potential vaginal pathogens into the lower urethra. However, in case–control studies, this strategy has not been shown to reduce the risk of recurrent UTIs. As with postcoital voiding, douching has not been shown to be effective in reducing recurrent UTIs. It has even been suggested that douching may increase the risk of recurrent UTIs. Further, douching can alter the vaginal flora and make users more susceptible to vaginal infections. D-mannose, a sugar substance available from health-food stores and through the Internet, theoretically works to block the adhesion of *E coli* bacteria to mannosylated receptors in the uroepithelium. However, D-mannose has not been evaluated for effectiveness in reducing UTIs in appropriately designed clinical trials.

Although the described patient has some reluctance to use this approach, antibiotics taken immediately after intercourse as a single dose constitute the most appropriate effective approach to reduce postcoital recurrent UTIs. In a randomized controlled trial of trimethoprim–sulfamethoxazole compared with placebo, the rate of recurrent UTIs per patient-year was reduced tenfold. Other single-dose regimens appear to be effective. Because the antibiotics are given as a single dose, the risk of developing monilial vaginitis as an adverse effect due to changes in the ecology of the vaginal flora is decreased.

Hooton TM. Clinical practice. Uncomplicated urinary tract infection. N Engl J Med 2012;366:1028–37.

Scholes D, Hooton TM, Roberts PL, Stapleton AE, Gupta K, Stamm WE. Risk factors for recurrent urinary tract infection in young women. J Infect Dis 2000;182:1177–82.

Schwarz RJ, Shrestha R. Needle aspiration of breast abscesses. Am J Surg 2001;182:117–9.

Stapleton A, Latham RH, Johnson C, Stamm WE. Postcoital antimicrobial prophylaxis for recurrent urinary tract infection. A randomized, double-blind, placebo-controlled trial. JAMA 1990;264:703–6.

Stapleton AE, Dziura J, Hooton TM, Cox ME, Yarova-Yarovaya Y, Chen S, et al. Recurrent urinary tract infection and urinary Escherichia coli in women ingesting cranberry juice daily: a randomized controlled trial. Mayo Clin Proc 2012;87:143–50.

World Health Organization Department of Child and Adolescent Health and Development. Mastitis: causes and management. Geneva: WHO; 2000. Available at: http://whqlibdoc.who.int/hq/2000/WHO_FCH_CAH_00.13.pdf. Retrieved June 6, 2013.

116

Dysmenorrhea in an adolescent patient

A 17-year-old patient has had dysmenorrhea for the past 2 years. In the first year after menarche, the dysmenorrhea was successfully managed with over-the-counter pain medications and heating pads. Subsequently, the dysmenorrhea worsened and was characterized by nausea, vomiting, and missed days from school. Despite treatment with extended-cycle oral contraceptive pills and prescription-strength nonsteroidal antiinflammatory drugs (NSAIDs), school absences consistently occurred with menses. She has no bowel or bladder problems and has never been sexually active. Pelvic ultrasonography yields normal results. The most appropriate next step is

        (A) dilation and curettage with hysteroscopy
        (B) pelvic magnetic resonance imaging (MRI)
   * (C) diagnostic laparoscopy
        (D) leuprolide acetate
        (E) empiric broad-spectrum antibiotics

Dysmenorrhea is a common condition in adolescent patients. The most common type, primary dysmenorrhea, is associated with varying degrees of monthly cramping, lower abdominal pain, backache, headache, nausea, vomiting, constipation, abdominal bloating, and diarrhea. Primary dysmenorrhea is associated with elevated levels of circulating prostaglandins produced in the endometrium and typically responds to medical intervention. Medical interventions involve several agents, such as hormonal contraceptives to thin the endometrium and decrease prostaglandin production, NSAIDs to relieve painful symptoms by blocking the prostaglandin receptors, and antiemetics to help with nausea.

This patient has dysmenorrhea refractory to standard medical interventions and significant enough to interrupt her attendance at school. Pelvic ultrasonography eliminates one diagnostic possibility in this scenario, an obstructed rudimentary müllerian remnant. The most appropriate next step is to perform a diagnostic laparoscopy to look for endometriosis.

Adolescents with dysmenorrhea that affects their ability to function despite good adherence to hormonal contraceptive agents and appropriate-dose NSAIDs may have endometriosis. In the absence of other etiologies of chronic pelvic pain, such as gastrointestinal disorders (constipation, irritable bowel syndrome, and inflammatory bowel disease), psychosocial factors (school avoidance behavior, somatization, and depression), musculoskeletal problems (sports injury, scoliosis, and leg length discrepancy), and urologic causes (chronic cystitis), a diagnostic laparoscopy should be considered. In appropriately chosen patients, more than one half will be identified with endometriosis at the time of laparoscopy. Adolescent endometriosis has a different appearance than adult endometriosis. Rather than the "classic" powder burn lesions, endometriomas, and adhesive disease, young women have clear vesicles and irregularities in the peritoneum. Because the changes are subtle, peritoneal biopsies should be used liberally.

A dilation and curettage with hysteroscopy is not indicated in this patient who has a normal appearing uterus on ultrasonography; it is unlikely that endometrial pathology is causing her symptoms. These procedures are not recommended at the time of diagnostic laparoscopy. Pelvic MRI is most useful in young women to explore suspected müllerian abnormalities or some adnexal masses. A pelvic MRI will not identify superficial endometriosis, which is most typically found in adolescent patients. Pelvic MRI is not required with a normal pelvic ultrasonography result.

Leuprolide acetate may be used in this patient if the diagnosis of endometriosis is confirmed with peritoneal biopsies at the time of diagnostic laparoscopy. It is imperative to use add-back therapy on initiation of leuprolide acetate to prevent bone demineralization and hot flushes. To date, no evidence supports empiric use of leuprolide acetate in adolescent patients with clinical suspicion of endometriosis.

The patient's symptoms are not consistent with either acute or chronic pelvic inflammatory disease. With chronic pelvic inflammatory disease, antibiotic therapy is not indicated.

The levonorgestrel IUD can be beneficial to treat primary dysmenorrhea and dysmenorrhea associated with endometriosis. However, in adolescents with refractory dysmenorrhea, a laparoscopy should be performed to address the diagnostic possibility of endometriosis.

Harel Z. Dysmenorrhea in adolescents and young adults: etiology and management. J Pediatr Adolesc Gynecol 2006;19:363–71.

Laufer MR. Helping "adult gynecologists" diagnose and treat adolescent endometriosis: reflections on my 20 years of personal experience. J Pediatr Adolesc Gynecol 2011;24:S13–S17.

Sanfilippo J, Erb T. Evaluation and management of dysmenorrhea in adolescents. Clin Obstet Gynecol 2008;51:257–67.

117

Ovarian cancer in *BRCA 1* and *BRCA 2* carriers

A 42-year-old woman, gravida 2, para 2, with an unremarkable past medical history recently received a diagnosis of a *BRCA 1* mutation. She is in good health and has a body mass index of 28 (calculated as weight in kilograms divided by height in meters squared). Her mother received a diagnosis of stage IIIC ovarian cancer at age 56 years. The best option to reduce the future risk of ovarian and breast cancer in this patient is

(A) combined estrogen–progesterone oral contraceptive (OC) use until age 50 years
* (B) prophylactic mastectomy and bilateral salpingo-oophorectomy
(C) biannual transvaginal ultrasonography, breast magnetic resonance imaging, and mammography
(D) bilateral tubal ligation

The American College of Obstetricians and Gynecologists recommends that women with a *BRCA* mutation undergo prophylactic surgery after age 40 years or after childbearing is complete. Up to 10% of women with ovarian cancer and up to 5% of women with breast cancer have a *BRCA 1* or *BRCA 2* mutation. The lifetime risk for development of breast and ovarian cancer in women with a *BRCA 1* mutation is approximately 65% and 39%, respectively, and the lifetime risk for women with a *BRCA 2* mutation for the is approximately 45% and 11%, respectively.

Combined OC use has been demonstrated to decrease the risk of ovarian cancer in the general population. However, the benefit for risk reduction with OC use in *BRCA* patients is unclear. Some reports have suggested a potential increased risk of breast cancer although these studies are limited by their sample size. Patients and clinicians need to weigh the risks and benefits of OC use before the initiation of use.

Current surveillance recommendations for women with *BRCA* mutations who desire future fertility and wish to avoid prophylactic surgery include biannual pelvic ultrasonography with CA 125 tests for ovarian cancer. These recommendations are based on expert consensus. Biannual evaluation by breast magnetic resonance imaging and mammography also are recommended for breast cancer surveillance. These surveillance recommendations are not meant for the general population.

Bilateral tubal ligation has been associated with decreased risk for ovarian cancer in the general population, and recent literature has suggested a potential role for salpingectomy in *BRCA* mutation carriers. Salpingectomy may be a reasonable option for women who wish to delay early surgical menopause and who are not interested in future fertility; however, at this time the benefits for this technique are not clear.

Prophylactic total mastectomy, defined as surgical removal of the entire breast tissue, areola, and nipple, can decrease the risk for subsequent breast cancer by more than 95%. Prophylactic bilateral salpingo-oophorectomy (BSO) reduces the risk of subsequent ovarian and fallopian tube cancer, but patients need to be made aware of the potential of peritoneal cancer. Hysterectomy at the time of BSO should be individualized based on patient risks and benefits of surgical intervention. The best option for the described patient is prophylactic mastectomy and BSO.

Brohet RM, Goldgar DE, Easton DF, Antoniou AC, Andrieu N, Chang-Claude J, et al. Oral contraceptives and breast cancer risk in the international BRCA1/2 carrier cohort study: a report from EMBRACE, GENEPSO, GEO-HEBON, and the IBCCS Collaborating Group. J Clin Oncol 2007;25:3831–6

Chivukula M, Niemeier LA, Edwards R, Nikiforova M, Mantha G, McManus K, et al. Carcinomas of distal fallopian tube and their association with tubal intraepithelial carcinoma: do they share a common "precursor" lesion? Loss of heterozygosity and immunohistochemical analysis using PAX 2, WT-1, and P53 markers. ISRN Obstet Gynecol 2011;2011:858647.

Hereditary breast and ovarian cancer syndrome. ACOG Practice Bulletin No. 103. American College of Obstetricians and Gynecologists and Society of Gynecologic Oncologists. Obstet Gynecol 2009;113:957–66.

Kaas R, Verhoef S, Wesseling J, Rookus MA, Oldenburg HS, Peeters MJ, Rutgers EJ. Prophylactic mastectomy in BRCA1 and BRCA2 mutation carriers: very low risk for subsequent breast cancer. Ann Surg 2010;251:488–92.

Kauff ND, Domchek SM, Friebel TM, Robson ME, Lee J, Garber JE, et al. Risk-reducing salpingo-oophorectomy for the prevention of BRCA1- and BRCA2-associated breast and gynecologic cancer: a multicenter, prospective study. J Clin Oncol 2008;26:1331–7.

Seidman JD, Yemelyanova A, Zaino RJ, Kurman RJ. The fallopian tube-peritoneal junction: a potential site of carcinogenesis. Int J Gynecol Pathol 2011;30:4–11.

Vicus D, Finch A, Rosen B, Fan I, Bradley L, Cass I, et al. Risk factors for carcinoma of the fallopian tube in women with and without a germline BRCA mutation. Hereditary Ovarian Cancer Clinical Study Group. Gynecol Oncol 2010;118:155–9.

118

Contraception in the morbidly obese patient

A 39-year-old woman, gravida 2, para 2, comes to the clinic and requests contraception. She has been in a monogamous relationship with a male sexual partner for the past 10 months and is not using any consistent contraceptive method. She reports a history of irregular menses that occur every 35–56 days without any intermenstrual spotting. On physical examination, her body mass index (BMI) is 33 (calculated as weight in kilograms divided by height in meters squared), blood pressure is 135 mm Hg systolic and 82 mm Hg diastolic, and pulse is 76 beats per minute. The abdominal and pelvic examinations are difficult to perform secondary to her body habitus, but no masses or point tenderness is noted. Urine pregnancy test and cultures for *Neisseria gonorrhoeae* and *Chlamydia trachomatis* yield negative results. You advise the patient that the best contraceptive option for her is

       (A) combination oral contraceptive
       (B) combination transdermal contraceptive patch
       (C) progestin-only contraceptive
*   (D) levonorgestrel IUD

Obesity is defined as a BMI of 30 or greater. The Centers for Disease Control and Prevention reported that in 2009–2010 approximately 41 million of women older than 20 years in the United States (40%) were obese. Obesity puts women at risk of medical and pregnancy-related complications and is linked to endometrial hyperplasia. Obese women who undergo bariatric surgery should not conceive for 12–24 months after the procedure.

Conflicting data exist in regard to obesity and the association with higher failure rates for hormonal contraceptive options, such as oral contraceptives, the contraceptive patch, and the vaginal contraceptive ring. It is important to note that previous research is limited by patient adherence issues and use of weight rather than BMI as a predictor of efficacy. To date, no randomized clinical trials have examined the question of the use of contraceptives among obese women. Data regarding the vaginal ring show similar efficacy and ovulation rates in women who have a BMI of up to 40. However, an increased likelihood of venous thromboembolism exists in obese women who use combined oral contraceptives. For obese women, a number of other contraceptive methods are available, eg, injectable, implantable, and intrauterine contraceptives. Either the hormonal or non-hormonal (copper) IUD is suitable. The progesterone-only methods also may be useful to prevent endometrial hyperplasia.

This patient has risk factors for endometrial hyperplasia because of oligomenorrhea and obesity. Oral contraceptives or the contraceptive patch could carry an increased risk of thromboembolism and decreased reliability because of obesity. Therefore, these methods would be less desirable than other listed methods. Progestin-only contraceptives may be a safer option but are less effective than combined contraceptives because of the narrow window of time for taking them and adverse effects, such as breakthrough bleeding. The levonorgestrel IUD would provide a safe, effective long-term option that would also prevent the development of endometrial hyperplasia.

Lopez LM, Grimes DA, Chen M, Otterness C, Westhoff C, Edelman A, et al. Hormonal contraceptives for contraception in overweight or obese women. Cochrane Database of Systematic Reviews 2013, Issue 4. Art. No.: CD008452. DOI: 10.1002/14651858.CD008452.pub3.

Ogden CL, Carroll MD, Kit BK, Flegal KM. Prevalence of obesity in the United States, 2009-2010. NCHS Data Brief 2012;(82):1–8.

Use of hormonal contraception in women with coexisting medical conditions. ACOG Practice Bulletin No. 73. American College of Obstetricians and Gynecologists. Obstet Gynecol 2006;107:1453–72.

Westhoff CL, Torgal AH, Mayeda ER, Petrie K, Thomas T, Dragoman M, et al. Pharmacokinetics and ovarian suppression during use of a contraceptive vaginal ring in normal-weight and obese women. Am J Obstet Gynecol 2012;207:39.e1–6.

119

Recurrent urinary tract infection

A 26-year-old nulligravid woman reports increased frequency and pain with urination for 3 days. In the past 3 years, she has called your office multiple times to report similar symptoms. Pelvic examination yields normal results. The prior urine culture result was positive for *Escherichia coli*. The current urine analysis yields positive results for nitrates and leukocytes esterase and negative results for blood. You treat the patient with antibiotics and send her urine for culture and sensitivity testing. After completion of the course of antibiotics, the best next step in management is to

       (A) refer the patient to a urologist
*   (B) perform a test of cure in 1–2 weeks
       (C) perform intravenous pyelography
       (D) perform renal ultrasonography
       (E) start daily prophylactic antibiotics

Urinary tract infections (UTIs) are common among adult women, and 11% of women will report at least one such infection per year. In addition, up to 50% of women will have a subsequent infection within 1 year. Classic symptoms include pain or burning with urination and an increased frequency. Many symptomatic women can be treated empirically with a short course of antibiotics.

Approximately 3–5% of women will suffer from frequent infections. *Recurrent UTIs* are commonly defined as either greater than or equal to two uncomplicated UTIs within 6 months or three or more positive results from urine cultures within 1 year. The first step in management is to confirm an actual infection. In women who present with recurrent symptoms, a urine culture and sensitivity testing should be performed when starting antibiotics to confirm appropriate treatment. After the patient is treated with a suitable antibiotic agent, a test of cure should be obtained in 1–2 weeks. This will help to assure that the patient has adhered to treatment, and the infection has been cleared. In addition, women should undergo a complete examination to evaluate for anatomic variation and evidence of sexually transmitted diseases.

Recurrent UTIs can be associated with pregnancy, diabetes mellitus, obesity, sickle cell disease, sexual activity, poor hygiene, spermicidal use, indwelling catheters, and anatomic abnormalities. Genitourinary abnormalities are more common in patients with a personal childhood history of UTIs or a family history of genital tract defects.

Prophylactic antibiotics are an appropriate option for women with recurrent UTIs once the current infection has been resolved and a test of cure yields a negative result. Daily suppression has been shown to decrease recurrent UTIs by 95%. Immediate referral to a urologist is not warranted for the described patient, but she can be referred once the test of cure is performed and the result is negative. Such a referral should be considered if she has evidence of an anatomic defect or urolithiasis or she is unresponsive to therapy. Any patients with a suspicion of genitourinary abnormalities or renal calculi should undergo an evaluation with imaging and cystoscopy. Patients with positive urine culture results for atypical bacteria, such as *Proteus, Enterobacter, Pseudomonas*, and *Klebsiella*, have an increased likelihood of a renal stone or anatomic variation. In addition, a thorough urologic workup is warranted in women with persistent hematuria.

Epp A, Larochelle A, Lovatsis D, Walter JE, Easton W, Farrell SA, et al. Recurrent urinary tract infection. Society of Obstetricians and Gynaecologists of Canada [published erratum appears in J Obstet Gynaecol Can 2011;33:12]. J Obstet Gynaecol Can 2010;32:1082–101.

Hooton TM. Clinical practice. Uncomplicated urinary tract infection. N Engl J Med 2012;366;11:1028–37.

Treatment of urinary tract infections in nonpregnant women. ACOG Practice Bulletin No. 91. American College of Obstetricians and Gynecologists. Obstet Gynecol 2008;111:785–94.

120

Role of hormone therapy in menopause

A 54-year-old woman is seeking therapy for worsening menopausal symptoms. The patient reports hot flushes, night sweats, vaginal dryness, breast tenderness, joint stiffness, and general aches and pains. She has been postmenopausal for 2 years and states that her symptoms are starting to affect her performance at work and her relationships at home. She is in good health and is not currently taking any medications. Her family history is negative for breast cancer and clotting disorders. The patient is interested in starting hormone therapy (HT). Of the symptoms described, HT is least likely to improve her

      (A) joint stiffness
      (B) vaginal dryness
   * (C) breast tenderness
      (D) general aches and pains
      (E) night sweats

Estrogen replacement has been shown to be the most effective treatment for postmenopausal hot flushes. Compared with placebo, estrogen decreases hot flushes by approximately 75%. In addition, estrogen replacement is effective at treating vaginal dryness and related dyspareunia.

The Women's Health Initiative study randomized more than 16,000 women aged 50–79 years to receive either placebo or combined continuous estrogen and progestin therapy. A separate arm of the study included approximately 11,000 women without a uterus who were randomized to receive either placebo or estrogen. The study was stopped early for patient safety concerns. Its primary objective was to determine if HT decreased the risk of coronary heart disease (CHD). However, the results indicated an increased risk of CHD in older women who took combination estrogen–progestin compared with women who took placebo. Women in the estrogen arm and the combined estrogen–progestin arm were noted to have an increased risk of venous thromboembolism. In addition, women who took combined estrogen–progestin HT were found to have a 26% increase in the risk of breast cancer. The findings of this large study indicated that candidates for HT should be selected judiciously and that therapy at the lowest dose for the shortest time should be administered.

A secondary analysis of the Women's Health Initiative study noted several other effects of postmenopausal HT.

Night sweats were reduced by 77.6%, and vaginal dryness was decreased by 74.1%. Joint stiffness and general aches and pains also were noted to be reduced in women who took HT compared with those who took placebo (47.1% versus 38%). In addition, women who took HT showed a 33% reduction in the risk of hip fractures. Compared with those who took placebo, women who took combined estrogen and progestin therapy were found to have six fewer cases of colorectal cancer per 10,000 women. For women who took estrogen alone, no statistical difference was present in the colorectal cancer rates. Women who took HT were more likely to develop breast tenderness than women who took placebo (9.3% versus 2.4%). Based on these findings and this patient's symptoms, HT is more likely to contribute to the breast tenderness than to alleviate the reported symptoms.

Barnabei VM, Cochrane BB, Aragaki AK, Nygaard I, Williams RS, McGovern PG, et al. Menopausal symptoms and treatment-related effects of estrogen and progestin in the Women's Health Initiative. Women's Health Initiative Investigators. Obstet Gynecol 2005;105: 1063–73.

North American Menopause Society. The 2012 hormone therapy position statement of: The North American Menopause Society. Menopause 2012;19:257–71.

Shifren JL, Schiff I. Role of hormone therapy in the management of menopause. Obstet Gynecol 2010;115:839–55.

121

Postoperative oliguria

A 45-year-old woman, gravida 2, para 2, with an unremarkable medical history underwent an uncomplicated total vaginal hysterectomy for adenomyosis. She has a body mass index of 22 (calculated as weight in kilograms divided by height in meters squared). On the night after the surgery, you are contacted by a nurse who reports new onset abdominal pain and oliguria in this patient. On evaluation, the patient is in moderate distress and her vital signs are significant for blood pressure of 140 mm Hg systolic and 90 mm Hg diastolic and a heart rate of 90 beats per minute. Examination reveals moderate suprapubic tenderness with abdominal distention and approximately 50 mL of clear urine in the Foley bag over the past 4 hours. The best next step in management is

      (A) complete blood count
      (B) intravenous bolus of 1,000 mL of isotonic fluids
      (C) computed tomography of abdomen and pelvis
  * (D) flushing the Foley catheter

Clinical evaluation of the patient is essential in postoperative care to help minimize unnecessary testing and to ensure effective outcomes. Postoperative evaluation in a patient with an unremarkable medical history is focused on identification of hypovolemia and anemia with acute blood loss. Subjective and objective data need to be considered to ensure a coherent assessment and a plan that is consistent with the clinical presentation.

To order an emergent complete blood count would be a reasonable step if the subjective and objective data supported acute blood loss anemia. Hypertension without tachycardia does not necessarily support acute blood loss, and a repeat surgery may not be indicated.

Increasing intravenous fluids is the first step in volume resuscitation in acute blood loss anemia but is not necessarily indicated in this patient. She has hypertension without tachycardia with suprapubic tenderness, which is more consistent with urinary retention than acute blood loss.

Computed tomography in a patient who is suspected to have acute blood loss but is clinically stable is reasonable, but it is important to emphasize the clinical presentation in this patient. Decreased urine output, suprapubic tenderness, and hypertension would point to blockage of the Foley catheter. Therefore, flushing the Foley catheter should be the first step in this patient's clinical evaluation. Multiple etiologies have been associated with urinary retention, including regional anesthesia and fibromas, but in a case of a patient with acute postoperative oliguria, evaluation should include flushing the Foley catheter.

Dolin SJ, Cashman JN. Tolerability of acute postoperative pain management: nausea, vomiting, sedation, pruritus, and urinary retention. Evidence from published data. Br J Anaesth 2005;95:584–91.

Mavromatidis G, Dinas K, Mamopoulos A, Delkos D, Rousso D. Acute urinary retention due to a uterine fibroid in a non-pregnant woman. Clin Exp Obstet Gynecol 2009;36:62–3.

Ramsey PS, Podratz KC. Acute pancreatitis after gynecologic and obstetric surgery. Am J Obstet Gynecol 1999;181:542–6.

122

Extended-cycle combined oral contraceptives

A 19-year-old female college athlete is considering trying extended-cycle combined oral contraceptives (OCs) for birth control and menstrual suppression. She has recently become sexually active and has used only condoms. You counsel her that the use of the extended-cycle formulation compared with the standard formulations will increase her risk of

   (A) contraceptive failure
   (B) breast cancer
   (C) deep vein thrombosis
   (D) weight gain
 * (E) unscheduled bleeding

The regimen of combined OCs, which consists of a 21-day course of estrogen–progestin (active) pills followed by a 7-day course of hormone-free (placebo) pills, remains the standard regimen for combined hormonal contraceptives. However, no medical reason exists for withdrawal bleeding, which occurs during the placebo week as a result of decreasing serum steroid levels. With extended-cycle regimens of combined OCs, patients take active pills for several weeks or months before a placebo interval. Some patients are motivated by cycle-dependent symptoms or menstrual-related disorders to use extended cycle regimens; others are attracted simply to avoid the inconvenience of withdrawal bleeding. Several patient surveys have shown that most patients prefer the extended regimens to suppress regular withdrawal bleeding and cycle-dependent problems and to improve the quality of life.

Some studies have shown that unscheduled intracyclic bleeding is more frequent in users of extended cycle combined OCs than in users of conventional combined OCs. Patients should be counseled regarding this increased risk of unscheduled bleeding with extended-cycle regimens. Unscheduled bleeding in patients who take combined OCs is a common reason cited for patient dissatisfaction and discontinuation of hormonal OCs. Patients should be informed that bleeding with extended-cycle regimens decreases with duration of use. Patients who are bothered by unscheduled bleeding may experience improvement if they stop their active pills for 4–7 days, allow for withdrawal bleeding, and then resume OCs. No evidence exists of increased contraceptive failure with extended-cycle combined OC regimens. The contraceptive efficacy between extended-cycle and conventional regimens is similar.

In a large survey, 14% of health care providers expressed concern regarding increased risk of deep vein thrombosis or pulmonary embolism with extended-cycle regimens. However, direct comparisons between extended-cycle and conventional regimens show no difference between various metabolic parameters, including hemostasis, carbohydrate metabolism, and lipid metabolism. Large-scale, extended-term trials did not show a higher risk of thromboembolic disease with the use of extended-cycle regimens compared with conventional regimens. Patients should be counseled that the risk of thromboembolic events is similar for extended-cycle regimens and conventional regimens.

No evidence has been found of increased complications with the use of extended-cycle regimen of combined OCs compared with conventional regimens. Similarly, no evidence has been found of increased risk of breast cancer. In addition, no differences have been demonstrated in weight gain between the two regimens.

Bitzer J, Simon JA. Current issues and available options in combined hormonal contraception. Contraception 2011;84:342–56.

Krishnan S, Kiley J. The lowest-dose, extended-cycle combined oral contraceptive pill with continuous ethinyl estradiol in the United States: a review of the literature on ethinyl estradiol 20 µg/levonorgestrel 100 µg + ethinyl estradiol 10 µg. Int J Womens Health 2010;2:235–9.

Seval DL, Buckley T, Kuehl TJ, Sulak PJ. Attitudes and prescribing patterns of extended-cycle oral contraceptives. Contraception 2011;84:71–5.

Wiegratz I, Stahlberg S, Manthey T, Sänger N, Mittmann K, Lange E, et al. Effect of extended-cycle regimen with an oral contraceptive containing 30 mcg ethinylestradiol and 2 mg dienogest on bleeding patterns, safety, acceptance and contraceptive efficacy. Contraception 2011;84:133–43.

123

Recurrent vaginal yeast infection

A 46-year-old woman, gravida 2, para 2, with type 2 diabetes mellitus comes to your office with recurrent itching and vaginal discharge. A wet preparation result confirms yeast. This is the fourth time she has had a confirmed vaginal yeast infection in the past 6 months. She received the diagnosis of diabetes mellitus 4 years ago and maintains her hemoglobin A_{1c} level at 5.1–5.5 g/dL. The most effective strategy to prevent recurrent yeast infections in this patient is

* (A) suppressive antifungal therapy
  (B) treatment of her sexual partner
  (C) improved glycemic control
  (D) oral antihistamine

Recurrent vulvovaginal candidiasis is defined as four or more symptomatic, acute episodes of *Candida* vaginitis in 1 year. The pathogenesis of this disease is complex and is based on genetic, behavioral, and biologic risk factors that predispose a woman to colonization and symptomatic states. The principles of treatment are as follows:

- Confirmation of microbiologic diagnosis
- Identification and treatment or removal of underlying causative factors
- Induction and maintenance of azole therapy

A trial of fluconazole given to women in three 72-hour intervals followed by weekly treatment for 6 months showed greater efficacy in preventing recurrence at 6 months compared with women who received a placebo. The proportions of women without recurrence at 6 months, 9 months, and 12 months in the fluconazole group were 90.8%, 73.2%, and 42.9%, respectively, compared with those in the placebo group with reported recurrences of 35.9%, 27.8%, and 21.9%, respectively. However, 50% of women initially without recurrences had a recurrence by 12 months after the start of treatment. Long-term therapy with fluconazole is effective for *Candida albicans* and has not been shown to lead to an increase in other *Candida* species in immunocompetent women. Oral ketoconazole is no longer used for the treatment of recurrent cases because of a higher risk of liver toxicity compared with fluconazole. Women who are unable to take fluconazole can use topical clotrimazole intermittently or a standard course of topical imidazole therapy. For women with unsuccessful azole therapy, daily or intermittent vaginal boric acid or nystatin suppositories can be prescribed. Culture and referral to a specialist should be considered in refractory cases.

Additional measures that can reduce the risk of recurrence include maintenance of euglycemia in women with diabetes mellitus and hygiene education. However, the described patient already has optimal glycemic control. Reassurance is a key part of the treatment plan. Treatment of sexual partners is unnecessary. An oral antihistamine will likely be of no use to decrease itching associated with *Candida* vaginitis.

Sobel JD. Management of recurrent vulvovaginal candidiasis: unresolved issues. Curr Infect Dis Rep 2006;8:481–6.

Sobel JD, Wiesenfeld HC, Martens M, Danna P, Hooton TM, Rompalo A, et al. Maintenance fluconazole therapy for recurrent vulvovaginal candidiasis. N Engl J Med 2004;351:876–83.

Viral hepatitis in pregnancy. ACOG Practice Bulletin No. 86. American College of Obstetricians and Gynecologists. Obstet Gynecol 2007;110:941–56.

124

Unplanned pregnancy

An 18-year-old woman, gravida 1, para 0, presented to your office with an unplanned pregnancy at 8 weeks of gestation. The patient opted to undergo pregnancy termination and stated that she does not want to become pregnant again anytime soon. In the recovery room, she is counseled regarding contraceptive options and refuses an implantable progestin rod. The best next step to prevent a repeat unplanned pregnancy is to

      (A) prescribe oral contraceptives
*   (B) administer depot medroxyprogesterone acetate
      (C) recommend condom use
      (D) schedule insertion of an intrauterine device (IUD)
      (E) prescribe the vaginal contraceptive ring

It is estimated that one half of all pregnancies in the United States are unplanned. Of those, approximately 40% are a result of not using birth control. The Centers for Disease Control and Prevention reported that approximately 800,000 abortions were performed in the United States in 2009. Additionally, data show that women who experience one unplanned pregnancy are at risk of a subsequent unplanned pregnancy.

After an abortion, because only approximately 50% of women return for postoperative care, many women miss a crucial opportunity for birth control. It is important that health care providers discuss appropriate birth control methods with the patient before the procedure. In one study of 865 women who underwent a first-trimester abortion, 21.4% of patients were pregnant again within 1 year and 52% of patients subsequently underwent a repeat termination. However, women who received depot medroxyprogesterone acetate at the time of the procedure were less likely (13%) to experience a subsequent pregnancy within 1 year. The other forms of birth control studied, including oral contraceptives, condoms, the vaginal contraceptive ring, and IUD, were shown to be less effective.

Oral contraceptives have up to 99% effectiveness with perfect use. However, the World Health Organization estimates that with typical use, oral contraception has only 92% effectiveness.

Although condoms are advocated as protection against risk of contracting sexually transmitted diseases, their use often provides inadequate birth control. Male condoms can be more than 97% effective with perfect use at preventing pregnancy; however, they have been reported to be 86% effective with typical use. Therefore, condoms should be combined with another form of birth control to achieve optimal protection against unplanned pregnancy.

The copper IUD and the levonorgestrel IUD are more than 99% effective in preventing pregnancy. Because such methods are not dependent on patient adherence, they offer excellent long-term reversible options. However, IUD insertion that is scheduled weeks after a pregnancy termination has been shown to be an inferior option to prevent repeat pregnancies because it is entirely dependent on the patient returning for follow-up care. Intrauterine devices can be placed at the time of an abortion. In a study of 308 women who requested an IUD after an abortion, insertion was achieved in 96% of the women who opted for immediate insertion versus only 23% of women who had planned on insertion at the postoperative visit. The expulsion rate for immediate insertion was 7% for second-trimester abortions and 3% for first-trimester abortions. Other studies have reported expulsion rates up to 10%. However, many health care providers are not yet experienced with postabortion insertion and, therefore, the method is not yet widely available.

The vaginal contraceptive ring provides patients with an option that is easily reversible and it needs to be inserted only once a month. However, adherence has been shown to be approximately 90%, comparable with adherence for oral contraceptive pills. In addition to proper insertion and removal, patients need to fill the prescription themselves.

Long-term subdermal progestin inserts have been shown to be highly effective for pregnancy prevention and should be considered at the time of pregnancy termination. However, the described patient has declined this option.

Fox MC, Oat-Judge J, Severson K, Jamshidi RM, Singh RH, McDonald-Mosley R, et al. Immediate placement of intrauterine devices after first and second trimester pregnancy termination. Contraception 2011;83:34–40.

Madden T, Westhoff C. Rates of follow-up and repeat pregnancy in the 12 months after first-trimester induced abortion. Obstet Gynecol 2009;113:663–8.

Matteson KA, Peipert JF, Allsworth J, Phipps MG, Redding CA. Unplanned pregnancy: does past experience influence the use of a contraceptive method? Obstet Gynecol 2006;107:121–7.

Pazol K, Creanga AA, Zane SB, Burley KD, Jamieson DJ; Centers for Disease Control and Prevention (CDC). Abortion surveillance—United States, 2009. MMWR Surveill Summ 2012;61(8):1–44.

125

Hydrosalpinx

A 28-year-old nulligravid woman with tubal factor infertility is preparing for her first cycle of in vitro fertilization (IVF). She was treated for pelvic inflammatory disease 9 years ago, and recent transvaginal ultrasonography suggests bilateral hydrosalpinges. She states that she does not have any abdominal pain, and her examination does not reveal adnexal tenderness. The most appropriate next step in management is

> (A) reassurance
> * (B) laparoscopic bilateral salpingectomy
> (C) broad spectrum oral antibiotics
> (D) laparoscopy with drainage of hydrosalpinges

Laparoscopic bilateral salpingectomy is the most appropriate next step in this patient's management. Favorable pregnancy outcomes in patients who undergo IVF are decreased in those with hydrosalpinx compared with those with other tubal factors. Any hydrosalpinx large enough in caliber to be visualized with pelvic ultrasonography is clinically relevant. Patients with hydrosalpinx who undergo IVF have approximately 50% the pregnancy and delivery rate and twofold the miscarriage rate compared with patients without hydrosalpinx who undergo IVF. The fluid from hydrosalpinx is theorized to be the causative agent, and interruption of communication between the fallopian tube and endometrium to prevent leakage of the fluid into the endometrium improves pregnancy rates. Tubal ligation, with proximal tubal occlusion, has been suggested as an alternative to salpingectomy when dense adhesions make salpingectomy difficult; however, the remaining hydrosalpinx may interfere with subsequent egg retrieval. Careful surgical technique at the time of salpingectomy is important. Care should be taken to avoid any damage to the nearby ovarian blood supply, which could compromise ovarian function. No consensus exists in the literature to suggest that salpingectomy alone limits ovarian function.

Whereas inpatient intravenous antibiotics and outpatient oral antibiotics are indicated in the treatment of acute pelvic inflammatory disease, no evidence exists that antibiotics are beneficial in improving outcomes of IVF in patients with hydrosalpinx. Therefore, antibiotics would not be a reasonable next step before initiation of IVF in this patient.

Ultrasonography-guided transvaginal aspiration of the fluid from hydrosalpinx has been advocated as a treatment option. When performed before ovarian stimulation, the fluid reaccumulates. Even when performed at the time of oocyte retrieval, the risk of reaccumulation is high at the time of embryo transfer. Two small retrospective studies failed to show improved prognosis with aspiration of the fluid from hydrosalpinx before IVF; therefore, this would not be the most appropriate next step for the described patient.

Reassurance is associated with decreased pregnancy and delivery rates and increased miscarriage rates. For this reason, reassurance would not be the most appropriate option for this patient who is preparing for IVF.

Omurtag K, Grindler NM, Roehl KA, Bates GW Jr, Beltsos AN, Odem RR, et al. How members of the Society for Reproductive Endocrinology and Infertility and Society of Reproductive Surgeons evaluate, define, and manage hydrosalpinges. Fertil Steril 2012;97:1095, 100.e1–2.

Salpingectomy for hydrosalpinx prior to in vitro fertilization. Practice Committee of American Society for Reproductive Medicine in collaboration with Society of Reproductive Surgeons. Fertil Steril 2008; 90:S66–S68.

Strandell A. Treatment of hydrosalpinx in the patient undergoing assisted reproduction. Curr Opin Obstet Gynecol 2007;19:360–5.

126

Beta-blocker therapy in perioperative care

A 70-year-old woman underwent an uncomplicated total laparoscopic hysterectomy and bilateral salpingo-oophorectomy for complex endometrial hyperplasia with atypia. Her medical history is remarkable for hypertension that requires multiple medications, including a calcium channel blocker, a β-blocker, and an angiotensin-converting enzyme (ACE) inhibitor. You are concerned about her risk of a postoperative myocardial infarction. The hypertension medication in the perioperative period that is most likely to help reduce her risk for postoperative myocardial infarction is

*   (A) β-blocker
     (B) ACE inhibitor
     (C) α-blocker
     (D) calcium channel blocker

Beta-blockers, such as metoprolol succinate, can help reduce risk of perioperative myocardial infarction (MI) and have been demonstrated to help with postoperative outcomes in patients with cardiac disease and patients who take long-term β-blocker therapy. It is important to note that the use of β-blockers in patients who have not used long-term therapy may be associated with an increased risk of postoperative morbidity and mortality, and particularly with an increased risk of postoperative stroke.

A large, randomized, multicenter, controlled trial on the effects of extended-release metoprolol in patients who underwent noncardiac surgery, the PeriOperative ISchemic Evaluation trial, was published in 2008. In this study of 8,351 patients, individuals who took metoprolol were less likely to have a perioperative MI compared with the patients in the placebo group (4.2% versus 5.7%; $P=.0017$). However, the overall mortality was increased in the metoprolol group compared with the placebo group (3.1% versus 2.3%; $P=.0317$). The stroke risk also was increased in the metoprolol group compared with the placebo group (1.0% versus 0.5%; $P=.0053$).

The ACE inhibitors, such as lisinopril, affect systemic vascular resistance and have not been directly associated with perioperative MI; ACE inhibitors do appear to have a role in perioperative hypotension. Communication with the anesthesia team is important regarding administration of this type of medication before surgery. In the postoperative period, the ACE inhibitor often can be withheld until the effects of anesthetic medications and systemic narcotics have cleared the patient's system, commonly on postoperative day 2 or postoperative day 3.

Alpha-agonists, such as clonidine, are centrally acting sympatholytic drugs. It is important to consider restarting the α-agonist as soon as possible to avoid the potential of rebound hypertension. Calcium channel blockers, also known as calcium channel antagonists, such as amlodipine, have been associated with perioperative bleeding through potential interaction with platelets. The use of calcium channel blockers has not been directly associated with perioperative MI.

Devereaux PJ, Yang H, Guyatt GH, Leslie K, Villar JC, Monteri VM, et al. Rationale, design, and organization of the PeriOperative ISchemic Evaluation (POISE) trial: a randomized controlled trial of metoprolol versus placebo in patients undergoing noncardiac surgery. POISE Trial Investigators. Am Heart J 2006;152:223–30.

Devereaux PJ, Yang H, Yusuf S, Guyatt G, Leslie K, Villar JC, et al. Effects of extended-release metoprolol succinate in patients undergoing non-cardiac surgery (POISE trial): a randomised controlled trial. POISE Study Group. Lancet 2008;371:1839–47.

Rupp H, Maisch B, Brilla CG. Drug withdrawal and rebound hypertension: differential action of the central antihypertensive drugs moxonidine and clonidine. Cardiovasc Drugs Ther 1996;10(Suppl 1):251–62.

Zuccalá G, Pahor M, Landi F, Gasparini G, Pagano F, Carbonin P, et al. Use of calcium antagonists and need for perioperative transfusion in older patients with hip fracture: observational study. BMJ 1997;314:643–4.

127

Carcinoma risk reduction

A 36-year-old woman, gravida 1, para 1, comes to the office for counseling regarding ovarian cancer risk reduction. She has a history of receiving four cycles of clomiphene citrate for ovulation induction to conceive. She tells you that her sister received a diagnosis of breast cancer at age 33 years, and that she and her sister have a *BRCA 1* mutation. The intervention that has the highest likelihood for reducing her risk for ovarian cancer is

     (A) tamoxifen citrate
     (B) oral contraceptives
*   (C) prophylactic bilateral salpingo-oophorectomy (BSO)
     (D) tubal ligation

Mutations of the *BRCA 1* and *BRCA 2* genes have been associated with the development of hereditary breast and ovarian cancer; both genes are categorized as tumor suppressors. In normal cells, *BRCA 1* and *BRCA 2* help ensure the stability of the cell's genetic material (DNA) and help prevent uncontrolled cell growth. The abbreviations *BRCA 1* and *BRCA 2* stand for *breast cancer susceptibility gene 1* and *breast cancer susceptibility gene 2*, respectively. The *BRCA* gene mutations are associated with a lifetime breast cancer risk of approximately 56–84% by age 70 years and also with an increased risk of ovarian cancer. The risk of ovarian cancer is 36–46% in women with *BRCA 1* mutations and 10–27% in women with *BRCA 2* mutations as compared with 1.8% in the general population.

Current strategies to reduce the risk of developing breast cancer in patients with *BRCA* mutations include surveillance, chemoprevention, and surgery. Ovarian cancer surveillance with CA 125 testing and screening ultrasonography has not been shown to be effective in reducing mortality or improving survival in high-risk populations. Nevertheless, consensus groups have advocated such periodic screening strategies, given the high risk for ovarian cancer in women beginning between ages 30 years and 35 years or 5–10 years earlier than the earliest age of diagnosis of ovarian cancer in the family.

The patient reports the use of clomiphene citrate for ovulation induction. Clomiphene is a synthetic compound with properties of a selective estrogen receptor modulator that is used for ovulation induction. A meta-analysis of the use of fertility drugs and ovarian cancer showed no significant increase in cancer risk compared with the general population. However, infertility for 5 years or longer compared with less than 1 year was associated with an increased risk, independent of fertility drug usage. Studies did show an association between fertility drug use and an increased risk of borderline tumors of the ovary (tumors of low-malignant potential). Although

a case–control study concluded that the use of fertility drugs does not increase the risk of breast cancer, conclusive evidence is lacking regarding breast cancer risk and use of fertility drugs in women with *BRCA* mutations. No studies have been conducted regarding the use of fertility drugs and risk of ovarian cancer in patients who have *BRCA* mutations.

Tamoxifen is a selective estrogen receptor modulator that is approved for the treatment and risk reduction of breast cancer in high-risk women. It is given for 5 years and has been shown to decrease the risk of breast cancer recurrence by approximately 40% and the annual mortality risk by 34%. Currently, tamoxifen is not indicated for chemoprophylaxis of ovarian cancer.

A cohort study that used data of more than 1 million women-years of observation showed that oral contraceptive (OC) use was associated with a 46% risk reduction in ovarian cancer compared with women who never used OCs. The protective effect was related to the duration of use; the effect persisted 15 years after cessation of OCs. Similarly, the risk of ovarian cancer in women with *BRCA* mutations who took OCs has been shown to be reduced by 40–50%.

Prophylactic BSO has been shown to reduce the risk of ovarian cancer in women with *BRCA* mutations by 80–88%. In this high-risk population, this procedure should be offered to women by age 40 years or when childbearing is complete. The procedure also has been shown to reduce the risk of breast cancer in patients with *BRCA* mutation by almost 50%, although the protection is mainly against estrogen receptor-positive tumors. Prophylactic BSO is the intervention that has the highest likelihood for reducing the described patient's risk for ovarian cancer.

In a recent meta-analysis, tubal ligation was shown to be protective against epithelial ovarian cancer in the general population. The study showed a risk reduction of 34%. The risk reduction was in endometrioid and serous tumors, but not in mucinous tumors. Similarly, a large cohort study that involved women with *BRCA* mutations showed that tubal ligation had a 58% reduction in the risk of ovarian cancer.

Parity has been shown to have a protective effect on the risk of ovarian cancer in the general population. In women with the *BRCA 1* mutation, parity was shown to decrease the risk of ovarian cancer by 44%; however, no conclusive data was found for women with the *BRCA 2* mutation, although some data suggested an increased risk.

Berek JS, Chalas E, Edelson M, Moore DH, Burke WM, Cliby WA, et al. Prophylactic and risk-reducing bilateral salpingo-oophorectomy: recommendations based on risk of ovarian cancer. Society of Gynecologic Oncologists Clinical Practice Committee. Obstet Gynecol 2010; 116:733–43.

Cibula D, Widschwendter M, Májek O, Dusek L. Tubal ligation and the risk of ovarian cancer: review and meta-analysis. Hum Reprod Update 2011;17:55–67.

Finch A, Beiner M, Lubinski J, Lynch HT, Moller P, Rosen B, et al. Salpingo-oophorectomy and the risk of ovarian, fallopian tube, and peritoneal cancers in women with a BRCA1 or BRCA2 mutation. Hereditary Ovarian Cancer Clinical Study Group. JAMA 2006;296: 185–92.

Fishman A. The effects of parity, breastfeeding, and infertility treatment on the risk of hereditary breast and ovarian cancer: a review. Int J Gynecol Cancer 2010;11(Suppl 2):S31–S33.

Hannaford PC, Selvaraj S, Elliott AM, Angus V, Iversen L, Lee AJ. Cancer risk among users of oral contraceptives: cohort data from the Royal College of General Practitioner's oral contraception study. BMJ 2007;335:651.

Kauff ND, Domchek SM, Friebel TM, Robson ME, Lee J, Garber JE, et al. Risk-reducing salpingo-oophorectomy for the prevention of BRCA1- and BRCA2-associated breast and gynecologic cancer: a multicenter, prospective study. J Clin Oncol 2008;26:1331–7.

128

Nonhormonal therapy for menopause

A 53-year-old woman, gravida 2, para 2, informs you that her last menstrual period was approximately 13 months ago and that since that time she has had significant hot flushes and sleep disturbance. She states that she wakes up several times a night sweating. Her medical history is significant for breast cancer diagnosed 3 years ago, for which she takes tamoxifen citrate. The best initial treatment for this patient is

    (A) black cohosh
    (B) ginseng
    (C) venlafaxine
    (D) combined estrogen and progestin therapy
*   (E) gabapentin

Traditionally, the most effective treatment for postmenopausal hot flushes has been estrogen therapy (with or without progestin). However, estrogen is not without risks. In 2002, the Women's Health Initiative study found that the use of combined hormone therapy (HT) has an increased risk of blood clots, stroke, coronary disease, and breast cancer. Since then, the number of women who used HT has decreased whereas the use of alternative therapies has increased. Such therapies include herbal medication, soy products, and behavior modification. In one survey of over 800 women, 76.1% of women reported using herbal medications. Women with breast cancer were six times more likely to try soy products to treat hot flushes.

Black cohosh is a popular herbal medication for the treatment of hot flushes. The herb has minimal adverse effects, mainly gastric upset. However, randomized trials have shown no benefit of black cohosh over placebo for the treatment of vasomotor symptoms. In addition, because of the potential estrogenic effects, some experts warn against the use of black cohosh in breast cancer patients.

Ginseng is commonly marketed to decrease stress, improve athletic performance, boost immunity, and decrease hot flushes. Data are lacking to support these claims; therefore, it is not an appropriate therapy for the described patient's vasomotor symptoms.

Venlafaxine, a serotonin norepinephrine reuptake inhibitor, was initially approved as an antidepressant. Research has since found that postmenopausal women who take venlafaxine report a decrease in severity and occurrence of hot flushes by up to 61%. Common adverse effects include dry mouth and constipation. However, venlafaxine decreases the conversion of tamoxifen citrate to its active metabolite, thus decreasing its benefits. The long-term effects of this combination on breast cancer survival and recurrence are unknown. Therefore, the concomitant use of venlafaxine and tamoxifen citrate should be avoided in breast cancer patients.

Combination of estrogen and progestin has numerous therapeutic and beneficial actions and is currently the only treatment approved by the U.S. Food and Drug Administration for vasomotor symptoms. Participants in the Women's Health Initiative study were noted to have a decreased risk of osteoporosis and colon cancer, in addition to a decrease in vasomotor symptoms. However, the medication is contraindicated in breast cancer patients. A randomized trial in Sweden monitored 442 breast cancer survivors for a median of 4 years. Cancer recurrence rates were 22.2% in women who took HT compared with 8% in patients in the control arm.

Gabapentin was originally approved as an antiseizure medication and for postherpetic neuralgia. A randomized double-blinded placebo controlled trial of 420 women with breast cancer showed a 46% reduction in hot flushes with high-dose gabapentin compared with a 15% reduction in patients who took a placebo. Common

adverse effects include headache and dizziness. Health care providers frequently start with a low dose and slowly increase the medication over a period of weeks. Gabapentin is the most appropriate initial medication for the described patient.

Bordeleau L, Pritchard KI, Loprinzi CL, Ennis M, Jugovic O, Warr D, et al. Multicenter, randomized, cross-over clinical trial of venlafaxine versus gabapentin for the management of hot flashes in breast cancer survivors. J Clin Oncol 2010;28:5147–52.

Guttuso T Jr, Kurlan R, McDermott MP, Kieburtz K. Gabapentin's effects on hot flashes in postmenopausal women: a randomized controlled trial. Obstet Gynecol 2003;101:337–45.

Newton KM, Buist DS, Keenan NL, Anderson LA, LaCroix AZ. Use of alternative therapies for menopause symptoms: results of a population-based survey [published erratum appears in Obstet Gynecol 2003;101:205]. Obstet Gynecol 2002;100:18–25.

Pandya KJ, Morrow GR, Roscoe JA, Zhao H, Hickok JT, Pajon E, et al. Gabapentin for hot flashes in 420 women with breast cancer: a randomised double-blind placebo-controlled trial. Lancet 2005;366: 818–24.

Use of botanicals for management of menopausal symptoms. ACOG Practice Bulletin No. 28. American College of Obstetricians and Gynecologists. Obstet Gynecol 2001;97(Suppl 1)1–11.

129

A patient with ductal carcinoma in situ

A 54-year-old postmenopausal woman, gravida 2, para 2, comes to your office for her well-woman examination. Her clinical breast examination is normal, but screening mammography shows an abnormal result. Her past medical history is significant for obesity and diabetes mellitus. Her father had colon cancer at age 71 years and her mother died of a heart attack at age 59 years. Diagnostic mammography and fine needle aspiration show ductal carcinoma in situ (DCIS) in the left breast. The best initial treatment option is

* (A) local surgical treatment
  (B) local radiation therapy
  (C) tamoxifen citrate
  (D) aromatase inhibitor

Ductal carcinoma in situ is a heterogeneous group of neoplastic disorders confined to breast tissue with a complex natural history. Histologically, it is characterized by proliferation of abnormal epithelial cells with an intact basement membrane and no stromal invasion. With increased breast cancer screening, the rate of diagnosis of DCIS has increased significantly over the past several decades.

In the treatment of DCIS, the goal for therapy is prevention of invasive breast cancer. Treatment strategies include surgery, radiation therapy, and adjuvant hormonal therapy. Surgical resection of diseased tissue is the primary treatment for DCIS, although the optimal surgical management strategy has been the subject of debate.

The best initial treatment option for the described patient is local surgical treatment. Two local surgical options are available: 1) mastectomy or 2) lumpectomy. Historically, mastectomy was the standard of care with 98–99% local recurrence-free survival at 10-year follow-up. However, it also may be considered overtreatment for the disease. Compared with mastectomy, lumpectomy with local radiation therapy is a reasonable breast-conserving option with lower morbidity and comparable years of survival, but has a higher risk of recurrence (7–15%). Research is ongoing to determine risk factors for recurrent invasive or noninvasive disease so that effective treatment with the least amount of morbidity can be offered to each patient. Systemic treatment with tamoxifen citrate or aromatase inhibitors would not be appropriate as primary treatment for the described patient. It may be considered after surgical treatment to prevent recurrence. Local radiation therapy would not be recommended for this patient.

Bijker N, Meijnen P, Peterse JL, Bogaerts J, Van Hoorebeeck I, Julien JP, et al. Breast-conserving treatment with or without radiotherapy in ductal carcinoma-in-situ: ten-year results of European Organisation for Research and Treatment of Cancer randomized phase III trial 10853—a study by the EORTC Breast Cancer Cooperative Group and EORTC Radiotherapy Group. EORTC Breast Cancer Cooperative Group and EORTC Radiotherapy Group. J Clin Oncol 2006;24:3381–7.

Petrelli F, Barni S. Tamoxifen added to radiotherapy and surgery for the treatment of ductal carcinoma in situ of the breast: a meta-analysis of 2 randomized trials. Radiother Oncol 2011;100:195–9.

Schmale I, Liu S, Rayhanabad J, Russell CA, Sener SF. Ductal carcinoma in situ (DCIS) of the breast: perspectives on biology and controversies in current management. J Surg Oncol 2012;105:212–20.

130

Eating disorders and irregular menstruation

A 21-year-old nulligravid woman comes to your office with menstrual irregularity. She has not had a menstrual cycle for 6 months. Her menses have been irregular since menarche at age 16 years. She has no medical problems and exercises daily. She has been a competitive cross-country runner since age 13 years. She keeps a strict vegan diet because she does not want to gain weight as many of her classmates have since they began college. Her body mass index is 17 (calculated as weight in kilograms divided by height in meters squared), blood pressure is 90 mm Hg systolic and 55 mm Hg diastolic, and pulse is 50 beats per minute. She is not interested in childbearing at this time. In addition to counseling about her menstrual irregularity, you tell her that her most significant health problem that needs to be addressed at this time is risk of

    (A) dental caries
*   (B) osteoporosis
    (C) ruptured ovarian cysts
    (D) facial hair growth

The *female athlete triad* is defined as follows:

1. Disordered eating compared with energy availability
2. Menstrual irregularity
3. Diminished bone mineral density

Traditionally, this diagnosis has been associated with activities, such as long distance running, ballet, and gymnastics. Diagnosis should be established after other causes of amenorrhea are ruled out and is based on history, physical examination, and laboratory findings. Testing may include assessment of β-hCG, prolactin, follicle-stimulating hormone, luteinizing hormone, and thyroid-stimulating hormone levels and bone mineral density determination.

Most women with exercise-induced amenorrhea have hypothalamic amenorrhea caused by decreased pulsatile secretion of gonadotropin-releasing hormone from the hypothalamus that leads to decreased secretion of follicle-stimulating hormone and luteinizing hormone. Lack of these hormonal stimuli leads to an estrogen-deficient state and disorders, such as osteopenia or osteoporosis, amenorrhea or oligomenorrhea, vaginal and breast atrophy, and infertility. Increased serum cholesterol levels and an increased risk of mortality also are associated with this condition.

Dental caries are of concern in amenorrheic women with eating disorders, such as bulimia nervosa. Ruptured ovarian cyst is uncommon in this population because of infrequent ovulation. Facial hair growth is a cosmetic issue that may occur in women with polycystic ovary syndrome or high testosterone levels and can be associated with menstrual irregularities.

Treatment for the female athlete triad is based on the woman's current reproductive goals. In reproductive-aged women who desire conception, low body mass index related to disordered eating should be addressed through behavioral therapy, increased nutritional intake, and reduction of energy expenditure. Women with the female athlete triad may need assessment of and treatment for infertility, if they desire pregnancy. If pregnancy is not desired, oral contraceptives can be used to regulate menses and protect the women from further bone loss. However, until body mass is increased, the underlying cause of the problem will not be addressed. Management and treatment for osteopenia or osteoporosis may be necessary, and women should be cautioned regarding their increased risk of musculoskeletal injury during athletic activities.

Loucks AB, Thuma JR. Luteinizing hormone pulsatility is disrupted at a threshold of energy availability in regularly menstruating women. J Clin Endocrinol Metab 2003;88:297–311.

Pollock N, Grogan C, Perry M, Pedlar C, Cooke K, Morrissey D, et al. Bone-mineral density and other features of the female athlete triad in elite endurance runners: a longitudinal and cross-sectional observational study. Int J Sport Nutr Exerc Metab 2010;20:418–26.

Thein-Nissenbaum JM, Carr KE. Female athlete triad syndrome in the high school athlete. Phys Ther Sport 2011;12:108–16.

131

Immunization

A 25-year-old woman, gravida 1, para 0, at 22 weeks of gestation comes to the emergency department after cutting her hand with a gardening tool. It has been 6 years since the patient's last tetanus shot, and she does not believe she has ever received vaccination for tetanus, diphtheria, and pertussis (Tdap). The wound is irrigated and sutured. The most appropriate next step in her management is to administer

(A) one dose of tetanus and diphtheria vaccine

(B) one dose of Tdap vaccine postpartum

* (C) one dose of Tdap vaccine immediately

(D) three-part series of Tdap vaccine

(E) one dose of tetanus and diphtheria vaccine today and pertussis vaccination postpartum

Tetanus vaccine should be given every 10 years. Tetanus vaccination also should be administered to individuals who present with a wound and who have not been vaccinated within the past 5 years. Pregnant women who have not been previously vaccinated for tetanus should receive a three-part vaccination at 0 months, 1 month, and 6–12 months. One of those doses should include pertussis. If only a tetanus booster is indicated and the patient has not been previously vaccinated for pertussis, Tdap vaccination is warranted.

Pertussis (also known as whooping cough) is a highly contagious respiratory infection. It is caused by the bacteria *Bordetella pertussis*, which attaches to pulmonary cilia and leads to uncontrollable coughing and even respiratory distress. Infants and children are at the highest risk of infection. Newborns can be infected by parents, older siblings, and caregivers. The overall incidence of pertussis has been increasing since 2007. For this reason, the Advisory Committee on Immunization Practices of the the Centers for Disease Control and Prevention has called for widespread vaccination.

Based on the review of safety profiles and the increasing incidence of the disease, the American College of Obstetricians and Gynecologists released new guidelines for pregnant women to be vaccinated against pertussis.

Before these recommendations, women were advised to undergo vaccination during the postpartum period. The 2012 protocol recommends vaccination after 20 weeks of gestation preferably in the third trimester or late second trimester. Vaccination during pregnancy is considered safe and allows for transfer of maternal antibodies to the newborn to increase neonatal protection. In addition, all members of the household and caregivers are recommended to undergo vaccination before having contact with the newborn.

The most common adverse effects of Tdap vaccination are a local reaction and injection site pain. Decreased intervals between vaccinations may increase the occurrence of local reactions. The Advisory Committee on Immunization Practices states that when pertussis vaccination is indicated it should be administered regardless of interval since the last tetanus or diphtheria toxoid vaccine. The Centers for Disease Control and Prevention also recommends that all women be vaccinated for pertussis after 20 weeks of gestation and during every pregnancy. The benefits of protection against pertussis exceed the potential adverse reaction.

The described patient is at 22 weeks of gestation and has not been vaccinated in more than 5 years. The most appropriate treatment is to administer a one-time dose of

Tdap vaccine. To give the patient a one-time dose of tetanus and diphtheria vaccine would cover her for potential tetanus infection, but would not provide her or her neonate with protection against pertussis. To delay vaccination until postpartum would be inappropriate because the patient would be at risk of a potential tetanus infection. In addition, Tdap vaccine has been shown to be safe after 20 weeks of gestation. Similarly, three doses of the vaccine would be unnecessary because the patient has received a prior tetanus vaccination.

General recommendations on immunization—recommendations of the Advisory Committee on Immunization Practices (ACIP). National Center for Immunization and Respiratory Diseases [published erratum appears in MMWR Recomm Rep 2011;60:993]. MMWR Recomm Rep 2011;60:1–64.

Update on immunization and pregnancy: tetanus, diphtheria, and pertussis vaccination. ACOG Committee Opinion No. 566. American College of Obstetricians and Gynecologists. Obstet Gynecol 2013;121:1411–4.

Updated recommendations for use of tetanus toxoid, reduced diphtheria toxoid, and acellular pertussis (Tdap) vaccine in adults aged 65 years and older—Advisory Committee on Immunization Practices (ACIP), 2012. Centers for Disease Control and Prevention [published erratum appears in MMWR Morb Mortal Wkly Rep 2012;61:515]. MMWR Morb Mortal Wkly Rep 2012;61:468–70.

Updated recommendations for use of tetanus toxoid, reduced diphtheria toxoid, and acellular pertussis vaccine (Tdap) in pregnant women—Advisory Committee on Immunization Practices (ACIP), 2012. Centers for Disease Control and Prevention. MMWR Morb Mortal Wkly Rep 2013;62:131–5.

132

Incomplete abortion in the second trimester

A 27-year-old woman comes to the emergency department with vaginal bleeding and pain. Her last menstrual period was 19 weeks ago and she reports delivering fetal tissue at home. Her vital signs are as follows: temperature, 38.9°C (102°F); pulse, 110 beats per minute; and blood pressure, 98 mm Hg systolic and 59 mm Hg diastolic. She is bleeding significantly. On bimanual examination, her uterus is tender and enlarged, the cervix is dilated 2 cm, the hematocrit is 25%, and the white blood cell count is 21,000 cells per microliter. Transvaginal ultrasonography reveals heterogeneous material in the uterus. In addition to initiating broad-spectrum intravenous antibiotics, the best option for her management is

     (A) misoprostol
*   (B) dilation and evacuation
     (C) blood transfusion
     (D) diagnostic laparoscopy

Women with incomplete abortion in the second trimester are at risk of retained products of conception and consequent complications of bleeding and septic abortion. Women who develop septic abortion have symptoms of fever, lower abdominal pain, and vaginal bleeding. Physical examination may show signs of peritonitis with guarding with or without rebound tenderness. Pelvic examination should include inspection for bleeding, pus, products of conception, or dilated cervix. After a surgical abortion, the vagina and cervix should be examined for lacerations and cellulitis. Laboratory testing may reveal leukocytosis and diminished hemoglobin or hematocrit levels. Blood culture results may indicate bacteremia. Ultrasonography is useful to evaluate for retained products of conception, parametrial abscess, or hematoma.

Treatment of septic abortion includes immediate treatment with intravenous broad-spectrum antibiotics after obtaining blood culture samples. It is inappropriate to wait for results of the blood culture before initiation of antibiotics. Because septic abortion is essentially a form of endometritis or pelvic inflammatory disease, the goal is to provide broad-spectrum antibiotics to treat aerobic and anaerobic Gram-negative and Gram-positive bacteria secondary to the polymicrobial nature of the infection.

Antibiotic administration should be initiated at the time of diagnosis of septic abortion. Removal of retained products of conception through manual vacuum aspiration or dilation and evacuation should occur simultaneously with antibiotic administration to remove the source of infection and prevent further complications. Removal of retained products of conception should occur expeditiously through dilation and evacuation regardless of the overall condition of the patient.

Diagnostic laparoscopy may be useful when uterine perforation or pelvic abscess after surgical abortion is of concern. A blood transfusion may be required in cases of severe anemia or active bleeding. In cases in which retained products of conception are observed in a stable patient with no evidence of serious injury, misoprostol may be administered. The described patient is medically unstable as indicated by heavy bleeding, anemia, hypotension, tachycardia, and infection (as demonstrated by fever, physical examination findings, and leukocytosis). Therefore, the most appropriate management would be concurrent immediate administration of intravenous antibiotics and dilation and evacuation.

Milingos DS, Mathur M, Smith NC, Ashok PW. Manual vacuum aspiration: a safe alternative for the surgical management of early pregnancy loss. BJOG 2009;116:1268–71.

Misoprostol for postabortion care. ACOG Committee Opinion No. 427. American College of Obstetricians and Gynecologists. Obstet Gynecol 2009;113:465–8.

Rahangdale L. Infectious complications of pregnancy termination. Clin Obstet Gynecol 2009;52:198–204.

Stubblefield PG, Grimes DA. Septic abortion. N Engl J Med 1994; 331:310–4.

133

End-of-life counseling

All adjuvant treatment was unsuccessful in an 82-year-old woman with a history of recurrent ovarian cancer. She agreed to hospice care after discussion with her oncologist last month but is admitted to the emergency department tonight with new onset nausea and vomiting. She remains mentally alert and can make decisions about her health. A computed tomography result is consistent with a multi-focal bowel obstruction indicative of progressive disease. You are contacted by the patient's daughter who wants everything possible done for her mother's care. The most reasonable next step in her care is

      (A) schedule for surgery
      (B) start total parenteral nutrition
      (C) reassure the daughter outside patient room
*   (D) schedule a meeting with the patient and family

End-of-life counseling care should involve the patient and any relevant members of the family to ensure a consistent message is conveyed to all. Communication is the most important medical care at this time with emphasis on support from the medical community to not "give up on the patient," even as active treatment for her medical condition, such as cancer treatment, has stopped.

It is important that communication between the oncologist and primary care physician be consistent so the patient and family do not get mixed messages regarding end-of-life care options. Studies show that primary care physicians report that they do not have an active role in the management of patients with terminal cancer. However, given their longstanding role in providing health care, they may find themselves in this situation. Such end-of-life care options include palliative therapy and other approaches to help support the patient and family during hospice care.

Ordering unnecessary tests, imaging, or medical interventions not only confuses the patient and family regarding the goals of care, but such procedures may also contribute to increased morbidity and potentially decreased overall survival. Studies that have evaluated total parenteral nutrition have demonstrated that overall survival was decreased for patients who underwent total parenteral nutrition.

A meeting with the patient and her family is important to reestablish the goals of care for those family members who have not been directly involved in the recent developments in the patient's medical condition. Meeting outside the room without the patient would not be appropriate. The clinician should anticipate some component of frustration and anger as family members grieve. He or she should be willing to offer support for the patient and family and be aware of the spiritual and cultural norms of those concerned.

Brard L, Weitzen S, Strubel-Lagan SL, Swamy N, Gordinier ME, Moore RG, et al. The effect of total parenteral nutrition on the survival of terminally ill ovarian cancer patients. Gynecol Oncol 2006;103: 176–80.

Brazil K, Sussman J, Bainbridge D, Whelan T. Who is responsible? The role of family physicians in the provision of supportive cancer care. J Oncol Pract 2010;6:19–24.

Chochinov HM, Kristjanson LJ, Breitbart W, McClement S, Hack TF, Hassard T, et al. Effect of dignity therapy on distress and end-of-life experience in terminally ill patients: a randomised controlled trial. Lancet Oncol 2011;12:753–62.

Keyser EA, Reed BG, Lowery WJ, Sundborg MJ, Winter WE 3rd, Ward JA, et al. Hospice enrollment for terminally ill patients with gynecologic malignancies: impact on outcomes and interventions [published erratum appears in Gynecol Oncol 2011;121:643]. Gynecol Oncol 2010;118:274–7.

Powazki RD, Palcisco C, Richardson M, Stagno SJ. Psychosocial care in advanced cancer. Semin Oncol 2000;27:101-8.

Zapka JG, Carter R, Carter CL, Hennessy W, Kurent JE, DesHarnais S. Care at the end of life: focus on communication and race. J Aging Health 2006;18:791–813.

134

Contraception in a patient with gastric bypass

A 33-year-old woman, gravida 2, para 2, comes to your office for contraception counseling. She underwent gastric bypass surgery 18 months ago and lost 45.4 kg (100 lb). Her current weight is 100.7 kg (222 lb). Her height is 1.75 m (69 in), and she has a body mass index of 32.7 (calculated as weight in kilograms divided by height in meters squared). She has a new partner and is interested in birth control options. She adheres to the weight management program and takes multivitamins daily. Her past medical history is otherwise unremarkable. The most suitable contraceptive option for this patient is

      (A) combined oral contraceptives
      (B) oral progestin-only contraceptives
      (C) transdermal contraceptive patch
      (D) diaphragm and contraceptive foam
*   (E) levonorgestrel IUD

Obesity is an epidemic in the United States; approximately 66% of adults are either overweight or obese. Obesity is associated with reduced fertility primarily related to anovulation or oligoovulation. After weight loss, fertility improves and the need for reliable birth control must be considered. The prevalence of bariatric surgical procedures has increased dramatically over the past decade and the procedure represents the most effective therapy for morbid obesity. Most bariatric procedures are performed in women, including reproductive-aged women and adolescents with morbid obesity.

Evidence is lacking regarding contraceptive effectiveness and safety in women with a history of bariatric surgery. Safety considerations include risk of thromboembolic disorders (especially perioperatively) and potential fracture risk with the use of depot medroxyprogesterone acetate, exacerbated by significant weight loss and nutritional deficiencies. Contraceptive effectiveness may be altered by drug distribution and half-life in women who are overweight or obese and altered absorption after bariatric surgery. The World Health Organization (WHO) identifies obesity as an independent risk factor for contraceptive use but does not specifically address the subject of bariatric surgery. The risks of unintended conception and pregnancy should be weighed against the risks associated with a particular contraceptive.

Because of the lack of data, it is unclear if malabsorptive procedures lead to reduced effectiveness of oral contraceptives. However, it is believed that postoperative complications, including diarrhea and vomiting, may contribute to decreased effectiveness. In addition, conflicting evidence exists regarding the effectiveness of combined oral contraceptives in obese women. Thus, oral formulations may not be the best contraception option for the described patient.

The American College of Obstetricians and Gynecologists suggests that if hormonal contraception is desired in women who have had malabsorptive bariatric surgery, non-oral forms should be considered. As with some oral contraceptive formulations, evidence shows that the contraceptive patch may be less effective in women with a body weight greater than 90 kg (198 lb). Although the described patient has lost considerable weight after undergoing gastric bypass surgery, her weight remains greater than 90 kg (198 lb).

Barrier methods have fewer side effects than hormonal contraception, but these event-based methods are more prone to user-related contraception failure and should be considered only in motivated women. A diaphragm requires appropriate fit and may need to be resized with ongoing weight changes after surgery to ensure correct fit.

No evidence exists of impaired contraceptive efficacy for obese women who use intrauterine contraception assuming appropriate insertion. Either the copper IUD or the levonorgestrel IUD offers an excellent option for women who desire effective contraception. The levonorgestrel IUD also may reduce the risk of endometrial hyperplasia and endometrial cancer, and thus would be the best option for the described patient.

Counseling women regarding their contraceptive options after bariatric surgery can be challenging. As weight loss ensues, fertility is likely to improve. Obese women who undergo bariatric surgery should not conceive for 12–24 months after the procedure so that the fetus is not exposed to a rapid maternal weight loss environment and the patient can achieve her full weight loss goals. Risks of comorbidities, various contraceptive options, and unintended pregnancy must be considered. The drug metabolism for many hormonal methods has not been evaluated in this population.

Bariatric surgery and pregnancy. ACOG Practice Bulletin No. 105. American College of Obstetricians and Gynecologists. Obstet Gynecol 2009;113:1405–13.

Murthy AS. Obesity and contraception: emerging issues. Semin Reprod Med 2010;28:156–63.

Paulen ME, Zapata LB, Cansino C, Curtis KM, Jamieson DJ. Contraceptive use among women with a history of bariatric surgery: a systematic review. Contraception 2010;82:86–94.

U.S. Medical Eligibility Criteria for Contraceptive Use, 2010. Centers for Disease Control and Prevention. MMWR Recomm Rep 2010;59: 1–86.

135–137
Patient safety in the office

For each scenario (135–137), select the patient safety approach (A–E) that would be the most cost-effective in addressing the described problem.

    (A) A fully stocked code cart
    (B) An emergency kit
    (C) Simulation training
    (D) An on-site anesthesiologist
    (E) Personnel certified in advanced cardiac life support available on site

135. E. Your practice is planning to institute office-based endometrial ablation procedures using conscious sedation.

136. C. An elderly patient who recently changed blood pressure medications faints in the waiting room. Transfer to a nearby emergency department does not go smoothly.

137. B. At the end of a loop electrosurgical excision procedure, a patient has a severe vasovagal reaction.

Annually in the United States, approximately 900 million office visits for medical care occur compared with 35 million hospitalizations. Thus, the volume of activity seen in the office certainly warrants that safety-related issues be addressed. Office safety poses different issues compared with safety in the inpatient setting. For example, most office-based or practitioner groups lack the level of safety and quality infrastructure found in a hospital, and fewer regulations govern safety in the office compared with a hospital. On a general basis, patients seen in the office will be less acutely ill compared with hospitalized patients. The three scenarios presented involve some of the issues that office-based practices should address in an effort to maintain a safe environment for their patients.

Scenario 135 involves introduction of a new procedure to the office that involves use of conscious sedation, also known as moderate sedation. Conscious sedation is defined as a drug-induced depression of consciousness during which patients respond purposefully to verbal commands either alone or accompanied by light tactile stimulation. (Reflex withdrawal from a painful stimulus is not considered a purposeful response.) No interventions are required to maintain a patent airway, and spontaneous ventilation is adequate. Cardiovascular function usually is maintained.

The Joint Commission, which certifies not only hospitals but also many ambulatory and office settings, requires that a health care professional who administers conscious sedation be competent to administer the medication. The professional must be able to rescue patients

from deep sedation, manage a compromised airway, and provide adequate oxygenation and ventilation. Such a standard seems reasonable even if an office does not operate under the auspices of the Joint Commission. Training in advanced cardiac life support would meet that requirement. Although having an anesthesiologist present also would suffice, it would not be cost effective in most office settings. Introduction of a new procedure to the office, such as endometrial ablation, should include the same credentialing as the hospital or surgical center procedure to ensure that the health care practitioner has the necessary skills and training to safely perform such procedures in an office setting.

Scenario 136 describes an incident in which the office experiences difficulty in handling an unexpected emergency. Such an incident usually is not experienced in most obstetrician–gynecologists' offices. The possibility that such an episode could occur provides an ideal situation for instituting a simulation drill. The drill should involve professional staff and support staff and will provide a good test on how they manage an emergency. It can help determine how knowledgeable the staff are about the location of emergency medications, how to access additional help, and how to rapidly and safely transfer a patient to a hospital setting, such as an emergency department. The use of a debriefing at the end of the drill often will identify problems and approaches to solve them. In addition to the scenario described, the office team also can conduct simulations of other emergencies, such as seizures or unanticipated bleeding.

For the patient in Scenario 137 who experiences a vasovagal response, an emergency kit that would include medications, such as atropine, would constitute the most cost-effective way to resolve the problem. Such a kit will also provide protocols with suggested dosages and contraindications to use. The protocols also should be part of the practice's policy and procedure manual. A fully stocked code cart would not be necessary; however, the kit must be checked regularly to ensure that perishable supplies have not expired.

The American College of Obstetricians and Gynecologist Presidential Task Force on Patient Safety in the Office Setting was convened to identify patient safety concerns, develop tools, and provide guidance. The task force has published a number of recommendations and the American College of Obstetricians and Gynecologists has established the Safety Certification in Outpatient Excellence program. This latter program assists practices in addressing safety issues in the office with a self-assessment tool and a site visit as part of a certification process.

Erickson TB, Kirkpatrick DH, DeFrancesco MS, Lawrence HC 3rd. Executive summary of the American College of Obstetricians and Gynecologists Presidential Task Force on Patient Safety in the Office Setting: reinvigorating safety in office-based gynecologic surgery. Obstet Gynecol 2010;115:147–51.

Gandhi TK, Lee TH. Patient safety beyond the hospital. N Engl J Med 2010;363:1001–3.

The Joint Commission. Comprehensive accreditation manual for hospitals: CAMH. Oakbrook Terrace (IL): The Commission; 2012.

The Joint Commission. Comprehensive accreditation manual for ambulatory care: CAMAC. Oakbrook Terrace (IL): The Commission; 2012.

Preparing for clinical emergencies in obstetrics and gynecology. ACOG Committee Opinion No. 487. American College of Obstetricians and Gynecologists. Obstet Gynecol 2011;117:1032–4.

Sclafani J, Levy B, Lawrence H, Saraco M, Cain JM. Building a better safety net: taking the safety agenda to office-based women's health [published erratum appears in Obstet Gynecol 2012;120:957]. Obstet Gynecol 2012;120:355–9.

Weiss PM, Swisher E. Patient safety in the ambulatory OB/GYN setting. Clin Obstet Gynecol 2012;55:613–9.

138–142

Cervical cancer screening and diagnosis

For the patient in each clinical scenario (138–142), match the best cervical cancer screening option (A–C).

(A) No screening recommended at this visit
(B) Cervical cytology with or without high-risk human papillomavirus testing.
(C) No further cervical cytology screening recommended.

138. A. A 26-year-old woman with a normal Pap test result 1 year ago

139. A. A 19-year-old woman who initiated vaginal intercourse 2 years ago

140. B. A 35-year-old morbidly obese female with diabetes mellitus and a normal Pap test result 3 years ago

141. C. A 46-year-old woman after total laparoscopic hysterectomy for stage 4 endometriosis with normal Pap test history

142. C. A 72-year-old postmenopausal woman with stress urinary incontinence and normal Pap test history

Current cervical cancer screening guidelines for healthy women recommend initiation of Pap test screening at age 21 years regardless of the time of initiation of sexual intercourse. Women aged 21–29 years should be screened every 3 years unless otherwise indicated because of abnormal Pap test findings or risk factors, such as human immunodeficiency virus (HIV) infection, immunosuppression, in utero diethylstilbestrol exposure, or history of cervical intraepithelial neoplasia (CIN) 2 or CIN 3. Human papillomavirus (HPV) testing should not be used as a screening method in these women. At age 30 years, low-risk women may be screened every 3 years with cytology alone or may increase their screening interval to every 5 years with the addition of a high-risk HPV co-test. Screening may be discontinued at age 65 years if the patient has had at least 3 consecutive negative cytology results or 2 negative co-tests results in the past decade, including one in the preceding 5 years. Women who have undergone hysterectomy for benign indications and who have no prior history of CIN 2 or CIN 3 may likewise discontinue Pap test screening; HPV testing alone is not recommended for routine screening. See Appendix H and Appendix I for complete cervical cancer screening recommendations.

For the patients in Scenario 138 and Scenario 139, the 26-year-old woman with a normal Pap test 1 year ago and the 19-year-old woman who initiated vaginal intercourse 2 years ago, respectively, no screening is needed at this visit. The patient in Scenario 140, the 35-year-old morbidly obese female with diabetes mellitus and a normal Pap test result 3 years ago, should undergo cervical cytology with or without high-risk HPV co-testing. For the patient in Scenario 141, the 46-year-old woman after total laparoscopic hysterectomy for stage 4 endometriosis with normal Pap test history, no further cervical cytologic screening is needed. Similarly, no further screening is needed for the patient in Scenario 142, the 72-year-old postmenopausal woman with stress urinary incontinence and normal Pap test history.

Massad LS, Einstein MH, Huh WK, Katki HA, Kinney WK, Schiffman M, et al. 2012 updated consensus guidelines for the management of abnormal cervical cancer screening tests and cancer precursors. 2012 ASCCP Consensus Guidelines Conference. Obstet Gynecol 2013;121: 829–46.

Saslow D, Solomon D, Lawson HW, Killackey M, Kulasingam SL, Cain JM, et al. American Cancer Society, American Society for Colposcopy and Cervical Pathology, and American Society for Clinical Pathology screening guidelines for the prevention and early detection of cervical cancer. J Low Genit Tract Dis 2012;16:175–204.

U.S. Preventive Services Task Force. Screening for cervical cancer: clinical summary of U.S. Preventive Services Task Force recommendations. Rockville (MD): USPSTF; 2013. Available at: http://www.uspreventiveservicestaskforce.org/uspstf11/cervcancer/cervcancersum.htm. Retrieved June 21, 2013.

143–146

Anterior abdominal wall anatomy and surgical complications

For the patient in each scenario (143–146), choose the likely diagnosis (A–E).

    (A) Injury of a patent urachus
    (B) Laceration of an inferior epigastric artery
    (C) Urinary sepsis
    (D) Ilioinguinal nerve entrapment
    (E) Occult injury of adherent bowel at the umbilicus

143. E. Twelve hours after she has undergone a laparoscopic hysterectomy, a patient with a history of prior cesarean delivery develops fever of 40°C (104°F), emesis, and abdominal rigidity and rebound with hyperactive bowel sounds.

144. A. Two days after laparoscopic Falope ring sterilization, a patient receives the diagnosis of urinary ascites. A midline suprapubic trocar–cannula site was used for ring application.

145. B. After insertion of a 12-mm trocar–cannula in the right lower abdomen, the patient has significant bleeding from the cannula.

146. D. Postoperatively, a patient experiences excruciating pain at the site of a 12-mm right lower quadrant cannula used for uterine morcellation. On examination, severe allodynia is observed to light touch medial to the incision.

Placement of a trocar–cannula to gain access to the abdominal or pelvic cavity presents a number of potential complications, particularly related to the anterior abdominal wall. Health care provider's knowledge of the anatomy at the site and of potential abnormalities of anatomy is crucial to minimize surgical complications.

The umbilicus is the most popular site for peritoneal access with laparoscopy. Its midline location minimizes the risk of abdominal wall vascular injury. It is the site of fusion of fascial layers with no muscle or subcutaneous fat, so it is thinner and more easily penetrated than other abdominal locations. However, in patients with prior surgery, adhesions may be present at the umbilicus. With a midline infraumbilical incision, the incidence of infraumbilical adhesions is approximately 50% and with a prior Pfannenstiel incision the incidence is approximately 25%. Patients who underwent such procedures have an increased risk of bowel injury during umbilical access to the abdominal cavity. If such injury occurs and is not immediately recognized, patients present with symptoms of sepsis and peritonitis, usually within 24 hours (the patient in Scenario 143). Open laparoscopic entry often is recommended in patients with prior laparotomy, but data have not confirmed that this decreases the risk of bowel injury. Also no data show that risk of injury is decreased by any specific type of trocar–cannula. An alternative entry site, such as the left upper quadrant, could be considered.

Knowledge and visualization of the anatomy of the lower and the lateral abdominal wall is crucial to safe placement of multiple trocar–cannulas to allow operative procedures. Midline suprapubic placement is relatively safe because the midline is devoid of major vessels and nerves. Injury to the bladder or to a patent urachus may occur at this site. The risk of bladder injury is greatly decreased by emptying the bladder with a catheter and by visualizing the position of bladder and ensuring that the trocar–cannula is inserted above its location. The patent urachus can readily be identified at the time of laparoscopy. Anomalies of the patent urachus are not always obvious, so it is best to penetrate under direct visualization with care to avoid the patent urachus if a suprapubic trocar–cannula needs to be inserted. A perforated patent urachus at the time of placement may lead to postoperative urinary ascites (the patient in Scenario 144).

Lateral placement of trocar–cannulas requires particular knowledge of the vessels, nerves, fascia, and muscles of the abdominal wall. One of the more frequent and potentially serious complications of lateral port placement is injury to the inferior epigastric vessels. The inferior epigastric vessels originate from the external iliac vessel just before the inguinal ligament and usually can be readily seen laparoscopically. Pressing the abdominal wall with a finger or instrument at the planned entry location usually will demonstrate that the planned insertion site is lateral to the vessels. Tracking at the planned insertion site with a needle also may be helpful. It is important that the trocar–cannula not be deviated medially during insertion because this may direct it to the epigastric vessels even after the maneuvers mentioned earlier. Sometimes, transillumination of the abdominal wall is helpful in identifying the location of the epigastric vessels. In a case of injury, heavy bleeding from the site may occur that is difficult to control (the patient in Scenario 145).

Another important aspect of the lateral lower abdominal wall anatomy is the location of the peripheral nerves, especially the ilioinguinal and iliohypogastric nerves. Transection injury of these nerves with trocar–cannula placement does not usually result in significant clinical sequelae. However, with larger trocar–cannulas that require fascial closure to avoid hernia formation, suture entrapment may occur in up to 5% of patients. Long-term neuropathic pain may occur in such cases if the nerve is not promptly released from the suture entrapment. When entrapment occurs, the patient experiences excruciating pain at the site that is not easily managed with usual postoperative analgesics. Examination reveals severe allodynia to light touch medial to the incision (the patient in Scenario 146).

Brill AI, Nezhat F, Nezhat CH, Nezhat C. The incidence of adhesions after prior laparotomy: a laparoscopic appraisal. Obstet Gynecol 1995;85:269–72.

Kumakiri J, Kikuchi I, Kitade M, Kuroda K, Matsuoka S, Tokita S, et al. Incidence of complications during gynecologic laparoscopic surgery in patients after previous laparotomy. J Minim Invasive Gynecol 2010;17:480–6.

Shin JH, Howard FM. Abdominal wall nerve injury during laparoscopic gynecologic surgery: incidence, risk factors, and treatment outcomes. J Minim Invasive Gynecol 2012;19:448–53.

147–149

Familial cancer syndromes

For the patient in each scenario (147–149), choose the likely diagnosis (A–E).

(A) *BRCA 1* gene mutation
(B) *BRCA 2* gene mutation
(C) Lynch II syndrome
(D) Li–Fraumeni syndrome
(E) Cowden disease

147. B.   A 48-year-old woman with breast cancer has a family history of breast cancer in her mother, her maternal grandmother, and her younger sister

148. A.   A 48-year-old woman with advanced ovarian cancer has a family history of breast cancer in her mother and ovarian cancer in a maternal aunt

149. C.   A 48-year-old woman with ovarian cancer has a family history of colon cancer in her father and brother

Although most types of solid tissue cancer occur sporadically, it is important for the practicing obstetrician–gynecologist to identify patients who might have a familial predisposition to breast, ovarian, endometrial, or colon cancer. If an individual has a genetic mutation for one of the heritable types of cancer, the risk of developing cancer increases approximately 5–10-fold over the general population.

Syndromes associated with inherited breast cancer include breast–ovarian cancer syndrome, Li–Fraumeni syndrome, Cowden disease, and mutated *ataxia telangiectasia* gene. Early onset breast and ovarian cancer occur through mutations in *BRCA 1* and *BRCA 2*. Either mutation confers a lifetime risk of breast cancer of approximately 56–87%. Mutations of *BRCA 1* and *BRCA 2* represent 90% of inherited breast cancer cases. The breast cancer and ovarian cancer that occurs in *BRCA 1* mutation carriers often occur in a younger age group than the same types of cancer in the general population, on average 10 years younger than noncarriers. The *BRCA 2* mutation is associated not only with early onset of breast and ovarian cancer, but also early onset of pancreatic, prostate, and male breast cancer.

It is important to distinguish clinically between *BRCA 1* and *BRCA 2* mutations primarily to define the risk of the associated cancer in *BRCA 2* mutation carriers. Inherited mutations in *BRCA 1* and *BRCA 2* predispose women to early onset ovarian cancer and involve 10% of all ovarian cancer cases. Many identified mutations with variable penetrance exist. The lifetime risk of ovarian cancer is 20–40% in *BRCA 1* mutation carriers and 10–20% in *BRCA 2* mutation carriers. The Ashkenazi Jewish population represents a high-risk group for mutations; such mutations occur in approximately 1 out of 40 individuals. Even with a *BRCA 2* mutation, the risk of ovarian cancer is low in individuals younger than 40 years. Other high-risk populations include Icelanders and some Norwegian and Dutch natives.

Two syndromes predispose to heritable colorectal cancer: 1) familial adenomatous polyposis and 2) hereditary nonpolyposis colorectal cancer (HNPCC), also known as Lynch syndrome. Familial adenomatous polyposis accounts for approximately 1% of colorectal cancer cases, but if a person inherits a mutation in the *adenomatous polyposis coli (APC)* gene, the risk of colon cancer by age 40 years is nearly 100%. Women with mutations in the *APC* gene usually will have greater than 100 adenomatous polyps on colonoscopy. Lynch syndrome or HNPCC accounts for 2–3% of colorectal cancer cases, and is caused by a mutation in a DNA mismatch repair gene. The syndrome is characterized by early onset colon cancer, with 70% of tumors occurring proximal to the splenic flexure; metachronous colon cancer; and extracolonic cancer, including cancer of the endometrium, ovary, small bowel, ureter, and renal pelvis.

The diagnosis of HNPCC is less obvious than familial adenomatous polyposis, and is based on clinical criteria. The revised Amsterdam criteria (Appendix K-1) require that the patient have three relatives with HNPCC-related cancer in two generations, ie, first- and second-degree relatives, with one case of colorectal cancer in an individual younger than 50 years. However, the Amsterdam criteria for the syndrome lack specificity. Only 60% of families who meet the Amsterdam criteria will have a mismatched repair gene mutation. The Amsterdam criteria require that the patient have three relatives with HNPCC-related cancer in two generations, ie, first- and second-degree relatives, with one case of colorectal cancer in an individual younger than 50 years. The revised Bethesda criteria (Appendix K-2) have higher specificity for identification of families with mismatch repair gene mutations. A patient suspected of having an HNPCC-related cancer can have the tumor evaluated for microsatellite instability. If present, the patient should undergo germline mutational analysis. Women with an HNPCC mutation have approximately an 80% lifetime risk of colorectal cancer, 43% risk of endometrial cancer, 19% risk of gastric cancer, 18% risk of urinary tract cancer, and 9% risk of ovarian cancer.

Inherited mutations in *BRCA 1* and *BRCA 2* predispose women to early onset ovarian cancer and comprise 10% of all cases of ovarian cancer. Many identified mutations with variable penetrance exist. The lifetime risk of ovarian cancer is 20–40% with a *BRCA 1* mutation and 10–20% in *BRCA 2* mutation carriers. The Ashkenazi Jewish population represents a high-risk group for mutations, and such mutations occur in approximately 1 out of 40 individuals. Even with a *BRCA* mutation, the risk of ovarian cancer is low in patients younger than 40 years.

It is important to clinically distinguish between *BRCA 1* and *BRCA 2* mutations primarily to define the risk for the associated cancers in *BRCA 2* mutation carriers. The patient in Scenario 147 has breast cancer and a family history of breast cancer, which suggests that *BRCA 2* is the likely diagnosis. The patient in Scenario 148 has advanced ovarian cancer and a family history of breast cancer and ovarian cancer. A lifetime risk of ovarian cancer with *BRCA 1* mutations is higher than the risk with *BRCA 2* mutations, making *BRCA 1* the likely diagnosis. The patient in Scenario 149 has ovarian cancer and a family history of colon cancer, which satisfies the Amsterdam criteria for HNPCC syndrome. Li–Fraumeni syndrome is characterized by soft tissue sarcomas and breast cancer, and is caused by the *p53* mutation. Cowden disease is inherited breast and thyroid cancer, and is caused by the *PTEN* mutation.

Erickson BK, Conner MG, Landen CN Jr. The role of the fallopian tube in the origin of ovarian cancer. Am J Obstet Gynecol 2013;209:409–14.

Guillem JG, Wood WC, Moley JF, Berchuck A, Karlan BY, Mutch DG, et al. ASCO/SSO review of current role of risk-reducing surgery in common hereditary cancer syndromes. ASCO and SSO. J Clin Oncol 2006;24:4642–60.

Lancaster JM, Powell CB, Kauff ND, Cass I, Chen LM, Lu KH, et al. Society of Gynecologic Oncologists Education Committee statement on risk assessment for inherited gynecologic cancer predispositions. Society of Gynecologic Oncologists Education Committee. Gynecol Oncol 2007;107:159–62.

150–153
Tumor markers

For the patient in each scenario (150–153), choose the most appropriate tumor marker (A–F).

(A) CA 125
(B) Alpha-fetoprotein (AFP)
(C) Inhibin B
(D) Follicle-stimulating hormone
(E) Carcinoembryonic antigen (CEA)
(F) Beta subunit of human chorionic gonadotropin (β-hCG)

150. B. A 16-year-old girl with a unilateral solid adnexal mass and regular menses

151. C. A 50-year-old woman with severe abdominal pain, a 14-cm unilateral complex adnexal mass, and hemoperitoneum

152. F. A 28-year-old woman at 5 months postpartum with bilateral 6-cm solid adnexal masses

153. A. A 50-year-old woman with pelvic pressure and a unilateral 8-cm cystic adnexal mass with mural nodularity

Tumor markers are biologic products of malignant tumors that are detectable in the blood. Current recognized tumor markers include enzymes, hormones, receptors, growth factors, and biologic response modifiers. To date, no tumor marker has been identified that has sufficient sensitivity and specificity to serve as a screening test for ovarian cancer in the general population, but these tests can be useful in the management of adnexal masses. Women with adnexal masses should undergo age-appropriate tumor marker testing to aid in the differential diagnosis and management of the mass.

Germ cell types of cancer are found in adolescent women and generally present with a rapidly expanding solid adnexal mass. Histologic subtypes of germ cell tumors are dysgerminoma, immature teratoma, endodermal sinus tumor, and choriocarcinoma. Useful tumor markers for germ cell tumors are AFP, β-hCG, lactate dehydrogenase, and placental alkaline phosphatase.

Stromal tumors of the ovary occur most commonly in the menopausal population. Granulosa cell tumor is the most common histologic subtype and presents with a unilateral solid adnexal mass. Granulosa cell tumors can present as an acute abdomen secondary to intratumoral hemorrhage and capsular rupture. Inhibin is the most useful tumor marker for granulosa cell tumor.

Epithelial ovarian cancer most commonly occurs in the form of bilateral, advanced cystic, and solid ovarian tumors in the perimenopausal or postmenopausal population. The most useful tumor marker for epithelial ovarian cancer is CA 125.

The patient in Scenario 150 has a unilateral solid mass. This is most likely to be a germ cell tumor. Alpha-fetoprotein and β-hCG are markers used in germ cell tumor cases, with endodermal sinus tumor much more common than ovarian choriocarcinoma. Her regular menses also suggests that she is not pregnant and is not at risk of trophoblastic disease. The most useful tumor marker for this patient is AFP.

The patient in Scenario 151 represents a classic presentation for granulosa cell tumor, and inhibin B would be the best marker for her case. The patient in Scenario 152 is a woman with bilateral adnexal masses postpartum. Highest on the differential for the patient in Scenario 152 is gestational trophoblastic disease, making β-hCG the most appropriate tumor marker for her case. The patient in Scenario 153 is a woman with epithelial ovarian cancer, making CA 125 the most appropriate tumor marker for her.

Marker CA 125 is a high molecular weight glycoprotein with an antigenic determinant recognized by the murine monoclonal antibody OC-125. The antigen is produced by coelomic and müllerian epithelium and epithelial ovarian tumors. Approximately 85% of women with epithelial ovarian cancer will have a CA 125 level greater than 21 units/mL. In the prediction of ovarian malignancy in premenopausal women, CA 125 has a sensitivity of approximately 50–74%, a specificity of 26–92%, and positive predictive value of 5–67%. By comparison, in the prediction of ovarian malignancy in postmenopausal women, CA 125 has a sensitivity of approximately 69–87%, a specificity of 81–100%, and a positive predictive value of 73–100%.

The American College of Obstetricians and Gynecologists recommends that a premenopausal woman with an adnexal mass and a CA 125 level greater than 200 units/mL be referred to a gynecologic oncologist. The College also recommends that a postmenopausal woman with an adnexal mass should be referred to a gynecologic oncologist if she has any elevation of CA 125 level.

Alpha-fetoprotein is an oncofetal protein produced by the fetal yolk sac, liver, and upper gastrointestinal tract. Elevations in serum levels of AFP are seen in pregnancy and benign and malignant liver disease. Elevated AFP levels also are seen in 100% patients with endodermal sinus tumors, 62% of those with immature teratomas, and 12% of those with dysgerminomas; AFP is a reliable marker for monitoring response to therapy and detecting recurrence of endodermal sinus tumors.

Inhibin is a heterodimeric glycoprotein with a common α subunit and one of two β subunits to become either inhibin A or inhibin B. Inhibin B levels have been associated with granulosa cell tumors and can be useful in evaluating response to treatment and recurrence. Follicle-stimulating hormone has not been shown to be overexpressed in ovarian cancer.

Carcinoembryonic antigen is an oncofetal protein found in small amounts in the adult colon. Increased levels of CEA are associated with colon and pancreatic carcinomas, benign disease of the liver, gastrointestinal tract, and lung. Elevated levels of CEA also are noted in smokers. Although elevated CEA level is not observed in patients with normal ovaries, CEA level can be elevated in approximately 25–50% of patients with ovarian cancer. However, statistical accuracy is low.

Serum β-hCG is made by the syncytiotrophoblast of pregnancy and is an ideal tumor marker for gestational trophoblastic neoplasia. Nontrophoblastic choriocarcinomas will also produce β-hCG, but these types of ovarian germ cell cancer are rare.

Barakat RR, Berchuck A, Markman M, Randall ME, editors. Principles and practice of gynecologic oncology. 6th ed. Philadelphia (PA): Wolters Kluwer/Lippincott Williams & Wilkins; 2013.

Miller RW, Ueland FR. Risk of malignancy in sonographically confirmed ovarian tumors. Clin Obstet Gynecol 2012;55:52–64.

154–158
Pediatric vaginitis

For the patient in each scenario (154–158), choose the likely diagnosis (A–E).

(A) Lichen sclerosus
(B) Streptococcal vaginitis
(C) Nonspecific vaginitis
(D) Physiologic discharge
(E) Retained foreign object

154. C. A 4-year-old girl has a 6-month history of intermittent dysuria, vulvar pruritus, and vaginal discharge. Physical examination reveals erythema of the vestibule and perineum and a yellow, foul-smelling discharge.

155. E. A 6-year-old girl has a persistent green, foul-smelling discharge often tinged with blood. Physical examination yields a normal result except for a thick green discharge noted at introitus.

156. A. A 7-year-old girl has constant vulvar pruritis, dysuria, and soreness. Physical examination shows skin changes in a figure-of-eight pattern around the vagina and anus with white sharply demarcated skin with fine wrinkles, fissures, and blood blisters.

157. D. A 9-year-old girl has thick, pasty clear to white vaginal discharge. The physical examination reveals Tanner 3 breast development and a normal perineum and introitus.

158. B. A 5-year-old girl has acute onset of green vaginal discharge. She has fever, chills, and ear pain. The physical examination reveals a green discharge and an erythematous introitus.

Nonspecific vaginitis is the most common cause of vaginal discharge in children. The patient in Scenario 154 has all the typical signs and symptoms of nonspecific vaginitis. As the symptoms have waxed and waned over several months, the patient has had dysuria (as the acidic urine touches the inflamed skin), pruritis, and foul-smelling discharge. On physical examination, the vulvar skin often is diffusely erythematous. Evidence of poor hygiene may be present with toilet paper or fecal matter on the perineum along with a malodorous discharge. Children are susceptible to nonspecific vaginitis because of anatomic, physiologic, and behavioral factors. In young children, the vulva is unprotected by pubic hair or labial fat pads. Based on the child's position, the labia minora may be opened, which allows exposure to pathogens. The combination of independent toileting, poor hygiene, and the close proximity of the anus and vulva present challenges. Improved hygiene, sitz baths, and use of inert barriers (such as petroleum jelly or diaper rash ointments) are the mainstay for improvement in symptomatology.

The patient in Scenario 155 presents with signs and symptoms that suggest a retained foreign object, most commonly toilet paper. Unlike the intermittent discharge associated with nonspecific vaginitis, this patient is experiencing a persistent discharge. The green color of the

discharge and the presence of blood raise the suspicion for a foreign object. Visualization and possibly irrigation of the vagina, either in the office or with vaginoscopy, are indicated. If a foreign object is identified and removed, the symptoms will resolve.

The patient in Scenario 156 has signs and symptoms consistent with lichen sclerosus. The combination of itching, dysuria, and soreness or pain is typical. Often, such patients are treated for urinary tract infections based on symptoms, but urine cultures will be sterile. Skin changes typically present in an hourglass or figure-of-eight configuration and involve the periclitoral area, labia, perineal body, and anus. Typically, the vagina is spared. Thin, white, and wrinkled skin and cracks, fissures, grooves, and "blood blisters" may be present. The appearance of the area sometimes raises concerns regarding genital trauma or abuse. Therapy should be directed toward the control of symptoms and preservation of normal anatomy. The use of sitz baths and topical corticosteroid ointments of mild to moderate potency along with avoidance of irritants will be beneficial. Pediatric lichen sclerosus improves with puberty.

The patient in Scenario 157 has physiologic vaginal discharge, secondary to the onset of puberty and increased estradiol production. Although some patients find the discharge irritating and worrisome, reassurance and consistent hygiene are the only required interventions. Supporting this diagnosis are the patient's age, thelarche, the color and nature of the discharge, and normal appearance of the vulvar skin and vaginal introitus.

The patient in Scenario 158 has streptococcal vaginitis, most likely secondary to autoinoculation. The fever, chills, and ear pain suggest an acute otitis media as the origin. Unlike the patient with nonspecific vaginitis, the erythema is limited to the introitus; this is typical for streptococcal vaginitis, as is the green discharge. A vaginal swab test would be indicated for diagnostic purposes and antibiotics to treat the offending organism. If symptoms resolve after antibiotic therapy, repeat vaginal culture for test of cure is not indicated.

Altchek A. Pediatric vulvovaginitis. J Reprod Med 1984;29:359–75.

Kass-Wolff JH, Wilson EE. Pediatric gynecology: assessment strategies and common problems. Semin Reprod Med 2003;21:329–38.

Koumantakis EE, Hassan EA, Deligeoroglou EK, Creatsas GK. Vulvovaginitis during childhood and adolescence. J Pediatr Adolesc Gynecol 1997;10:39–43.

Smith YR, Quint EH. Clobetasol propionate in the treatment of premenarchal vulvar lichen sclerosus. Obstet Gynecol 2001;98:588–91.

159–162

Human papillomavirus vaccination

For the patient in each scenario (159–162), indicate the appropriate human papillomavirus (HPV) vaccination (A–C).

   (A) Human papillomavirus vaccine not recommended
   (B) Full (three-dose) course of the HPV vaccine
   (C) One dose of HPV vaccine

159. A.   A 42-year-old woman with a new sexual partner and a history of normal Pap test results

160. B.   A 12-year-old girl who is not sexually active

161. B.   A 14-year-old boy who is sexually active with a history of two lifetime partners

162. C.   A 19-year-old woman who received the scheduled first two doses of HPV vaccination 2 years ago

Human papillomavirus is a causal agent for cervical cancer and other types of anogenital tract cancer. Two types of HPV vaccine are available: 1) the bivalent vaccine for HPV serotype 16 and HPV serotype 18 and 2) the quadrivalent vaccine for HPV serotype 6, HPV serotype 11, HPV serotype 16, and HPV serotype 18. The original target population for HPV vaccination in the United States was young women. However, evidence exists that HPV vaccination reduces risk of genital warts, anal HPV infection, and dysplasia in men. The predominant HPV serotypes associated with risk of other types of anogenital tract cancer and oropharyngeal cancer are serotype 16 and serotype 18. Current recommendations support vaccination of girls and boys aged 11–12 years for protection against HPV infection with the quadrivalent vaccine. The bivalent vaccine is approved for use in girls only.

Individuals may be vaccinated as early as at age 9 years and up to age 26 years. Although less effective, individuals who have already engaged in sexual activity or have received the diagnosis of HPV infection may still be vaccinated. Individuals whose three-dose series is incomplete may receive the remaining doses without restarting the series. At this time, insufficient data are available to support the efficacy of the vaccine in preventing HPV-related disease in individuals older than 26 years.

For the patient in Scenario 159, the 42-year-old woman with a new sexual partner and no evidence of prior HPV infection, vaccination would not be recommended because she is older than 26 years. For the patients in Scenario 160 and Scenario 161, the 12-year-old girl and 14-year-old boy, the full three-dose vaccination series should be recommended because they are in the target age range regardless of any history of sexual activity. The patient in Scenario 162, the 19-year woman whose three-part vaccination series is incomplete, should receive the last dose of HPV vaccine despite the delayed time interval since her second dose.

Elbasha EH, Dasbach EJ. Impact of vaccinating boys and men against HPV in the United States. Vaccine 2010;28:6858–67.

Giuliano AR, Palefsky JM, Goldstone S, Moreira ED Jr, Penny ME, Aranda C, et al. Efficacy of quadrivalent HPV vaccine against HPV Infection and disease in males. N Engl J Med 2011;364:401–11.

Human papillomavirus vaccination. Committee Opinion No. 467. American College of Obstetricians and Gynecologists. Obstet Gynecol 2010;116:800–3.

Palefsky JM, Giuliano AR, Goldstone S, Moreira ED Jr, Aranda C, Jessen H, et al. HPV vaccine against anal HPV infection and anal intraepithelial neoplasia. N Engl J Med 2011;365:1576–85.

163–165
Vulvar vestibulitis

For the patient in each scenario (163–165), choose the best treatment option (A–E).

(A) Pelvic floor physical therapy
(B) Vestibulectomy
(C) Trigger point injection
(D) Oral anticonvulsant
(E) Local corticosteroid

163. B. A 27-year-old nulligravid woman has localized vestibulodynia that has not responded to previous therapy that included oral tricyclic antidepressant, oral antiepileptic, topical lidocaine, compounded topical antiepileptic, and cognitive behavioral counseling.

164. A. A 20-year-old nulligravid woman with vaginismus requests treatment to facilitate tampon use for swimming during menstruation. Ultimately, she desires vaginal intercourse.

165. D. A 51-year-old nulligravid woman has generalized vulvodynia unresponsive to local skin care guidelines, trial of topical anesthetic, and prescribed cognitive behavioral counseling. Also, she notes night sweats and sleep disruption.

Sexual pain is an underrecognized and poorly treated constellation of disorders that significantly affects women and their partners. Sexual pain disorders are heterogeneous and include dyspareunia, vaginismus, vulvodynia, vestibulodynia, and noncoital sexual pain disorder. The lack of standard criteria and the overlapping descriptors for sexual pain disorders negatively affect our understanding of the pathophysiology. However, evidence suggests vulvar pain syndromes represent heterogeneous disorders because of multifactorial processes in which the end result is neuropathically mediated pain. Often, the management is based on anecdotal experience of other neuropathic pain disorders (eg, fibromyalgia, migraines, diabetic neuropathy, and postherpetic neuropathy), descriptive studies, and reports of expert committees.

Vulvodynia, including generalized and localized vestibulodynia, will affect approximately 15–20% of U.S. women during their lifetime. Conflicting evidence exists about whether generalized and localized vulvar pain syndromes represent two distinct disorders or a single disorder. Vulvodynia is a diagnosis of exclusion. Thus, careful history and evaluation should be initiated to exclude an identifiable etiology. Multiple treatments have been used, including vulvar care measures; topical, oral, and injectable medications; biofeedback; physical therapy; dietary modification; cognitive behavioral therapy; sexual counseling; and surgery. Additional treatments employed include acupuncture, hypnotherapy, nitroglycerin, and botulinum toxin.

It is important to note that only estrogen therapy is approved by the U.S. Food and Drug Administration (FDA) for dyspareunia and other vulvar pain syndromes. Commonly prescribed topical medications include local anesthetics, estrogen cream, and tricyclic antidepressants or anticonvulsants compounded into topical form. Oral therapies targeted toward neuropathic pain are commonly prescribed and include tricyclic antidepressants and anticonvulsants. Trigger point injections have been successful for some patients with localized vulvodynia. Topical steroids generally do not help patients with vulvodynia.

Biofeedback and physical therapy are used in the treatment of localized and generalized vulvodynia. Vestibulectomy has been helpful for many patients with localized pain that has not responded to previous treatments. Patients should be evaluated for vaginismus and, if present, treated before vestibulectomy.

The patient in Scenario 163 is a woman with refractory localized vestibulodynia. She has tried multiple therapies with inadequate pain resolution. Vestibulectomy should be considered. The procedure involves excision of the vulvar vestibule and is successful in up to 85% of women. Although vestibulectomy has the highest success rate for localized vestibulodynia, it is generally reserved until other (noninvasive) treatments have proved inadequate.

The patient in Scenario 164 is a young woman with vaginismus. She is motivated and will likely respond well with physical therapy and gradual desensitization.

The patient in Scenario 165 is a menopausal woman with generalized vulvodynia. A systemic anticonvulsant medication may address her neuropathic pain and vasomotor symptoms.

Andrews JC. Vulvodynia interventions—systematic review and evidence grading. Obstet Gynecol Sur 2011;66:299–315.

Boardman LA, Stockdale CK. Sexual pain. Clin Obstet Gynecol 2009;52:682–90.

Haefner HK, Collins ME, Davis GD, Edwards L, Foster DC, Hartmann ED, et al. The vulvodynia guideline. J Low Genit Tract Dis 2005;9: 40–51.

Tommola P, Unkila-Kallio L, Paavonen J. Surgical treatment of vulvar vestibulitis: a review. Acta Obstet Gynecol Scand 2010;89:1385–95.

Appendix A
Normal Values for Laboratory Tests*

Analyte	Conventional Units
Alanine aminotransferase, serum	8–35 units/L
Alkaline phosphatase, serum	15–120 units/L
Menopause	
Amniotic fluid index	3–30 mL
Amylase	20–300 units/L
Greater than 60 years old	21–160 units/L
Aspartate aminotransferase, serum	15–30 units/L
Bicarbonate	
Arterial blood	21–27 mEq/L
Venous plasma	23–29 mEq/L
Bilirubin	
Total	0.3–1 mg/dL
Conjugated (direct)	0.1–0.4 mg/dL
Newborn, total	1–10 mg/dL
Blood gases (arterial) and pulmonary function	
Base deficit	Less than 3 mEq/L
Base excess, arterial blood, calculated	–2 mEq/L to +3 mEq/L
Forced expiratory volume (FEV_1)	3.5–5 L
	Greater than 80% of predicted value
Forced vital capacity	3.5–5 L
Oxygen saturation (So_2)	95% or higher
Pao_2	80 mm Hg or more
Pco_2	35–45 mm Hg
Po_2	80–95 mm Hg
Peak expiratory flow rate	Approximately 450 L/min
pH	7.35–7.45
Pvo_2	30–40 mm Hg
Blood urea nitrogen	
Adult	7–18 mg/dL
Greater than 60 years old	8–20 mg/dL
CA 125	Less than 34 units/mL
Calcium	
Ionized	4.6–5.3 mg/dL
Serum	8.6–10 mg/dL
Chloride	98–106 mEq/L
Cholesterol	
Total	
Desirable	140–199 mg/dL
Borderline high	200–239 mg/dL
High	240 mg/dL or more
High-density lipoprotein	40–85 mg/dL
Low-density lipoprotein	
Desirable	Less than 130 mg/dL
Borderline high	140–159 mg/dL
High	Greater than 160 mg/dL
Total cholesterol-to-high-density lipoprotein ratio	
Desirable	Less than 3
Borderline high	3–5
High	Greater than 5
Triglycerides	
20 years and older	Less than 150 mg/dL
Less than 20 years old	35–135 mg/dL

*Values listed are specific for adults or women, if relevant, unless otherwise differentiated.

(continued)

Normal Values for Laboratory Tests* (*continued*)

Analyte	Conventional Units
Cortisol, plasma	
8 AM	5–23 micrograms/dL
4 PM	3–15 micrograms/dL
10 PM	Less than 50% of 8 AM value
Creatinine, serum	0.6–1.2 mg/dL
Dehydroepiandrosterone sulfate	60–340 micrograms/dL
Erythrocyte	
Count	3,800,000–5,100,000/mm³
Distribution width	10 plus or minus 1.5%
Sedimentation rate	
Wintrobe method	0–15 mm/hour
Westergren method	0–20 mm/hour
Estradiol-17β	
Follicular phase	30–100 pg/mL
Ovulatory phase	200–400 pg/mL
Luteal phase	50–140 pg/mL
Child	0.8–56 pg/mL
Ferritin, serum	18–160 micrograms/L
Fibrinogen	150–400 mg/dL
Follicle-stimulating hormone	
Premenopause	2.8–17.2 mIU/mL
Midcycle peak	15–35 mIU/mL
Postmenopause	24–170 mIU/mL
Child	0.1–7 mIU/mL
Glucose	
Fasting	70–105 mg/dL
2-hour postprandial	Less than 120 mg/dL
Random blood	65–110 mg/dL
Hematocrit	36–48%
Hemoglobin	12–16 g/dL
Fetal	Less than 1% of total
Hemoglobin A$_{1c}$ (nondiabetic)	5.5–8.5%
Human chorionic gonadotropin	0–5 mIU/mL
Pregnant	Greater than 5 mIU/mL
17α-Hydroxyprogesterone	
Adult	50–300 ng/dL
Child	32–63 ng/dL
25-Hydroxyvitamin D	10–55 ng/mL
International Normalized Ratio	Greater than 1
Prothrombin time	10–13 seconds
Iron, serum	65–165 micrograms/dL
Binding capacity total	240–450 micrograms/dL
Lactate dehydrogenase, serum	313–618 units/L
Leukocytes	
Total	5,000–10,000/cubic micrometer
Differential counts	
Basophils	0–1%
Eosinophils	1–3%
Lymphocytes	25–33%
Monocytes	3–7%
Myelocytes	0%
Band neutrophils	3–5%
Segmented neutrophils	54–62%

*Values listed are specific for adults or women, if relevant, unless otherwise differentiated.

(*continued*)

Normal Values for Laboratory Tests* (*continued*)

Analyte	Conventional Units
Lipase	
60 years or younger	10–140 units/L
Older than 60 years	18–180 units/L
Luteinizing hormone	
Follicular phase	3.6–29.4 mIU/mL
Midcycle peak	58–204 mIU/mL
Postmenopause	35–129 mIU/mL
Child	0.5–10.3 mIU/mL
Magnesium	
Adult	1.6–2.6 mg/dL
Child	1.7–2.1 mg/dL
Newborn	1.5–2.2 mg/dL
Mean corpuscular	
mCH Hemoglobin	27–33 pg
mCHC Hemoglobin concentration	33–37 g/dL
mCV Volume	80–100 cubic micrometers
Partial thromboplastin time, activated	21–35 seconds
Phosphate, inorganic phosphorus	2.5–4.5 mg/dL
Platelet count	140–400 × 10^3 per microliter
Potassium	3.5–5.3 mEq/L
Progesterone	
Follicular phase	Less than 3 ng/mL
Luteal phase	2.5–28 ng/mL
On oral contraceptives	0.1–0.3 ng/mL
Secretory phase	5–30 ng/mL
Older than 60 years	0–0.2 ng/mL
First trimester	9–47 ng/mL
Second trimester	16.8–146 ng/mL
Third trimester	55–255 ng/mL
Prolactin	0–17 ng/mL
Pregnant	34–386 ng/mL by 3rd trimester
Prothrombin time	10–13 seconds
Reticulocyte count	Absolute: 25,000–85,000 cubic micrometers
	0.5–2.5% of erythrocytes
Semen analysis, spermatozoa	
Antisperm antibody	% of sperm binding by immunobead technique; greater than 20% = decreased fertility
Count	Greater than or equal to 20 million/mL
Motility	Greater than or equal to 50%
Morphology	Greater than or equal to 15% normal forms
Sodium	135–145 mEq/L
Testosterone, female	
Total	6–86 ng/dL
Pregnant	3–4 × normal
Postmenopause	One half of normal
Free	
20–29 years old	0.9–3.2 pg/mL
30–39 years old	0.8–3 pg/mL
40–49 years old	0.6–2.5 pg/mL
50–59 years old	0.3–2.7 pg/mL
Older than 60 years	0.2–2.2 pg/mL
Thyroid-stimulating hormone	0.2–3 microunits/mL
Thyroxine	
Serum free	0.9–2.3 ng/dL
Total	1.5–4.5 micrograms/dL

*Values listed are specific for adults or women, if relevant, unless otherwise differentiated.

(*continued*)

Normal Values for Laboratory Tests* (*continued*)

Analyte	Conventional Units
Triiodothyronine uptake	25–35%
Urea nitrogen, blood	
Adult	7–18 mg/dL
Older than 60 years	8–20 mg/dL
Uric acid, serum	2.6–6 mg/dL
Urinalysis	
Epithelial cells	0–3/HPF
Erythrocytes	0–3/HPF
Leukocytes	0–4/HPF
Protein (albumin)	
Qualitative	None detected
Quantitative	10–100 mg/24 hours
Pregnancy	Less than 300 mg/24 hours
Urine specific gravity	
Normal hydration and volume	1.005–1.03
Concentrated	1.025–1.03
Diluted	1.001–1.01

*Values listed are specific for adults or women, if relevant, unless otherwise differentiated.

Appendix B

Categories of Medical Eligibility Criteria for Contraceptive Use

1. A condition for which there is no restriction for the use of the contraceptive method
2. A condition for which the advantages of using the method generally outweigh the theoretical or proven risks
3. A condition for which the theoretical or proven risks usually outweigh the advantages of using the method
4. A condition that represents an unacceptable health risk if the contraceptive method is used

Adapted from U.S. Medical Eligibility Criteria for Contraceptive Use, 2010. Centers for Disease Control and Prevention. MMWR Recomm Rep 2010;59 (RR-4):1–86.

Appendix C

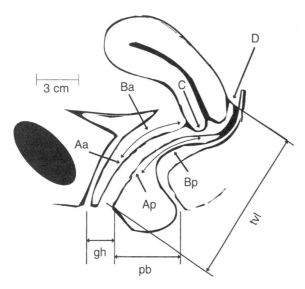

FIG. C-1. Six sites (points Aa, Ba, C, D, Bp, and Ap), genital hiatus (gh), perineal body (pb), and total vaginal length (tvl) used for pelvic organ prolapse quantification (POP-Q) score. (Bump RC, Mattiasson A, Bø K, Brubaker LP, DeLancey JO, Klarskov P, et al. The standardization of terminology of female pelvic organ prolapse and pelvic floor dysfunction. Am J Obstet Gynecol 1996;175: 10–7. Copyright 1996 by Elsevier.)

Anterior wall **Aa**	Anterior wall **Ba**	Cervix or cuff **C**
Genital hiatus **gh**	Perineal body **pb**	Total vaginal length **tvl**
Posterior wall **Ap**	Posterior wall **Bp**	Posterior fornix **D**

FIG. C-2. Three-by-three grid for recording quantitative description of pelvic organ support. (Bump RC, Mattiasson A, Bø K, Brubaker LP, DeLancey JO, Klarskov P, et al. The standardization of terminology of female pelvic organ prolapse and pelvic floor dysfunction. Am J Obstet Gynecol 1996;175:10–7. Copyright 1996 by Elsevier.)

Appendix D

World Health Organization Fracture Risk Assessment Tool (FRAX).

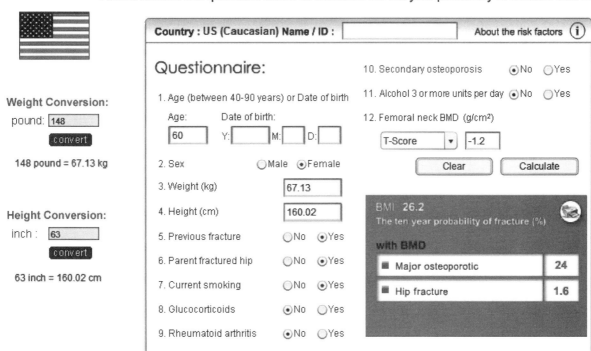

World Health Organization Collaborating Centre for Metabolic Bone Diseases. WHO Fracture Risk Assessment Tool (FRAX). Sheffield, United Kingdom: University of Sheffield; 2013. Available at: http://www.shef.ac.uk/FRAX/tool.aspx?country=9. Retrieved October 2, 2013.

Appendix E

European Society for Gynaecologic Endoscopy Classification of Submucosal Myomas

---

Type 0
Entirely within endometrial cavity
No myometrial extension (pedunculated)

Type I
Less than 50% myometrial extension (sessile)
Less than 90-degree angle of myoma surface to uterine wall

Type II
50% or greater myometrial extension (sessile)
90-degree or greater angle of myoma surface to uterine wall

AAGL practice report: practice guidelines for the diagnosis and management of submucous leiomyomas. American Association of Gynecologic Laparoscopists (AAGL): Advancing Minimally Invasive Gynecology Worldwide. Reprinted from Journal of Minimally Invasive Gynecology, Vol. 19, Pages 152–71, Copyright 2012, with permission from Elsevier.

Appendix F

Venous Thromboembolism Risk Factors

- Surgery
- Trauma (major trauma or lower extremity injury)
- Immobility and lower extremity paresis
- Malignancy
- Cancer (active or occult)
- Cancer therapy (hormonal, chemotherapy, angiogenesis inhibitors, or radiotherapy)
- Venous compression (tumor, hematoma, or arterial normality)
- Previous venous thromboembolism
- Increasing age
- Pregnancy and the postpartum period
- Estrogen-containing oral contraception or hormone therapy
- Selective estrogen receptor modulators
- Erythropoiesis-stimulating agents
- Acute medical illness
- Inflammatory bowel disease
- Nephrotic syndrome
- Myeloproliferative disorders
- Paroxysmal nocturnal hemoglobinuria
- Obesity
- Central venous catheterization
- Inherited or acquired thrombophilia

Geerts WH, Bergqvist D, Pineo GF, Heit JA, Samama CM, Lassen MR, et al. Prevention of venous thromboembolism: American College of Chest Physicians Evidence-Based Clinical Practice Guidelines (8th Edition). American College of Chest Physicians. Chest 2008;133:381S–453S. Reproduced with permission from the American College of Chest Physicians.

Appendix G

Considerations for the Gynecologic Surgeon in Choosing Which Antibiotic Agents to Use in the Preoperative Period

The antibiotic agent selected must fulfill the following criteria:

- Be of low toxicity
- Have an established safety record
- Not be routinely used for the treatment of serious infections
- Have a spectrum of activity that includes the microorganisms most likely to cause infection
- Reach a useful concentration in relevant tissues during the procedure
- Be administered for a short duration
- Be administered in a manner that will ensure it is present in surgical sites at the time of the incision

Appendix H

Summary of Recommendations for Screening for Cervical Cancer

Population	Recommended screening method*	Management of screening results	Comments
Younger than 21 years	No screening	Not applicable	HPV testing should not be used for screening or management of patients with ASC-US in this age group
Aged 21–29 years	Cytology alone every 3 years	HPV-positive ASC-US[†] results or cytology results of LSIL or more severe: refer to ASCCP guidelines Negative cytology or HPV-negative ASC-US[†] results: rescreen with cytology in 3 years.	Testing for HPV should not be used for screening in this age group
Aged 30–65 years	HPV and cytology co-testing every 5 years (preferred) Cytology alone every 3 years (acceptable)	HPV-positive ASC-US[†] or cytology results of LSIL or more severe: refer to ASCCP guidelines Human papillomavirus-positive and cytology negative results: • Option 1—12-month follow-up with co-testing • Option 2—Test for HPV-16 or HPV-16/18 genotypes If HPV-16 or HPV-16/18-positive results: refer for colposcopy. If HPV-16 or HPV-16/18-negative results: 12-month follow-up with cotesting in 5 years is recommended Human papillomavirus-positive ASC-US[†] or cytology results of LSIL or more severe: refer to ASCCP guidelines Cytology negative or HPV-negative ASC-US[†] results: rescreen with cytology in 3 years	
Older than 65 years	No screening after adequate negative prior screening	Not applicable	Women with a history of CIN 2 or a more severe diagnosis should continue routine screening for at least 20 years
After hysterectomy	No screening	Not applicable	Applies to women without a cervix and without a history of CIN 2 or a more severe diagnosis in the past 20 years or cervical cancer ever
HPV vaccinated	Follow age-specific recommendations (same as unvaccinated women)		

Abbreviations: ASCCP indicates American Society for Colposcopy and Cervical Pathology; ASC-US, atypical squamous cells of undertermined significance; CIN 2, cervical intraepithelial neoplasia grade 2; HPV, human papillomavirus; LSIL, low grade squamous intraepithelial lesion.

*Women should not be screened annually at any age by any method.

[†]Cytology result of ASC-US with secondary HPV testing for management decisions

Saslow D, Solomon D, Lawson HW, Killackey M, Kulasingam SL, Cain J, et al. American Cancer Society, American Society for Colposcopy and Cervical Pathology, and American Society for Clinical Pathology screening guidelines for the prevention and early detection of cervical cancer. American Cancer Society, American Society for Colposcopy and Cervical Pathology, and American Society for Clinical Pathology. Am J Clin Pathol 2012;137:516–42.

Appendix I

Essential Changes From Prior Management Guidelines for Cervical Cancer Screening*

- Cytology reported as negative but lacking endocervical cells can be managed without early repeat.

- Cervical intraepithelial neoplasia (CIN) 1 on endocervical curettage should be managed as CIN 1, not as a positive endocervical curettage result.

- Cytology reported as unsatisfactory requires repeat even if the result is negative for human papillomavirus (HPV) negative.

- Genotyping triages HPV-positive women with HPV type 16 or type 18 to earlier colposcopy only after negative cytology result; colposcopy is indicated for all women with HPV and atypical squamous cells of undetermined significance (ASC-US), regardless of genotyping result.

- For ASC-US cytology result, immediate colposcopy is not an option. The serial cytology option for ASC-US cytology result incorporates cytology at 12 months, not 6 months and 12 months, and then if result is negative, cytology every 3 years.

- An HPV-negative and ASC-US-positive result should be followed with cotesting at 3 years rather than 5 years.

- An HPV-negative and ASC-US-positive result is insufficient to allow exit from screening at age 65 years.

- The pathway to long-term follow-up of treated and untreated CIN higher than grade 2 is increasingly clearly defined by incorporating co-testing.

- Many strategies incorporate co-testing to reduce follow-up visits. Pap-test only strategies are now limited to use in women younger than age 30 years, but co-testing is expanded even to women younger than 30 years in some circumstances. Women aged 21–24 years are managed conservatively.

*Prior management guidelines were published in Wright TC Jr, Massad LS, Dunton CJ, Spitzer M, Wilkinson EJ, Solomon D; 2006 ASCCP-Sponsored Consensus Conference. 2006 consensus guidelines for the management of women with abnormal cervical screening tests. J Low Genit Tract Dis 2007;11:201–22. Prior guidelines not changed were retained.

Massad LS, Einstein MH, Huh WK, Katki HA, Kinney WK, Schiffman M, et al. 2012 updated consensus guidelines for the management of abnormal cervical cancer screening tests and cancer precursors. 2012 ASCCP Consensus Guidelines Conference. Obstet Gynecol 2013;121:829–46.

Appendix J

Recommended Parenteral Regimen for Antibiotic Management of Pelvic Inflammatory Disease

Cefotetan, 2 g intravenously, every 12 hours, or

Cefoxitin, 2 g intravenously, every 6 hours, plus

Doxycycline, 100 mg orally or intravenously, every 12 hours

Workowski KA, Berman S. Sexually transmitted diseases treatment guidelines, 2010. Centers for Disease Control and Prevention [published erratum appears in MMWR Morb Mortal Wkly Rep 2011;60:18]. MMWR Recomm Rep 2010;59:1–110.

Appendix K-1

Revised Amsterdam Criteria (Amsterdam II) for Hereditary Nonpolyposis Colorectal Cancer-Associated Cancer

- At least three relatives with hereditary nonpolyposis colorectal cancer (HNPCC)-associated cancer
- One relative with HNPCC-associated cancer should be a first-degree relative of other two relatives
- At least two successive generations affected
- At least one relative received the diagnosis of HNPCC-associated cancer before age 50 years
- Familial adenomatous polyposis excluded
- Tumors should be verified by pathologic examination

Modified from Bonis PA, Trikalinos TA, Chung M, Chew P, Ip S, DeVine D, et al. Hereditary ponpolyposis colorectal cancer: diagnostic strategies and their implications. Evidence Report/Technology Assessment No. 150 (Prepared by Tufts–New England Medical Center Evidence-based Practice Center under Contract No. 290-02-0022). AHRQ Publication No. 07-E008. Rockville, MD: Agency for Healthcare Research and Quality; May 2007.

Appendix K-2

Revised Bethesda Criteria for Hereditary Nonpolyposis Colorectal Cancer-Associated Cancer

- Colorectal cancer diagnosed in a patient before age 50 years
- Presence of synchronous, metachronous colorectal, or other hereditary nonpolyposis colorectal cancer (HNPCC)-associated tumors regardless of age
- Colorectal cancer with the microsatellite instability-high-like histology* diagnosed in a patient before age 60 years
- Colorectal cancer diagnosed in a patient with one or more first-degree relatives with an HNPCC-related tumor, with one type of cancer diagnosed before age 50 years
- Colorectal cancer in a patient with two or more first or second-degree relatives with HNPCC-related tumors, regardless of age

*Microsatellite instability-high refers to changes in two or more of the five National Cancer Institute-recommended panels of microsatellite markers.

Modified from Bonis PA, Trikalinos TA, Chung M, Chew P, Ip S, DeVine D, et al. Hereditary ponpolyposis colorectal cancer: diagnostic strategies and their implications. Evidence Report/Technology Assessment No. 150 (Prepared by Tufts–New England Medical Center Evidence-based Practice Center under Contract No. 290-02-0022). AHRQ Publication No. 07-E008. Rockville, MD: Agency for Healthcare Research and Quality; May 2007.

Index

A

Abdominal surgery, 101
Abdominal wall, 143–146
Ablation, 90
Abnormal uterine bleeding
  in adolescent, 4, 81
  chronic, 40
  in reproductive-aged woman, 40
Abortion(s)
  Centers for Disease Control and Prevention
    on, 124
  incomplete, 132
  septic, 132
Abscess(es)
  breast, 87
  pelvic, 66
ACC/AHA. *See* American College of
  Cardiology/American Heart Association
Acute pulmonary embolus, 96
Adenocarcinoma in situ (AIS)
  with positive margins, 14
  versus cervical intraepithelial neoplasia,
    14
Adnexal masses, 150–153
  in older reproductive-aged woman, 25
  in postmenopausal woman, 95
Adolescent(s)
  abnormal uterine bleeding in, 4, 81
  dysmenorrhea in, 81, 116
  endometriosis in, 81
  ovarian mass in, 2
Advisory Committee on Immunization
  Practices, 131
AFP. *See* Alpha-fetoprotein
AGC–NOS. *See* Atypical glandular cells, not
  otherwise specified
AIS. *See* Adenocarcinoma in situ
Allen stirrups, 8
Allergy, 67
Alpha-fetoprotein (AFP), 150–153
American Cancer Society
  on ovarian cancer screening, 59
  revised cervical cancer screening guidelines
    of, 71
  on vaginal cancer screening after hysterec-
    tomy, 68
American College of Cardiology/American
  Heart Association (ACC/AHA)
  Guidelines on Perioperative Cardiac
    Evaluation and Care for Noncardiac
    Surgery, 38
  stepwise approach to perioperative cardiac
    assessment, 38
American College of Obstetricians and
  Gynecologists
  on adnexal mass, 150–153
  Committee on Patient Safety and Quality
    Improvement of, 23
  on contraception, 134
  on motivational interviewing for changes in
    behavior, 22
  on newly diagnosed pelvic mass in post-
    menopausal woman, 95
  on pregnant women with active recurrent
    genital herpes, 107

American College of Obstetricians and
  Gynecologists (*continued*)
  Presidential Task Force on Patient Safety in
    the Office Setting of, 135–137
  Safety Certification in Outpatient Excellence
    program of, 135–137
  statement on the ethical importance of
    informed consent, 51
  on vaccination in pregnant women, 131
  on vaginal cancer screening after hysterec-
    tomy, 68
  on women with *BRCA* mutations, 117
American Society for Colposcopy and Cervical
  Pathology
  on cervical cancer prevention and early
    detection, 94
  revised cervical cancer screening guidelines
    of, 71
Androgen therapy, 58
Anovulation
  in adolescent, 81
  causes of, 40
Anovulatory bleeding, 40
Anterior abdominal wall
  anatomy of, 143–146
  surgical complications of, 143–146
Antibiotic(s)
  for abdominal surgery, 101
  in penicillin-allergic surgical patients, 67
  in perioperative period, 101
Anticholinergic(s), 61
Anticoagulant(s), 63
Antiestrogen therapy, 102
Antiincontinence procedure, 3
Antiviral agents, 78
Arrhythmia(s), 42
Assault, 56
Atypical glandular cells, not otherwise specified
  (AGC–NOS), 34

B

Bacterial vaginosis
  complications of, 36
  recurrent, 36
Bariatric surgery, 24, 134
Barrier contraception, 134
Behçet disease, 46
Beta-blockers, 126
Beta subunit of human chorionic gonadotropin,
  150–153
Bilateral salpingo-oophorectomy (BSO), 35
  hysterectomy with, 98
  laparoscopic, 125
  prophylactic, 117
  as risk reduction factor for ovarian cancer,
    27
  site of injury during, 41
Bilateral tubal ligation, 27
Bisphosphonate therapy, 97
Black cohosh, 128
Bladder, 61
Bladder emptying, 3
Bleeding
  abnormal uterine, 4
  anovulatory, 40

Bleeding (*continued*)
  heavy menstrual. *See* Heavy menstrual
    bleeding
  postmenopausal, 26, 85
  uterine, 77
Blood test, 59
BMD. *See* Bone mineral density
Bone fracture(s)
  osteopenia and, 33
  osteoporosis and, 33
Bone loss, 33
Bone mineral density (BMD)
  in osteoporosis, 97
  screening for, 33
Bradycardia, 42
BRCA 1 gene mutation, 147–149
  in hereditary breast and ovarian cancer, 127
  ovarian cancer in women with, 27, 11
BRCA 2 gene mutation, 117, 147–149
  in hereditary breast and ovarian cancer, 127
  ovarian cancer in women with, 27
Breast abscess, 87
Breast cancer
  genetic risk assessment for, 95
  risk reduction for, 127
Breast disease
  fibrocystic, 105
  premalignant, 102
  in situ, 102
Breast mass, 30
Breast pain, 105
Breast tenderness, 120
BSO. *See* Bilateral salpingo-oophorectomy
Burnout in physicians, 9

C

CA 125
  level, 95, 150–153
  testing, 59
Calcium-rich diet, 97
Cancer
  breast, 95, 127
  cervical, 1, 94, 138–142
  colon, 98
  colorectal, 39, 98
  endometrial, 26, 76
  hereditary nonpolyposis colorectal, 39
  ovarian, 27, 59, 117, 127
  uterine, 76
  vaginal, 68
Candidiasis, 123
Carbamazepine, 7
Cardiac arrhythmias, 42
CDC. *See* Centers for Disease Control and
  Prevention
Cefazolin, 67
Ceftriaxone, 74
Centers for Disease Control and Prevention
  (CDC)
  on abortions, 124
  on human immunodeficiency virus exposure
    and prevention, 18
  on human immunodeficiency virus prophy-
    laxis in cases of sexual assault, 56

NOTE: Numbers refer to questions, not pages.

Centers for Disease Control and Prevention (CDC) *(continued)*
on human papillomavirus vaccine, 52
on pertussis vaccination, 131
on pelvic inflammatory disease, 74, 84
Cervical cancer
cytology in, 1
diagnosis of, 138–142
early detection of, 94
prevention of, 94
screening for, 138–142
Cervical cytology, 1, 71
Cervical intraepithelial neoplasia (CIN), 14, 50
Cervix, 50
Children, 154–158
Chronic abnormal uterine bleeding, 40
Chronic pelvic pain, 29
conditions causing, 29
defined, 29
irritable bowel syndrome and, 88
CIN. *See* Cervical intraepithelial neoplasia
Clindamycin
for recurrent bacterial vaginosis, 36
in surgical patients with penicillin allergy, 67
Clobetasol propionate, 92
Clomiphene citrate
in cancer risk reduction, 127
in ovulation induction, 43
Cold knife cone biopsy, 14
Colon cancer, 98
Colonoscopy, 64
Colorectal cancer
disorders associated with, 98
hereditary nonpolyposis, 39, 98
Colposacropexy, 70
Colposcopy, 50
Committee on Patient Safety and Quality Improvement, 23
Communication, 21
Complex endometrial hyperplasia, 104
Computed tomography (CT), 47
Condom(s), 124
Condyloma, 86
Confidentiality, 21
Consent, 51
Contraception. *See also specific methods*; Contraceptive(s)
barrier, 134
depot medroxyprogesterone acetate, 33
emergency, 11, 112
in morbidly obese patient, 118
in patient with gastric bypass, 134
single-rod implantable, 19
thrombophilias and, 106
Contraceptive(s)
in abnormal uterine bleeding management, 40
oral. *See* Oral contraceptives
for woman with diabetes mellitus and seizure disorder, 7
Copper intrauterine device, 11, 124, 134
Counseling
end-of-life, 133
for sterilization, 60
"Critical timing hypothesis," 48
CT. *See* Computed tomography (CT)
Current Procedural Terminology codes, 79
Cyst(s), 2
Cystic teratoma, 2, 12
Cystitis, 29, 88
Cytology, 1

D
DCIS. *See* Ductal carcinoma in situ
Delirium
defined, 109
postoperative, 109
Dental caries, 130
Depot medroxyprogesterone acetate (DMPA), 33
Depression, 45
Dermoid(s), 2
Desquamative inflammatory vaginitis, 10, 46
Diabetes mellitus
gestational, 7
perioperative care of patient with, 89
seizure disorder with, 7
Dilation and evacuation, 132
Discriminatory zone, 93
Distention media, 82
DMPA. *See* Depot medroxyprogesterone acetate
Doxycycline, 74
Dual-energy X-ray absorptiometry, 97
Ductal carcinoma in situ (DCIS), 129
ipsilateral recurrent, 102
treatment of, 129
Dysmenorrhea
in adolescent, 81, 116
management of, 13
Dyspareunia
conditions associated with, 10
estrogen therapy for, 163–166
severe, 46
sexual dysfunction caused by, 10

E
E-mail communication, 21
Eating disorders, 130
Ectopic pregnancy, 2, 44, 93
Elderly patient
oliguria in, 49
postoperative delirium in, 109
Electronic communication, 21
Embolization
complications of, 55
uterine artery, 55, 80
Embolus, 96
Emergency contraception, 11, 112
End-of-life counseling, 133
Endometrial ablation, 90
Endometrial biopsy, 26
Endometrial cancer, 26, 76
Endometrial cells
evaluation of, 1
in Pap test, 1
Endometrial hyperplasia
atypical, 76
complex, 104
Endometrioma(s), 2
Endometriosis, 88
in adolescent patient, 81
chronic pelvic pain and, 29
defined, 69
hysterectomy for, 69
Estrogen therapy
after hysterectomy for endometriosis, 69
in one mineral density improvement, 97
for dyspareunia, 163–166
Ethic(s), 51
Etonogestrel subdermal implants, 77
Exercise(s)
Kegel, 61
in polycystic ovary syndrome management, 43
strength-building, 97

Exogenous gonadotropin therapy, 43
Extended-cycle combined oral contraceptives, 122

F
Factor V Leiden mutation, 106
Familial adenomatous polyposis, 147–149
Familial cancer syndromes, 147–149
Female athlete triad, 130
Femoral neurapraxia, 8
Fibrocystic breast disease, 105
Fibroid(s). *See* Myoma(s)
FIGO. *See* International Federation of Gynecology and Obstetrics
First-trimester pregnancy loss, 114
Fistula(s), 32, 108
"5 A's" intervention model, in smoking cessation, 22
Fluconazole, 123
Foreign object, 154–158
Fractional excretion of sodium, 49
Fracture(s)
bone, 33
hip, 97
Fracture Risk Assessment Tool (FRAX), 33
FRAX. *See* Fracture Risk Assessment Tool
French Cancer Genetics Network, 98

G
Gabapentin, 128
Gastric bypass, 134
GDM. *See* Gestational diabetes mellitus
Genital herpes
prevalence of, 107
recurrent, 78
sexual partner with, 107
Genital warts, 86
Gestational diabetes mellitus (GDM), 7
Gestational trophoblastic neoplasia (GTN), 54
Ginseng, 128
Glandular cells, 34
Glycemic index, 103
Gonadotropin therapy, 43
GTN. *See* Gestational trophoblastic neoplasia
Guidelines on Perioperative Cardiac Evaluation and Care for Noncardiac Surgery, 38
Gynecologic Oncology Group study, 104
Gynecologic procedures, 42

H
Heart, 83
Heavy menstrual bleeding, 113
defined, 62, 83
levonorgestrel intrauterine device for, 83
in patient with low platelet count, 62
Heparin, 63
Hereditary nonpolyposis colorectal cancer (HNPCC), 39, 98, 147–149. *See also* Lynch syndrome
Herpes simplex virus type 1 (HSV-1), 78
Herpes simplex virus type 2 (HSV-2), 78
Hip fractures, 97
HIV infection. *See* Human immunodeficiency virus infection
HNPCC. *See* Hereditary nonpolyposis colorectal cancer
Hormone therapy (HT)
after hysterectomy, 48, 69
menopausal, 48, 120

NOTE: Numbers refer to questions, not pages.

Hormone therapy (HT) *(continued)*
  postmenopausal, 120
  postmenopausal bleeding with, 85
Hospital patients, 63
Hot flushes, 128
HPV. *See* Human papillomavirus
HSV-1. *See* Herpes simplex virus type 1
HSV-2. *See* Herpes simplex virus type 2
HT. *See* Hormone therapy
Human chorionic gonadotropin (hCG)
  beta subunit of, 150–153
  in ectopic pregnancy, 93
Human immunodeficiency virus (HIV) infection
  after sexual assault, 56
  exposure and prophylaxis, 18
Human papillomavirus (HPV), 86
  prevention of, 52
  testing for, 34
  vaginal intraepithelial neoplasia and, 94
  vaccine, 52, 159–162
Hydrosalpinx, 2, 125
Hypoactive sexual disorder, 58
Hypotension, 96
Hysterectomy
  age at, 99
  bilateral salpingo-oophorectomy with, 98
  for complex endometrial hyperplasia, 104
  for endometriosis, 69
  hormone therapy after, 48
  for myomas, 37
  oophorectomy at time of, 99
  ovarian preservation or removal at time of, 99
  prevalence of, 99
  vaginal cancer screening after, 68
Hysteroscopic myomectomy, 37
Hysteroscopic sterilization, 60
Hysteroscopy
  complications of, 82
  office-based, 65

I

IBS. *See* Irritable bowel syndrome
Ilioinguinal nerve entrapment, 143–146
Immunization, 131
Implant(s). *See specific types*
In situ breast disease, 102
Incomplete abortion, 132
Incomplete bladder emptying, 3
Incontinence. *See specific types*
Infection(s)
  human immunodeficiency virus, 18
  urinary tract, 115
  wound, 5
  yeast, 53
Inferior epigastric artery, 143–146
Infertility, 43
Informed consent, 51
Inhibin B, 150–153
Institute of Medicine, 23
Intermittent self-catheterization, 3
International Federation of Gynecology and
    Obstetrics (FIGO), 54
Interstitial cystitis
  chronic pelvic pain and, 29
  defined, 88
Intestinal obstruction, 47
Intrauterine devices (IUDs)
  copper, 11, 124, 134
  levonorgestrel, 110, 118, 134.
Intrinsic sphincter deficiency, 100

Ipsilateral recurrent ductal carcinoma in situ, 102
Iron supplementation, 4
Irregular menstruation, 130
Irritable bowel syndrome (IBS)
  chronic pelvic pain and, 29, 88
  Rome III criteria for, 29
IUDs. *See* Intrauterine devices

K

Kegel exercises, 61

L

Laparoscopic bilateral salpingectomy, 125
Laparoscopic salpingostomy, 44
Laparoscopy, 13, 116
LARC methods. *See* Long-acting reversible
    contraceptive methods
Le Fort partial colpocleisis, 31
LEEP. *See* Loop electrosurgical excision proce-
    dure (LEEP)
Levonorgestrel
  in emergency contraception, 11, 112
  intrauterine device, 7, 11, 83, 110, 118, 124,
    134
Liability suits, 23
Libido, 58
Lichen
  planus, 10, 46
  sclerosus, 10, 53, 92, 154–158
  simplex chronicus, 53
Long-acting reversible contraceptive (LARC)
    methods, 77
Loop electrosurgical excision procedure
    (LEEP), 15
Low-grade squamous intraepithelial lesion
    (LSIL), 50
LSIL. *See* Low-grade squamous intraepithelial
    lesion
Lynch II syndrome, 39, 98, 147–149
Lynch syndrome, 147–149. *See also* Hereditary
    nonpolyposis colorectal cancer

M

Magnetic resonance imaging-guided focused
    ultrasound ablation, 37
Major depressive disorder, 45
Mammography, 30
Mass(es)
  adnexal, 25, 95, 150–153
  breast, 30
  ovarian, 2, 25
Mastalgia, 30, 105
Mastectomy, 117
Mastitis, 87
Mature cystic teratoma, 2, 12
*Medical Eligibility Criteria for Contraception
    Use*, 112
Medical errors
  disclosure of, 23
  discussion of, 23
Medical records, 21
Menopausal women, 10
Menopause
  hormone therapy in, 120
  nonhormonal therapy in, 128
Menstrual bleeding, 62, 83, 113
Menstruation
  eating disorders effects on, 130
  irregular, 130
Metformin hydrochloride, 43

Methotrexate
  contraindications to, 44
  for ectopic pregnancy, 44, 93
Metoprolol succinate, 126
Metronidazole, 36
Mifepristone, 11
Misoprostol, 114
Modified lithotomy position, 8
Molar pregnancy, 54
Motivational interviewing technique, 22
Multiple pregnancies, 27
Myoma(s)
  alternatives to hysterectomy for, 37
  asymptomatic, 72
  defined, 37
  prolapsed submucosal, 80
  treatment of, 37
  uterine, 55
Myomectomy, 37

N

National Cancer Comprehensive Network
    (NCCN)
  on ovarian cancer screening, 59
  on recurrent breast mass, 30
  on screening, 98
NCCN. *See* National Cancer Comprehensive
    Network
Nerve injury, 8
Neurapraxia, 8
Nonhormonal therapy, 128
Nonspecific vaginitis, 154–158
North American Menopause Society, 48

O

Obesity, 24, 103, 118
  management of, 24
  morbid, 118
  prevalence of, 134
Office-based procedures
  coding for, 79
  hysteroscopy, 65
  patient safety-related, 135–137
Older reproductive-aged woman, 25
Oliguria
  defined, 49
  in the elderly, 49
  postoperative, 121
Omentectomy, 6
Oophorectomy, 99
Oophoropexy, 28
Operative complications, 57
Oral contraceptives
  in cancer risk reduction, 127
  effectiveness of, 124
  extended-cycle combined, 122
  as risk reduction factor for ovarian cancer, 27
  venous thnromboembolism caused by, 106
Osteopenia, 33
Osteoporosis, 33, 97
Ovarian cancer
  blood test in, 59
  in *BRCA 1* and *BRCA 2* carriers, 117
  risk factors for, 27, 59, 127
  screening for, 59
Ovarian cyst, 2
Ovarian mass
  in adolescent patient, 2
  in older reproductive-aged woman, 25
Ovarian preservation or removal, 99
Ovarian remnant syndrome, 17, 64

NOTE: Numbers refer to questions, not pages.

Ovarian torsion
    management of, 28
    prevention of recurrence of, 28
Ovarian tumor, 6
Overactive bladder, 61
Ovulation induction
    clomiphene citrate in, 43
    exogenous gonadotropin therapy in, 43

P
Paget disease, 53
Pain
    breast, 105
    pelvic, 29, 88
    sexual, 163–166
    vulvar, 73
Pap test
    atypical glandular cells, not otherwise speci-
        fied on, 34
    in cervical cancer, 138–142
    endometrial cells in, 1
    in loop electrosurgical excision procedure
        follow-up, 15
    low-grade squamous intraepithelial lesion
        on, 50
    in ovarian cancer screening, 59
    in vaginal intraepithelial neoplasia screening,
        75
Papanicolaou, G.N., 1
Parity, 127
Patient privacy, 21
Patient safety, 135–137
PCOS. See Polycystic ovary syndrome
Peer review, 57
Pelvic abscess, 66
Pelvic floor, 41
Pelvic inflammatory disease (PID)
    described, 84, 90
    diagnosis of, 84
    outpatient management of, 84
    treatment of, 74
Pelvic organ prolapse, 70
Pelvic Organ Prolapse Quantification (POP-Q)
        technique, 31, 70
Pelvic pain, 29, 88
Pelvic Pain and Urgency/Frequency Patient
        Symptom Scale, 88
Pelvic surgery, 8
Pelvis, 91
Penicillin allergy, 67
Percutaneous injuries, 18
Perforation, uterine, 65
Perioperative Ischemic Evaluation trial, 126
Perioperative period
    anticoagulants in, 63
    beta-blockers in, 126
    cardiac complications in, 38
    cardiac evaluation in, 38
    diabetic patient care during, 89
    prophylactic antibiotics in, 101
    pulmonary complications in, 35
Peroneal nerve injury, 8
Pertussis vaccine, 131
Pessary, 70
Physical therapy, 8
Physician burnout, 9
Physiologic discharge, 154–158
PID. See Pelvic inflammatory disease
Platelet count, 62
Polycystic ovary syndrome (PCOS)
    described, 43

Polycystic ovary syndrome (PCOS) *(continued)*
    metformin hydrochloride and, 43
    Rotterdam criteria for, 43
Postembolization syndrome, 55
Postmenopausal bleeding, 26, 85
Postmenopausal hot flushes, 128
Postmenopausal woman
    adnexal mass in, 95
    hormone therapy in, 120
Postoperative delirium, 109
Postoperative intestinal obstruction, 47
Postoperative pelvic abscess, 66
Pregnancy
    ectopic, 2, 44, 93
    molar, 54
    multiple, 27
    unplanned, 124
    vaccination during, 131
Pregnancy loss, 114
Premalignant breast disease, 102
Presidential Task Force on Patient Safety in the
        Office Setting, 135–137
Progestins, 104
Prolapse, 31
Prolapsed submucosal myomas, 80
Prophylactic total mastectomy, 117
Pruritis, 53
Psoriasis, 53
Puerperal mastitis, 87
Pulmonary embolus, 96
Pulmonary issues, 35
Pyomyoma, 80

R
Radiography, 110
Recalcitrant condyloma, 86
Recurrent bacterial vaginosis, 36
Recurrent breast mass, 30
Recurrent genital herpes, 78
Recurrent urinary incontinence, 100
Recurrent urinary tract infections, 115, 119
Recurrent vaginal yeast infection, 123
Recurrent vulvovaginal candidiasis, 123
Recurrent yeast infections, 53
Reproductive-aged woman, 40
Risk-reducing surgery, 98
Rome III criteria, 29
Rotterdam criteria, 43

S
Safety Certification in Outpatient Excellence
        program, 135–137
Saline sonohysterography, 26
Salpingo-oophorectomy. See Bilateral salpingo-
        oophorectomy
Salpingostomy, 44
Second trimester, 132
Seizure disorder, 7
Selective estrogen receptor modulators
        (SERMs), 97
Selective serotonin reuptake inhibitors (SSRIs),
        45
Self-catheterization, 3
Septic abortion, 132
SERMs. See Selective estrogen receptor modu-
        lators
Severe reactions, 67
Sexual assault, 56
Sexual dysfunction, 10, 58
Sexual interest and arousal disorder, 58
Sexual pain, 163–166

Sexual partner, 107
Sexually transmitted diseases, 74
SGO. See Society of Gynecologic Oncologists
Single-rod implantable contraception, 19
Smoking cessation, 22
Society of Gynecologic Oncologists (SGO)
    on newly diagnosed pelvic mass in post-
        menopausal woman, 95
    on ovarian cancer screening, 59
Squamous dysplasia, 50
SSRIs. See Selective serotonin reuptake
        inhibitors
Sterilization
    counseling for, 60
    hysteroscopic, 60
Strength-building exercise, 97
Streptococcal vaginitis, 154–158
Stress incontinence, 3, 108
Stroke, 109
Subdermal progestin inserts, 124
Submucosal myomas, 80
Suburethral sling procedure
    after pelvic organ prolapse, 70
    for urinary stress incontinence, 3, 100
Surgical Care Improvement Project, 101
Surgical Wound Classification System, 101

T
Tamoxifen, 127
Tamoxifen citrate, 102
Tdap vaccine, 131
Tension-free vaginal tape (TVT) procedure,
        91, 100
Teratoma(s), 2, 12
Testosterone therapy, 58
Tetanus vaccine, 131
3 Incontinence Questions (3-IQ) questionnaire,
        20
Thromboembolism
    in hospital patients, 63
    venous, 106
Thrombophilia(s), 106
Tinidazole, 36
Tobacco use, 22
Total laparoscopic hysterectomy, 41
Tranexamic acid, 113
Transobturator tape procedures, 100
Transvaginal ultrasonography, 59
Tumor(s), 6. See also specific types
Tumor markers, 150–153
TVT procedure. See Tension-free vaginal tape
        procedure
2001 Bethesda System, 1
2012 Consensus Guidelines for the Management
        of Abnormal Cervical Cancer Screening
        Tests and Cancer Precursors, 1

U
Ulipristal acetate, 11
Ultrasonography
    in adnexal mass evaluation, 95
    in chronic pelvic pain evaluation, 29
    of dermoid, 2
    in recurrent breast mass evaluation, 30
    transvaginal, 59
Umbilicus, 143–146
Unexpected surgical findings, 51
Unfractionated heparin, 63
Unplanned pregnancy, 124
Urachus, 143–146
Ureteral injury, 41

NOTE: Numbers refer to questions, not pages.

Urinary incontinence
    evaluation of, 20
    recurrent, 100
    stress, 3, 108
Urinary tract infections (UTIs)
    prevalence of, 115, 119
    recurrent, 115, 119
Urination, 108
U.S. Food and Drug Administration
    on estrogen therapy for dyspareunia and
        other vulvar pain syndromes, 163–166
    on hormone therapy, 128
U.S. Preventive Services Task Force, 59
Uterine artery embolization, 55, 80
Uterine bleeding
    abnormal, 4, 40, 81
    etonogestrel subdermal implants and, 77
Uterine cancer, 76
Uterine myomas, 55
Uterine perforation, 65
Uterine vessels, 41
Uterosacral ligament suspension, 16
Uterovaginal prolapse, 31
UTIs. *See* Urinary tract infections

V
Vaccination. *See* Immunization; Vaccine(s)
Vaccine(s), 131. *See also specific types*
    human papillomavirus, 52, 159–162
    pertussis, 131
    Tdap, 131
    tetanus, 131
Vaginal atrophy, 10

Vaginal cancer screening, 68
Vaginal contraceptive ring, 124
Vaginal intraepithelial neoplasia (VAIN), 94
    human papillomavirus infection infection
        and, 94
    screening for, 75
Vaginal prolapse, 16
Vaginal yeast infection, 123
Vaginismus, 163–166
Vaginitis
    defined, 36
    desquamative inflammatory, 10, 46
    nonspecific, 154–158
    pediatric, 154–158
    streptococcal, 154–158
Vaginosis, 36
VAIN. *See* Vaginal intraepithelial neoplasia
Venlafaxine, 128
Venous thromboembolism (VTE)
    combined oral contraceptives and, 106
    risk factors for, 106
Vesicovaginal fistula, 32, 108
Vestibulectomy, 163–166
Vestibulitis, 163–166
Voiding diary, 20
Voiding dysfunction, 3
VTE. *See* Venous thromboembolism
Vulva, 53
Vulvar epithelial neoplasia, 53
Vulvar lichen simplex chronicus, 53
Vulvar pain, 73
Vulvar pruritus, 53
Vulvar psoriasis, 53

Vulvar vestibulitis, 163–166
Vulvodynia, 73, 163–166
Vulvovaginal candidiasis, 123
Vulvovaginal disorders, 46

W
Wart(s), 86
Weight loss
    in infertility management, 43
    in obesity management, 103
    in polycystic ovary syndrome management,
        43
    steps in promoting, 24
WHO. *See* World Health Organization (WHO)
Whooping cough vaccine, 131
Women's Health Initiative study, 120, 128
World Health Organization (WHO)
    on disease screening, 59
    on endometrial hyperplasia, 104
    FRAX of, 33
    *Medical Eligibility Criteria for Contraception
        Use* of, 112
    on obesity, 134
Wound dehiscence, 111
Wound infections, 5
Wound separation, 111

X
X-ray absorptiometry, 97

Y
Yeast infections, 53, 123

NOTE: Numbers refer to questions, not pages.

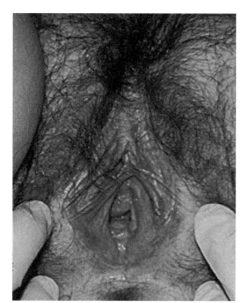

FIG. 10-1

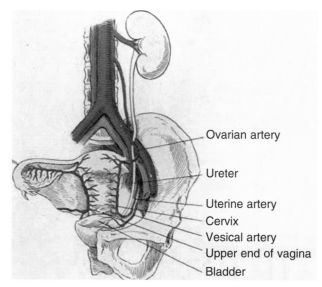

Ovarian artery

Ureter

Uterine artery

Cervix

Vesical artery

Upper end of vagina

Bladder

FIG. 41-1. Schematic showing the ureters. (Davis GG. Applied anatomy: the construction of the human body. 2nd ed. Philadelphia, PA: JB Lippincott Co; 1913. Available at: http://chestofbooks.com/health/anatomy/Human-Body-Construction/index.html. Retrieved August 27, 2013.)

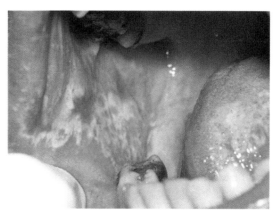

FIG. 46-2

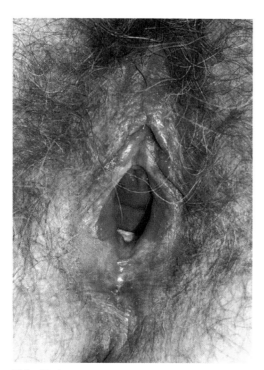

FIG. 46-1

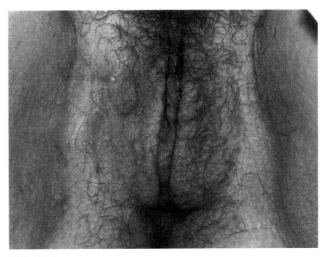

FIG. 53-1

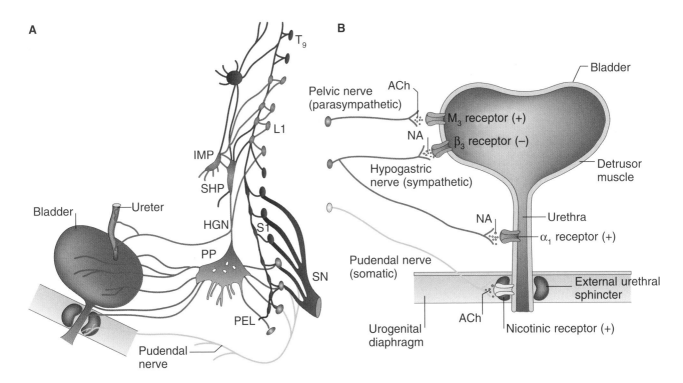

FIG. 61-1. Efferent pathways of the lower urinary tract. Abbreviations: ACh, acetylcholine; HGN, hypogastric nerve; IMP, inferior mesenteric plexus; L1, first lumbar root; M, muscarinic receptor; NA, noradrenaline; PEL, pelvic nerves; PP, pelvic plexus; S1, first sacral root; SHP, superior hypogastric plexus; SN, sciatic nerve. (Reprinted by permission from Macmillan Publishers Ltd: Fowler CJ, Griffiths D, de Groat WC. The neural control of micturition. Nat Rev Neurosci 2008;9:453–66, copyright 2008.)

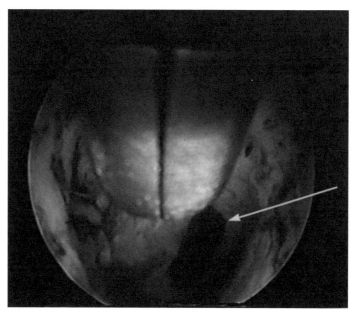

FIG. 65-1. Hysteroscopic view of uterine perforation. Arrow indicates perforation. (Image courtesy of Ceana Nezhat, MD.)

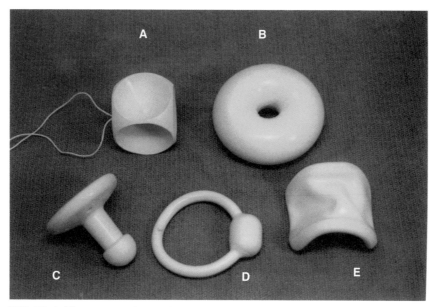

FIG. 70-1. Five commonly used pessaries: **A.** cube, **B.** donut, **C.** Gellhorn, **D.** ring, and **E.** Gehrung.

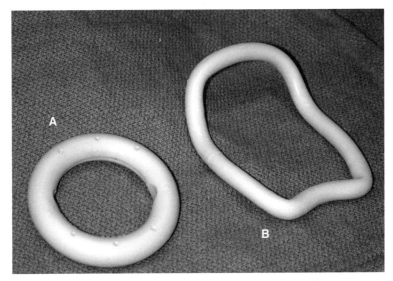

FIG. 70-2. Two commonly used pessaries: **A.** ring and **B.** Risser.

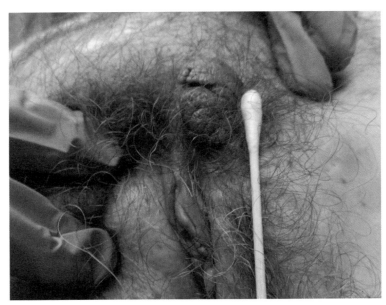

FIG. 86-1

Acknowledgments

Fig. 2-1, Fig. 2-2, Fig. 2-3, Fig. 2-4, Fig. 2-5, Fig. 6-1, and Fig. 25-1. Images provided by Task Force Co-Chair James M. Shwayder, MD.

Fig. 10-1. Image courtesy of Gloria A. Bachmann, MD.

Fig. 46-1, Fig. 46-2, and Fig. 53-1. Images were originally published in Edwards L, Lynch PJ. Genital dermatology atlas. First edition. Philadelphia (PA): Lippincott Williams & Wilkins; 2004.

Fig. 47-1. Figure is reprinted with permission from "Abdominal wall hernias: imaging features, complications, and diagnostic pitfalls at multi-detector row CT" by DA Aguirre, AC Santosa, G Casola, and CB Sirlin. *Radiographics* 2005;25:1501–20. Copyright 2005, Radiological Society of North America.

Fig. 86-1. Image provided by Task Force member Colleen K. Stockdale, MD.

Fig. 95-1. Image courtesy of Ghada Mansour, MD.